LASER APPLICATIONS

Volume I

CONTRIBUTORS

FREDERICK ARONOWITZ   BRIAN J. THOMPSON

JAMES C. OWENS   LELLAND A. WEAVER

MONTE ROSS

LASER APPLICATIONS

Edited by MONTE ROSS

McDonnell Douglas Astronautics Company
St. Louis, Missouri

VOLUME I

ACADEMIC PRESS   New York and London   1971

ACADEMIC PRESS, INC.
111 Fifth Avenue, New York, New York 10003

United Kingdom Edition published by
ACADEMIC PRESS, INC. (LONDON) LTD.
Berkeley Square House, London W1X 6BA

LIBRARY OF CONGRESS CATALOG CARD NUMBER: 79-154380

PRINTED IN THE UNITED STATES OF AMERICA

CONTENTS

0748

Machining and Welding Applications

LELLAND A. WEAVER

Laser Communications

MONTE ROSS

LIST OF CONTRIBUTORS

Numbers in parentheses indicate the pages on which the authors' contributions begin.

FREDERICK ARONOWITZ, Systems and Research Center, Honeywell Inc., Minneapolis, Minnesota (133)

JAMES C. OWENS, Research Laboratories, Eastman Kodak Company, Rochester, New York (61)

MONTE ROSS, McDonnell Douglas Astronautics Company, St. Louis, Missouri (239)

BRIAN J. THOMPSON, The Institute of Optics, University of Rochester, Rochester, New York (1)

LELLAND A. WEAVER, Westinghouse Research Laboratories, Churchill Borough, Pittsburgh, Pennsylvania (201)

PREFACE

Lasers are finding new applications at a rapid rate, and these applications are, in many cases, in quite diverse areas. However, there yet exists a gap between laser research and development and laser applications which restricts the growth of laser systems. The purpose of this volume and of future volumes is to help close this gap by providing basic review articles addressed to personnel in application areas. These volumes will not deal with highly specific applications. Each article will be designed to provide a base of understanding for a common group of applications.

The five articles in this first volume deal with five rapidly growing areas of interest: guidance via laser gyros, holography, machining and welding, metrology and geodesy, and communications. Future volumes will cover medical uses of lasers, laser systems as monitors of the environment, laser recording and displays, and laser radar and tracking systems.

There is no way of knowing which of the many potential applications of lasers may ultimately become the most significant. Perhaps holographic movies, precision mass machining of previously unmachinable parts, or the global village concept due to wideband satellite communications will first have massive impact on our society. In the interim, laser applications of a smaller scale will be developed, special systems will come into being, and specialized products produced.

I wish to thank Washington University and Dr. G. Esterson of the Continuing Education Department for their being the catalyst for this series through a short course in laser applications which I directed in April, 1969. I also wish to express appreciation to the individual contributors and their respective affiliations, in addition to the help provided by McDonnell Douglas Astronautics Company.

MONTE ROSS

May, 1971

APPLICATIONS OF HOLOGRAPHY

Brian J. Thompson

The Institute of Optics, University of Rochester
Rochester, New York

I. Introduction

Holography was invented with a specific application in mind. In the late 1940s electron microscopy was limited by the quality of electron lenses to a resolution of about 5 Å; hence Gabor (1948) suggested a method of overcoming this limitation in a short paper entitled "A New Microscopic Principle." He

1

later followed this up with a detailed discussion on "Microscopy by Recon-structed Wave-Fronts" (Gabor, 1949, 1951). The method was a two-step coherent image forming process in which a record is made of the interference pattern produced by the interaction of the radiation diffracted by the object of interest and a coherent background or reference wave. The intensity distribu-tion in the interference pattern is recorded and constitutes the hologram. This hologram has the property that when it is illuminated coherently the original wavefront is reconstructed; therefore, an image can be formed of the original diffracting object. The suggested application was to make the holo-gram with an electron beam, and then use that hologram illuminated with light to form an aberration free image, by providing a light beam that had exactly the same aberration as the original electron beam. The experimental procedure consisted of illuminating the specimen with an electron beam; the electrons diffracted by the specimen interfered with the undiffracted beam passing through the specimen. A photographic record was made of the result-ing electron intensity distribution. Before using the hologram to form an image of the specimen it was magnified by a factor determined by the ratio of the wavelengths of the optical and the electron beams. The hologram was then illuminated by a light beam that had the same aberrations as the electron beam again magnified by the ratio of the wavelengths. Despite very determined efforts by a number of workers (Haine and Dyson, 1950; Haine and Mulvey, 1952a,b) this application never developed and the hoped for resolution of 1 Å were not obtained. It is interesting to note that work has recently started again on holographic electron microscopy (Tonomura *et al.*, 1968). The major factor that hindered progress was the presence of the two images formed when the hologram was illuminated—when one image was viewed the other image produced a component of the total field in that plane as an out-of-focus coherent contribution. Much of the early work in holog-raphy was devoted to eliminating the unwanted image (Bragg and Rogers, 1951; Gabor, 1951; El Sum, 1952). Other problems were concerned with film resolution and vibrational stability.

The roots of holography go back further than indicated above. Of par-ticular interest is the experiment of Michelson (1927) in forming an image of a slit from its recorded Fraunhofer diffraction pattern by adding the necessary known phase component as an additional optical element. Bragg's X-ray microscope was another excellent example of a coherent two-step image form-ing process; here the method was deliberately limited to crystal structures that had a center of symmetry so that the diffraction pattern is wholly real. This technique was later extended to noncentrosymmetrical structures (Buerger, 1950; Hanson, 1952; Harburn and Taylor, 1962). It was quickly recognized that the X-ray diffraction problem was very closely related to the electron-diffraction proposals, and X-ray holography became an early application for serious consideration (Haine and Mulvey, 1952a; El Sum, 1952; Baez, 1952; Baez and El Sum, 1957). Again no significant progress has been made although the problem has not been completely abandoned (Tollin *et al.*, 1966).

The disappointment over the lack of success of these original applications certainly slowed progress in the technological advances of the subject, but work did continue on the further understanding of the subject in a number of laboratories. The current impetus in holographic research and development came about with the work of Leith and Upatnieks who exploited the off-axis reference beam technique (Leith and Upatnieks, 1962), which eliminated the overlap of the two images, and then showed the experimental importance of the gas laser (Leith and Upatnieks, 1963) as a light source for holography. At about this same time the pulsed laser was introduced into holography, and a new application was developed for particle size analysis using a hologram formed in the far field of the individual particle (Thompson, 1963, 1964a,b; Parrent and Thompson, 1964a; B. J. Thompson *et al.*, 1965; B. J. Thompson *et al.*, 1967). This technique minimized the problems associated with the second image. Thus the new phase of research and development in holography became the glamour queen of optics and electronics.

In the 22-year history of holography some 800 papers have been written involving some 500 authors. The principles of the subject are therefore well understood and documented with several books devoted to the subject (Stroke, 1966; DeVelis and Reynolds, 1967; Smith, 1969; Kock, 1969). Two conferences have been held on the subject and the proceedings are extremely valuable records of the state-of-the-art (Society of Photo-Optical Instrumentation Engineers Seminar-in-Depth 1968; Engineering Applications of Holography 1968). To guide the reader to this mass of literature a number of bibliographies are available (Chambers and Courtney-Pratt, 1966a,b; Latta, 1968; Kallard, 1969; Anonymous, 1968). Finally it may be noted that some attempts have been made to critically analyze the literature (Thompson, 1969a,b, 1970).

This review is devoted to a discussion of the applications of holography. It is necessary, however, to provide a basis for this discussion by first defining a terminology and notation that can be used throughout, without reviewing the science and technology in any depth.

The applications are discussed in three sections that relate to the basic use of the process rather than grouping them by specific holographic technique. The first group involves those applications involving image formation when, for a variety of reasons, normal incoherent or coherent image formation is not satisfactory. Clearly it is not sufficient merely to replace a normal imaging process by a holographic technique unless there is some significant gain, i.e., the required record can be obtained more easily or more accurately.

In some instances the record cannot be obtained in any other way. It is fair to state that holographic image formation should not be used unless it is a necessity. Applications which fall into this category are particle size analysis (for a recent review see Thompson, 1968b); holographic microscopy (for a recent review, see Van Ligten, 1968); high-speed photography of various types, particularly of gas flows; data storage and retrieval, including displays; image formation through a random medium; nonoptical holography, particularly acoustic holography (Metherell *et al.*, 1969).

The second group of interest are those applications which are non-image forming. One of the very real and exciting applications is holographic interferometry and its applications to nondestructive testing. The basic technique involves recording a hologram of the object of interest and then interfering the image produced from this hologram with the coherently illuminated object itself (or an image formed from a second hologram) at a later time. Another technique uses a time averaged hologram to study vibrating objects. An interesting brief review of the subject was recently given by Powell (1969), one of the originators of this area of holography. Hence the realm of interferometry is extended to whole new classes of objects. In a similar but separate effort, interference microscopy has been developed using holographic methods (Snow and Vandewarker, 1968).

The third and final group are those applications which use the hologram as an optical element in its own right. Good possibilities exist for the manufacture of accurate specialized gratings. Of significant value could be the application of holographic filters in coherent optical data processing.

II. Basic Systems Concepts

There is always a great danger in yielding to the temptation of classifying various areas of a subject since this inevitably leads to arguments, especially with respect to those techniques that do not clearly fall into any one of the chosen categories. However, it is necessary to set up some terminology that can be used as a basis for the discussion of the applications of known holographic techniques. Two broad categories will be used here. First, those that are in-line, meaning that the coherent background radiation is coaxial with the diffracted radiation associated with the field of interest. The in-line systems are conveniently divided along the classical line of Fresnel and Fraunhofer diffraction. Thus we would define in-line Fresnel holograms and in-line Fraunhofer (or far field) holograms. The second and more important category are those techniques that use a separate off-axis reference beam to make the hologram. Again we can define a Fresnel region and a Fraunhofer (far field) region associated with the object. This technique also allows the hologram to be formed by interfering the Fraunhofer diffraction pattern of the object formed by a lens with a reference beam, leading to a so-called Fourier transform (or generalized) hologram. Finally in this category we can form an image hologram by interfering a coherent image of an object in a plane with a coherent reference. The justification (if one is needed) for this classification is that it depends only on the diffracted field of the object. It is not dependent upon whether the reference beam is plane or spherical or upon how the reference beam is produced. Subclassification based on properties of the reference beam could be considered if required.

A hologram, then, is the recorded interference pattern obtained between the optical field of interest and the known coherent reference field. Hence the hologram is a recorded intensity distribution. All detectors of optical radiation are responsive to the intensity of radiation incident upon them. The quantity that is normally called intensity is the long time average of the optical field times its complex conjugate. Let the complex amplitude of an optical field be $V(x, t)$. The instantaneous intensity $I(x, t)$ is then given by $V(x, t)V^*(x, t)$, where the asterisk denotes a complex conjugate. The observable intensity is defined as

$$I(x) = \langle I(x, t) \rangle = \langle V(x, t)V^*(x, t) \rangle \tag{1}$$

When two optical fields, $V_1(x, t)$ and $V_2(x, t)$ are added, the resultant intensity becomes

$$I(x) = \langle V_1(x, t)V_1^*(x, t) \rangle + \langle V_2(x, t)V_2^*(x, t) \rangle$$
$$+ \langle (V_1(x, t)V_2^*(x, t) \rangle + \langle V_1^*(x, t)V_2(x, t) \rangle \tag{2}$$

The first two terms are the intensities associated with the individual fields $I_1(x)$ and $I_2(x)$. The remaining two terms are the cross-correlations functions of the two fields at two points at the same time. The value of these last two terms depends upon the coherence relationships of the two fields. For incoherent fields they are both zero in the time average, and the resultant recorded intensity is not a hologram.

Ideally in holography the two optical fields to be added are coherent and will therefore interfere. If we assume a time harmonic field then the optical field may be written as

$$V(x, t) = \psi(x) \exp - (2\pi i \bar{v}t) \tag{3}$$

where $\bar{v}$ is the frequency of the wave, $\psi(x)$ is the spatial variation of amplitude $a(x)$ and phase $\phi(x)$, i.e.,

$$\psi(x) = a(x) \exp [i\phi(x)] \tag{4}$$

The intensity of such a field is then given by

$$I(x) = \psi(x)\psi^*(x) = |a(x)|^2 \tag{5}$$

Hence, Eq. (2) becomes

$$I(x) = a_1^2(x) + a_2^2(x) + a_1(x)a_2(x)$$
$$\times \{\exp i[\phi_1(x) - \phi_2(x)] + \exp i[\phi_2(x) - \phi_1(x)]\} \tag{6}$$

The record of the intensity distribution of Eq. (6) is a hologram where $a_1(x) \exp [i\phi_1(x)]$ is the optical field of interest and $a_2(x) \exp [i\phi_2(x)]$ is the known reference field. The classification now relates to exactly how the hologram is formed and the nature of the diffracted field.

A. IN-LINE HOLOGRAPHY

1. *Near Field Fresnel Holograms*

In the original systems devised by Gabor (1948, 1949) the hologram was a record of the interference between the light diffracted by the object and a colinear background. This automatically restricts the class of objects to those that have considerable areas that are transparent. Consider, for example, the arrangement shown in Fig. 1(a)—the light diffracted by the letter "E" interferes with the undiffracted light. The record of this interference pattern is the hologram. Hence Eq. (6) is applicable with $a_1(x) \exp [i\phi_1(x)]$ being the diffracted field associated with the letter "E" and $a_2(x) \exp [i\phi_2(x)]$ is the undiffracted field. In the original systems and most subsequent ones using this principle, the hologram was recorded in the near field of the object of interest, and thus the hologram is formed between the Fresnel diffraction pattern of the object and the background.

The second part of the image forming process is accomplished by illuminating the hologram with the original beam (or some other known beam)—see Fig. 1(b). The resulting amplitude transmittance $\Psi(x)$ is then given by

$$\Psi(x) = a(x) \exp [i\phi(x)]\{a_1^2(x) + a_2^2(x) + a_1(x)a_2(x)$$
$$\times \{\exp i[\phi_1(x) - \phi_2(x)] + \exp i[\phi_2(x) - \phi_1(x)]\} \tag{7}$$

In writing this result we have assumed that the hologram was recorded with a photographic gamma of -2 and that the linear portion of the film's characteristic curve was used. The terms in Eq. (7) that are of interest here are the last two, which represent the original optical field in the hologram plane and that same field with the phase of the field of interest, ϕ_2, shifted by 180°. Thus the original optical field is reconstructed together with a second field that has similar properties except for the phase shift noted above. These two reconstructed fields give rise to two images [see Fig. 1(b)]. Under the circumstances described here one image is real and the other virtual—the virtual

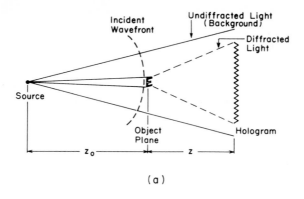

(a)

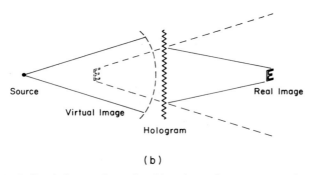

(b)

FIG. 1. In-line hologram formation (a) and wavefront reconstruction (b).

image corresponding to the original object. The radiations associated with these two images are propagating in the same direction and hence when the real image is viewed the virtual image is superimposed but well out of focus; a similar situation exists when the virtual image is viewed. This type of holo-gram is usually referred to as an in-line Fresnel hologram and has the serious disadvantages discussed above plus the added problem of photographic gamma control and the difficulty of providing sufficient light for the coherent background wave.

2. Far Field Fraunhofer Holograms

The problem of the degradation of the image by the presence of a second image that is out of focus can be overcome for certain classes of object by forming the hologram in the far-field of the object (Thompson, 1963, 1964a; Parrent and Thompson, 1964a; DeVelis et al., 1966). The arrangement for forming the hologram is identical to that discussed in the last section except that the hologram is recorded in a plane that is in the far field of the object defined by the inequalities

$$z_0 \quad \text{and} \quad z > d^2/\lambda \tag{8}$$

where λ is the wavelength of the illumination, z_0 is the distance of the object from the source of illumination, z is the distance of recording plane from the object, and d is the maximum dimension of the object. It appears then that this method can only be applied when small objects are under consideration. However, much larger objects can be handled by demagnification before forming the hologram (Thompson, 1967).

When this type of hologram is illuminated, two wavefronts are reconstructed producing the two images as before. However, the contribution of the one image in the plane of the other is not only small but is also essentially a constant.

This technique has found application in microscopy, particularly particle size analysis (Thompson et al., 1967), measurement of glass fibers (Lomas, 1969), and electron microscopy (Tonomura et al., 1968).

B. OFF-AXIS HOLOGRAPHY

1. Transmission

One of the major advances in the development of holography came with the exploitation of the off-axis reference beam technique (Leith and Upatnieks, 1962, 1963). This method solves many of the problems associated with in-line systems; the two images can be separated, and the object does not have to allow the reference beam to pass through it. Figure 2(a) shows one version of the technique; clearly there are many ways in which the coherent reference beam can be produced and, of course, it can be plane or have any other known or reproducible wavefront. Part of the original wavefront is used to illuminate the object and produce the diffracted light field, the other part of the wavefront is refracted by the prism to produce the reference beam. The hologram is formed in the region of overlap of the diffracted and reference beams.

The reference beam wavefront is tipped with respect to the diffracted wavefront and hence is described by a term $a_1(x) \exp(ik\alpha x)$ where α is the angle between the two wavefronts which is assumed small. Thus, the intensity distribution of the resultant interference pattern which is recorded as the hologram is

$$I(x) = |a_1(x) \exp(ik\alpha x) + a_2(x) \exp[i\phi(x)]|^2 \tag{9}$$

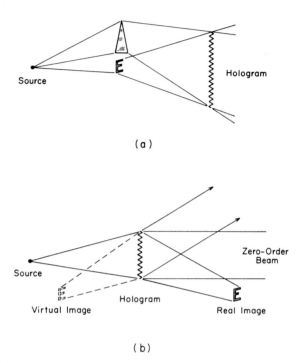

(a)

(b)

FIG. 2. Off-axis reference beam hologram formation (a) and reconstruction (b).

and hence the resulting amplitude transmittance of the hologram is

$$\Psi(x) = C\{a_1(x)^2 + a_2{}^2(x) + 2a_1(x)a_2(x) \cos [k\alpha x - \phi(x)]\} \qquad (10)$$

where C is a constant determined by the photographic process. Again a linear relationship between Ψ and I is strived for which is readily obtained if a_1/a_2 is made large. A good summary of the transfer characteristics of emulsion when used for holography can be found in a review article by Leith and Upatnieks (1967). Kozma (1966) has treated the problem in detail with special reference to the effects of nonlinearity. It is important to note here that linear recording is obtained in a single-step process (rather than the two-step method required to obtain a gamma of -2). Furthermore, the negative slope of the amplitude transmittance versus exposure curve has the effect of reversing the phase of the cos $k\alpha x$ term which is only acting as a carrier that is phase modulated by $\phi(x)$.

When this hologram is illuminated three beams are formed [see Fig. 2(b)], a zero-order beam and two first-order beams. It is these two first-order beams that are important; they give rise again to real and virtual images.

However, the two image beams do not now overlap in the region of the images providing, of course, that a suitable α is chosen.

The distinction between the near-field (Fresnel) and the far-field (Fraunhofer) diffraction region of the object are no longer of any consequence experimentally. However, a detailed analysis would be simplified by noting this difference. In most circumstances, it is the near-field that will be used and indeed most of the work done with this method is certainly of the type that would be called off-axis Fresnel holography. The off-axis Fraunhofer holography has been recognized and described (Rose, 1965; Thompson, 1967), but it is of little consequence.

A further virtue of this method is that improved "cosmetic" quality of the final image may be obtained by diffusing the light which illuminates the object (Leith and Upatnieks, 1964). The technique is, of course, accompanied by an increased spatial-frequency bandwidth.

2. *Reflection*

Now that the concept of a separate non object-dependent reference has been introduced, it is an easy step to apply the technique to three-dimensional diffusely reflecting objects. The hologram is formed by the light scattered by the object of interest and a known reference beam (see Fig. 3). The remainder

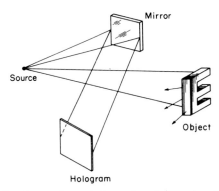

FIG. 3. Off-axis reference beam holography of diffusely reflecting object.

of the process is the same as before. The images formed from the reconstructed wavefronts now have the three-dimensionality of the object and normal parallax is observed. Usually the virtual image is used by looking through the hologram; a faithful reproduction of the object is seen, and the result is equivalent to the aerial image formed by more conventional optical systems. The real image, however, has a number of unusual properties since it cannot be viewed from the hologram plane (Meier, 1965).

3. *Fourier Transform Holograms*

In previous sections we have examined the formation of the Fraunhofer hologram formed in the far field of the object. There is, of course, another condition to produce the characteristic Fraunhofer diffraction pattern of an object. The Fraunhofer pattern is formed in the image plane of the point source that illuminates the object. Often collimated illumination of the object is used so that the appropriate diffraction pattern is formed in the focal plane of the lens. The Fraunhofer diffraction field is, of course, the Fourier transform of the object field. Clearly, a hologram can be formed by adding a suitable reference wave to this diffraction field. This idea was introduced by Leith and Upatnieks (1962) as a generalized hologram. However, it is now most usually called a Fourier transform hologram (Stroke *et al.*, 1965).

A variety of techniques are available for producing this type of hologram. The reference beam may or may not pass through the lens and again the reference wavefront may be varied. Figure 4(a) shows an often used system that produces a collimated reference beam.

The hologram is formed as the interference pattern between the Fourier transform of the object field and the reference field. Hence, if we write

$$b(\xi) \exp [i\theta(\xi)] = \int a(x) \exp [i\phi(x)] \exp (ikx\xi/f) \, dx \qquad (11)$$

and the reference beam as $a_1 \exp (ik\alpha\xi)$ then the intensity in the hologram plane is

$$I(\xi) = \Psi(\xi)\Psi^*(\xi)$$

where

$$\Psi(\xi) = a_1 \exp (ik\alpha\xi) + b(\xi) \exp [i\theta(\xi)] \qquad (12)$$

Conceptually, we can see that each point in the object, together with the point reference, produces a set of cosine fringes in the transform plane. Thus, when the hologram is illuminated, say with a collimated beam, then each cosine function will produce a zero-order and two first-order diffracted beams. Hence, a lens can collect these diffracted orders and produce two real images on either side of the zero-order image.

Another way to form an exact Fourier transform hologram would be to use a system shown in Fig. 4(c) and form the hologram in the far field of the object. Approximate forms of this arrangement have been very successfully used by Stroke and Falconer (1964) and Stroke, Brumm, and Funkhouser (1965). The advantage of this type of holographic process is that the resolution requirements are considerably eased since the reference wavefront and the diffracted wavefront have approximately the same sphericity and hence the

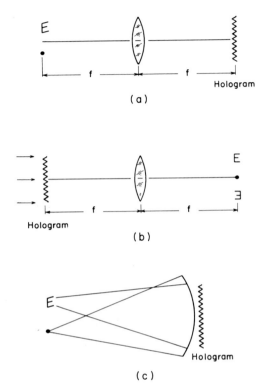

FIG. 4. Fourier transform hologram formation (a) and wavefront reconstruction (b). Approximate method (c) of hologram formation.

resultant fringes have a relatively large period (Winthrop and Worthington, 1965).

In concluding this section on off-axis reference beam techniques, we must note their importance in the development of applications. The majority of applications that will be discussed here will make use of this technology.

III. Applications of Holographic Image Formation

Since holography is basically a two-step coherent image forming process, it is not surprising that the first useful applications were in image formation. Clearly there are problems in image formation that cannot be solved by conventional techniques in a satisfactory manner. Hence, it is realistic to determine whether holography can help in these areas to obtain an image that previously could not be obtained or perhaps record an image of an event more easily or more accurately. The first of the real applications of holography certainly falls into this category. We will use this application as an example of the statements made above. Consider the problem of trying to form an image of a number of small dynamic objects whose positions are not known. By conventional means it is possible to focus an imaging system on only a few of these objects which happen to be in or near a given plane. Information about the other objects in other planes cannot be recorded without refocusing the system. However, it is possible to record a hologram of these objects made with a short enough exposure time that the hologram provides a record of these objects at a given instant. A stationary image can now be formed of these objects so that they may be studied in detail. (We will return to a discussion of this application in Section III,B.)

A. MICROSCOPY

Several approaches have been tried to devise schemes for microscopy and to obtain resolution comparable to the conventional microscope. The advantages here would be to obtain a larger field of view at this high resolution and also to increase the depth of field. The hologram can serve as its own optical element and so lensless microscopes were considered with the magnification then obtained by the use of divergent beams and wavelength changes, as discussed by several authors including Baez (1952), El-Sum (1952), and Rogers (1952). The aberrations inherent in such processes have also received attention (Rogers, 1952; Armstrong, 1965; Meier, 1965; Leith et al., 1965a). Good results by these lensless techniques have been described with resolution of a few microns (e.g., see Leith and Upatnieks, 1965). The fly's wing result is now a classic!

A detailed discussion of the analysis of the magnification and aberrations of lensless holographic microscopy is not warranted here, but for the interested reader an excellent review is given by Smith (1969). After Smith, we write the magnification M as

$$M = m/[1 \pm m^2 z_0/\mu z_c - z_0/z_r] \tag{13}$$

where z_0 is the distance from the object to the hologram plane z_r the distance from the point reference to the hologram plane (see Fig. 5), z_c is the distance from the point source to the hologram in the wavefront reconstruction step, μ is the ratio of the wavelength of the beams used to form the hologram and reconstruct the wavefronts, and m is the linear magnification of the hologram. The resolution of the image is determined by the effective aperture of the hologram and the wavelength of the incident illumination.

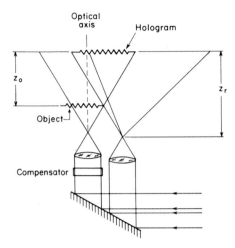

FIG. 5. Schematic diagram of system for "lensless" microscopy (after Leith and Upatnieks, 1965).

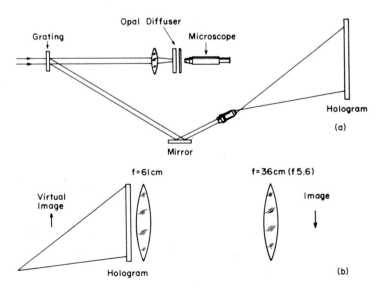

FIG. 6. Holographic microscopy and image formation (after Carter *et al.*, 1966).

Holographic microscopy has been pursued in a very different way by modifying a conventional microscope so that the process is no longer lensless. This idea was developed almost simultaneously by two groups of workers (Van Ligten and Osterberg, 1966; Van Ligten, 1967; Carter *et al.*, 1966; Carter and Dougal, 1966).

Figure 6(a) shows the arrangement used by Carter in his work. A grating beam splitter is used to produce the illumination and reference beams. The object is illuminated and the diffracted light allowed to pass through a conventional microscope. The reference beam is reflected from a mirror and then focused to a point reference. To form an image from the hologram, the system shown in Fig. 6(b) was used. The spatial filter removes the unwanted components of the reconstructed wavefront. The field of view cannot be extended over that obtained by the normal use of the microscope. However, resolution up to the limit set by the microscope can be obtained and appreciable depth of field can be recorded. This depth of field is limited by the coherence of the reference beam and the resolution of the photographic emulsion. Figure 7(a) shows the image of a three bar target formed by this technique but with the diffuser removed. Resolution of about 1 μ is obtained. However, the overall appearance of the image leaves much to be desired. The use of the fine opal glass diffuser discussed earlier can remove some of these defects, but at high resolution this causes other problems apart from the resolution loss [(Fig. 7(b)]. This noise in the image is a result of the coherent nature of the image formation. A great deal of concentrated effort has gone into solving this problem, but there still is no good solution. As Leith (1970) recently pointed out, one method is to use a numerical aperture greater than that needed for the required resolution. Together with the use of the diffuser this can achieve desired results, but not when resolution of a few microns is required. There is a possibility that a purely random phase diffuser in contact with the object could help (Upatnieks, 1969). However, phase objects do have unusual effects in coherent image formation because of the nonlinearity of the process.

This work just described was laboratory experimentation and no attempt was made to use these results in any instrument. However, Van Ligten has pursued his original work to the point that a holographic microscope is a reality. Figure 8 shows the instrument developed by Van Ligten together with a schematic diagram. Figure 9 shows a typical result of the image of neurons. It is possible to see small fibers about a micron wide and, of course, to follow the structure in depth and make counts of crossovers of fibrous structures.

Van Ligten has also pointed out some other advantages of holographic microscopy, including the fact that both amplitude and some phase information is contained in the hologram. Furthermore, the advantage gained if the

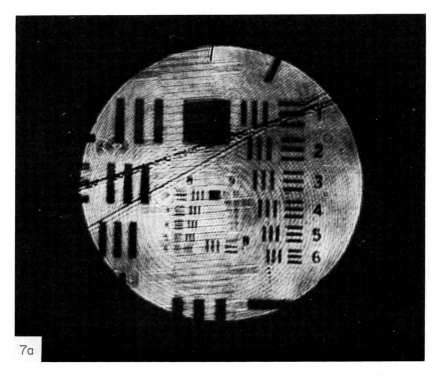

FIG. 7. Holographic microscope image (a) without and (b) with a diffuser (after Carter, 1969).

specimen is changing with time is enormous since a whole range of diagnostic techniques are available to study the image at leisure; these would include Schlieren system viewing, dark and bright field analysis, and interferometry.

B. MICROSCOPY USING FRAUNHOFER HOLOGRAPHY

The microscopy discussed in the last section used the off-axis reference beam techniques to advantage. There is, however, a separate branch of microscopy that developed from a specific requirement. This requirement was particle size analysis in dynamic situations; the discovery of the special properties of Fraunhofer holograms came directly from studies attempting to meet this requirement (Thompson, 1964a; Parent and Thompson, 1964a). Initially, the technique was used for recording droplets of water in naturally occurring fog, but has since been used to solve a variety of other problems.

The basic principles of this type of holography were stressed in an earlier section.

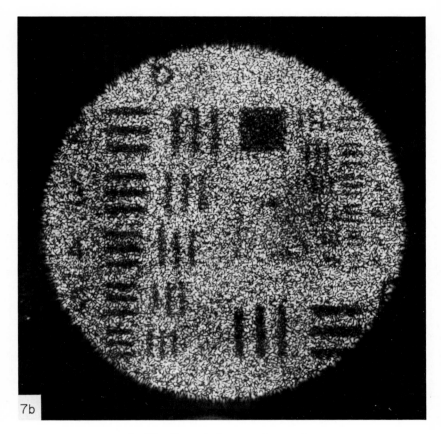

See Fig. 7a on facing page for caption.

1. Particle Size Analysis

A number of papers on this application have appeared in the literature (Silverman *et al.*, 1964; Thompson *et al.*, 1966, 1967). The discussion here is similar to portions of a recent review article (Thompson, 1968b).

a. Fog Droplet Camera. The hologram camera (laser fog disdrometer) system was designed and fabricated as a customized instrumentation system for recording size and relative position of naturally occurring fog droplets in the 5 to 100 μ diameter size range. This system is based on a two-step imaging technique using Fraunhofer holograms; consequently, the system is composed of two subsystems: the recording subsystem and the reconstructing subsystem.

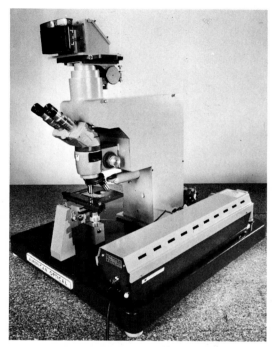

FIG 8. The van Ligten holographic microscope (courtesy of American Optical Corp.).

In the recording subsystem, a Q-switched ruby laser illuminates the sample volume and forms a hologram. The short time laser pulse stops the motion of the fog particles and instantaneously records the size and relative position of the particles in the sample volume with considerable resolution and depth of field.

In the reconstructing subsystem, the hologram record is illuminated with a helium–neon cw gas laser. This illumination reconstructs the wavefronts and a three-dimensional visual image of the original fog particle sample is formed. A closed-circuit video system with appropriate optical systems provides a two-dimensional display of selected planes through the sample volume for viewing and measuring particle size and relative position.

The first system was put together in the summer of 1963 (Silverman *et al.*, 1964), and the basic principles verified. This system, however, employed a spatial filter to remove the background light so that the recording showed typical Airy patterns.

Two laser fog disdrometer units were fabricated and operated in the field at Otis Air Force Base, Cape Cod during the summer of 1964. Figure 10 is a

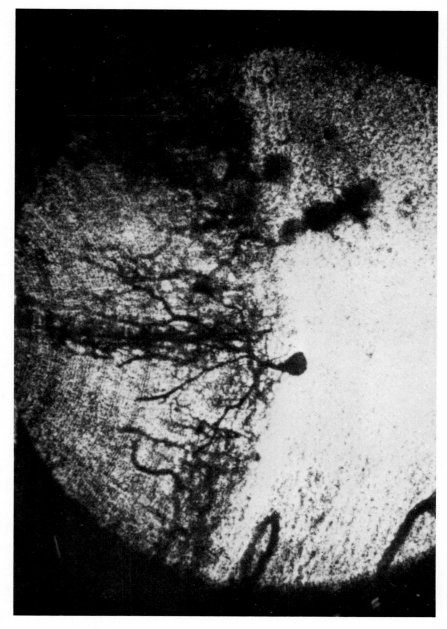

FIG. 9. Image formed from a hologram made with the microscope of FIG. 8 of a specimen of neurons (courtesy of American Optical Corp.).

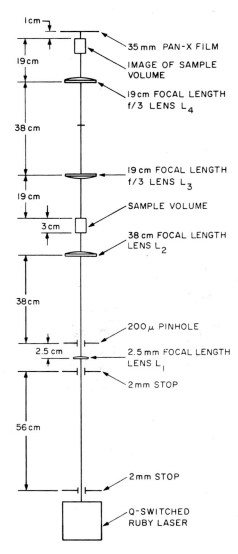

1 cm

35 mm PAN-X FILM

IMAGE OF SAMPLE
VOLUME

19 cm

19 cm FOCAL LENGTH
f/3 LENS L$_4$

38 cm

19 cm FOCAL LENGTH
f/3 LENS L$_3$

19 cm

SAMPLE VOLUME

3 cm

38 cm FOCAL LENGTH
LENS L$_2$

38 cm

200 μ PINHOLE

2.5 cm

2.5 mm FOCAL LENGTH
LENS L$_1$

2 mm STOP

56 cm

2 mm STOP

Q-SWITCHED
RUBY LASER

FIG. 10. Optical schematic of holographic particle size analyzer in 1964 (after B. J. Thompson *et al.*, 1965, 1967).

schematic diagram of this disdrometer. The *Q*-switched ruby laser beam was provided with two 2-mm diameter aperture stops, 56 cm apart. This removed off-axis laser modes and selected a relatively uniform area of the beam as the input to the collimator collector lens. Lenses L$_1$ and L$_2$ were used to expand and collimate the laser beam; the beam diameter could be expanded approximately $20 \times$. Fog droplets were allowed to flow through the sample volume, which was 3 cm in depth along the optic axis. Two 19-cm focal length, $f/3$ lenses (L_3 and L_4) were arranged with coincidental focal points; these imaged the fog droplets to a volume directly in front of the 35-mm film plane. The film used was Kodak Panatomic-X. The film plane was 1 cm beyond the nearest boundary of the imaged sample volume.

This unit was designed to be installed in a field instrument trailer. The laser head and collimator are suspended vertically below the 1/2 inch aluminum plate. The two dishlike plates shown in the photograph (Fig. 11) define

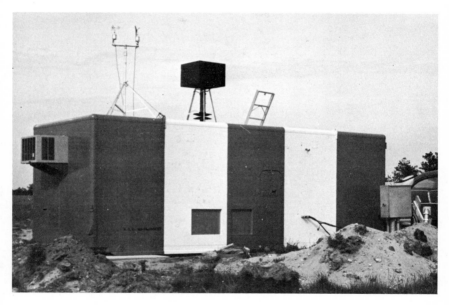

FIG. 11. Holographic particle size analyzer installed in trailer and ready for operation at Otis Air Force Base, Cape Cod.

the sample volume. The imaging optics and shutters are in the top vertical tube. There are two additional components in the top section: a solenoid to actuate the shutter and a clock that was imaged into the corner of each data frame; the entire top section was enclosed.

For several reasons, the laser fog disdrometer constructed in 1964 was limited to recording particles 30 μ in diameter and larger. Neither the resolution of Panatomic-X film nor the imaging lenses were capable of recording particles less than 20 μ in diameter. The laser fog disdrometer systems were redesigned and data were reduced by measuring the diameter of reconstructed droplet images.

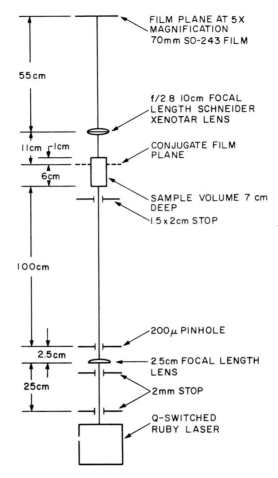

FILM PLANE AT 5X
MAGNIFICATION
70mm SO-243 FILM

55 cm

f/2.8 10cm FOCAL
LENGTH SCHNEIDER
XENOTAR LENS

CONJUGATE FILM
PLANE

11cm ⌐1cm

6cm

SAMPLE VOLUME 7 cm
DEEP

1.5 x 2cm STOP

100cm

200 μ PINHOLE

2.5cm

2.5cm FOCAL LENGTH
LENS

25cm

2mm STOP

Q-SWITCHED
RUBY LASER

FIG. 12. Optical schematic of particle size analyzer as modified in 1965 (after Thompson *et al.*, 1967).

During the summer of 1965, the two laser fog disdrometer units described above were modified and reinstalled at the Otis Air Force Base site. Figure 12 is an optical schematic of the modified instrument. A typical hologram of droplets is shown in Fig. 13.

Figure 14 is an optical schematic of the laser fog disdrometer readout instrument. Holograms are reconstructed with illumination from a collimated He–Ne gas laser of 3×10^{-4} W output power. The laser light is first converged by a positive collecting lens and then passed through a pinhole, which acts as a low-pass spatial-frequency filter smoothing out small-scale intensity

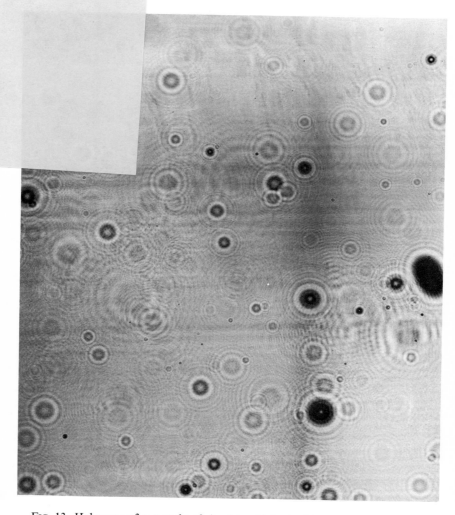

FIG. 13. Hologram of a sample of droplets obtained with system shown in Fig. 12 (after Thompson, 1968b).

variations in the cross section of the laser beam. The hologram is placed on a traveling carriage, and the reconstructed real images are imaged onto the face of a vidicon tube in a closed-circuit video system. Focused droplet images are then sized visually by measuring them with a reticle inked onto the face of the video monitor. The closed circuit video system permits magnification at an increase in brightness, but without loss of contrast.

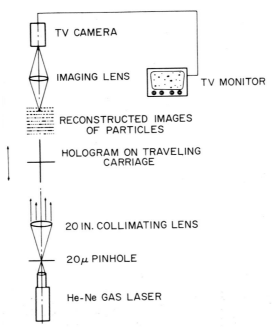

FIG. 14. Optical schematic of a readout device for measurement of particle size.

The readout instrument magnifies 65 ×. This gives the system an overall geometric magnification from droplet to video monitor image of 325 ×. The scale on the face of the video monitor is divided into 0.064-in. intervals corresponding to 5 μ increments. Drops are sized to the nearest 5 μ diameter.

Several schemes for fully automatic data reduction have been studied. The most difficult step in data reduction is to find and focus the real images of individual droplets. Although some positive results were obtained for droplet diameters 25 μ and larger, feasibility could not be demonstrated for the small droplet sizes. In the size range below 25 μ, film noise and out-of-focus images of larger drops can give signal levels (intensities) on the same order as the intensity in the focused image of small droplets. However, nonautomatic visual techniques allow sizing down to a few microns.

The readout instrument was designed to facilitate reduction of field data in a manner as convenient for the operator as possible. The optical system design was kept simple so it could accommodate any changes made in possible future disdrometer units that would reduce droplet data of other size ranges. Electrically driven mechanical scanning in the x, y, and z directions was used in order that a fully automatic data reduction scheme might be incorporated if and when an automatic technique becomes available.

Figure 15 is a photograph of a readout instrument. A joy-stick controls the motion of the film carriage along the z axis. Since the laser fog disdrometer magnifies the hologram $5 \times$, length of the reconstructed sample volume is expanded $25 \times$. The carriage travels 168 cm along the track. A four position toggle switch controls the x, y direction film scan. The x, y, z scans have continuously variable scanning speed. The matrix of panel lights identifies the particular area of the hologram data frame being viewed on the video monitor.

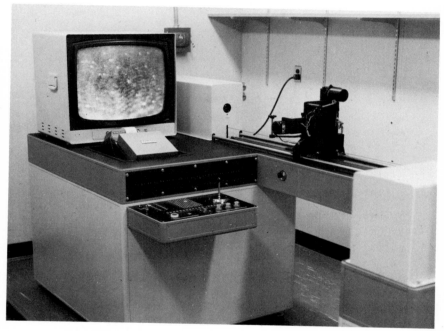

Fig. 15. Photograph of the instrument shown schematically in Fig. 14.

The operator punches the diameters of the droplets into the row of size buttons on the control panel, and a tape printer records the x, y, z position coordinates along with these diameters. The row of counters on the face of the console above the control panel shows the number of recorded particles in each $5~\mu$ size range. The printer will record these totals on command of the operator. Data are reduced by first scanning the focused image of the hologram data frame and searching for the hologram patterns of individual droplets. When a pattern is found, the operator drives the carriage along the optic axis to focus the real image. A lock-in control in the y-scan direction prevents the operator from counting droplets more than once, and to provide a regular scanning pattern.

The resolution limit of the readout, which is set by the imaging lens magnification and the raster resolution in the vidicon tube, is approximately 25 μ. A 25 μ spot size was chosen to correspond to the resolution limit of the disdrometer and to give the readout instrument the largest possible field of view without degrading the reconstructed images.

This same scheme can be used for objects other than droplets. Lomas (1969) has used the method to dynamically measure the shape changes along glass fibers produced in the continuous filament process. Since the glass fibers are transparent, a modification of the hologram takes place caused by an extra interference pattern obtained from the transmitted beam. When the image is formed, a set of interference fringes are seen down the middle of the fiber. These fringes relate directly to diameter changes in the fiber which tapers as it is drawn and allows shape changes to be followed and measured.

b. Dynamic Aerosol Camera. An entirely new system was designed and fabricated for evaluation of highly dynamic aerosols. Clearly, the environment can provide special problems in this application. The schematic of this system is shown in Fig. 16 with detailed annotation.

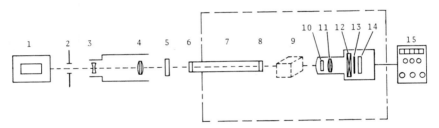

FIG. 16. Schematic diagram of aerosol assessment camera. (1) Ruby laser, Lear Seigler, LS-100, 10 mW peak, pulse duration 20×10^{-9} sec. (2) Stop 2.2 mm, 31.75 cm from laser port. (3) Collimator lens: 33 mm E.F.L. (4) Colimator objective glass flat, 6 mm thick. (7) Light tube, 12.75 cm diam $\times$ 2.4 cm long (helim filled). (8) Protective flat, 6 mm thick. (9) Picture volume 1.37 $\times$ 2.05 $\times$ 6 cm (for particles 22μ and larger). (10) Flat, 6 mm thick. (11) Camera lens, 5 cm E.F.L., $f/1.6$. (12) Shutter, Hex No. 5 or Graflex Focal Plane. (13) Filter, Wratten No. 70. (14). Film, SO-243, 70 mm. (15) Shutter and magazine control (after Thompson *et al.*, 1967).

c. Application to Larger Particles. The extension of this technique to larger particles of many hundreds of microns and upwards can be achieved. (The off-axis reference beam method will always be useful in principle except that in practice it is not always possible to provide the reference beam because of the configuration of the system.) However, the system can be used if slightly modified; the modification is necessitated since the far field for big particles rapidly becomes prohibitively large. Unless the far field is used the reconstruction is adversely affected by the virtual image term. Before the hologram is recorded the particles are demagnified and the far field is then calculated from the demagnified image size. This technique could find important applications in such fields as raindrop sizing where sample volumes several meters in depth could be handled in a single exposure.

d. Bubble-Chamber Photography. Welford (1966) suggested that holography might be used in getting increased focal depth in bubble chamber photography. Recently feasibility tests (Thompson and Ward, 1967; Ward and Thompson, 1967) have been conducted to determine the applicability of holographic techniques to bubble chamber recording. Typically, the bubbles are about 400 μ in diameter and the chamber may be as large as 132 cm or even 200 cm. Furthermore, because of the magnet yoke it is not possible to go straight through the chamber, it is necessary to come out the same side as the source of illumination. A scheme was devised where this could be accomplished using a mirror at the rear end of the simulated chamber. In the tests, a variety of fixed wires and injected aerosols were used to determine the parameters of the system. The resolution ($\pm 3\%$) of individual particles can readily be obtained over sample depths in excess of those required. The location accuracy in depth is not so great being approximately 20 particle diameters; angular accuracy of tracks can be $\pm 4°$.

To simulate the effects of bubbles, a quantity of glass beads of 150 μ diameter were allowed to fall freely through a cell containing polyglycol. The index of the glass beads was 1.52 and the index of the liquid was 1.45. Excellent resolution was obtained with the reconstruction of these holograms, the diameter being determined to about 3% accuracy. The positional accuracy was again 10–20 particle diameters, which is poorer than that obtained by current triangulation techniques applied to pairs of bubble chamber photographs. The limitation is essentially fundamental to this type of holography since it arises from the effective lens size of the hologram record. The diameter of the effective lens is determined by the diameter of the hologram associated with an individual particle. This can be readily calculated, and agrees with the experimental results already quoted. To increase the positional accuracy would require going to a much higher resolution film—a direction to be avoided in bubble chamber recording.

Further experimental work has been carried out by Murata, Fujiwara, and Asakura (1968). In this work optical spatial filtering was used to suppress undesirable beam tracks.

e. Very Small Particles. A number of developments in this subject have occurred recently. Hickling (1968) has produced Fraunhofer holograms on a computer and has successfully reconstructed them. In this work a cathode-ray tube linked to a computer is used to synthesize holograms of spherical liquid droplets illuminated by plane waves of monochromatic linearly polarized light. The classical Mie solution is employed to determine the far-field radiation pattern of the light waves scattered by the droplets. The most distinctive maxima and minima in the radiation pattern of a droplet are found to occur in the side scattering adjacent to the forward lobe, when the droplet is viewed in a plane that is perpendicular to the direction of polarization of the incident waves. Typical examples of these maxima and minima were recorded on the computed holograms. The reference source was an electric dipole with its axis of polarization parallel to the direction of polarization of the light waves incident on the droplets. Reconstructed images were obtained from the computed holograms using a low power He–Ne laser source. The reconstructed images were found to show all of the appropriate maxima and minima in the radiation pattern. A holographic method is suggested by Hickling for determining the size of spherical liquid droplets in the range of diameters from about 0.5 to 20 μ. This method is based on the techniques used in the construction of the computed holograms and depends on the relation between the angles of the maxima and minima, the wavelength and the size.

Recently, the possibility of detecting the presence of submicron particles, and hence determining the concentration and spatial position of submicron objects in a three-dimensional sample has been demonstrated (Thompson and Zinky, 1969).

Small particles which are less than a micron in mean diameter act essentially as point scatterers, and hence the hologram is formed by the addition of a spherical wave from the point scatterer and the undiffracted background plane wave. When the hologram of submicron objects is transilluminated to reconstruct the image, an image intensity distribution is formed that is essentially the impulse response of the overall system put down at the location in space of the original point object. Results using a latex hydrosol containing a dispersion of 0.365 μ mean diameter latex spheres on a microscope cover glass have been shown.

f. Electron Beam Particle Size Analysis. Perhaps the most exciting development was the recent work of Tonomura *et al.* (1968), on the optical reconstruction of images from Fraunhofer electron holograms. Opaque particles of gold 100 Å in diameter were illuminated with a collimated beam of quasimonochromatic electrons of $\lambda_{el} = 0.037$ Å. The reconstruction is accomplished with light from a He–Ne laser and excellent results are demonstrated.

C. PARTICLE SIZING USING OFF-AXIS REFERENCE BEAM HOLOGRAPHY

The field of particle size analysis is a very difficult one from the experimentalist's point of view. Hence, it is not surprising that approaches to the problem other than those described above have been taken. Thus Brooks *et al.* (1965)

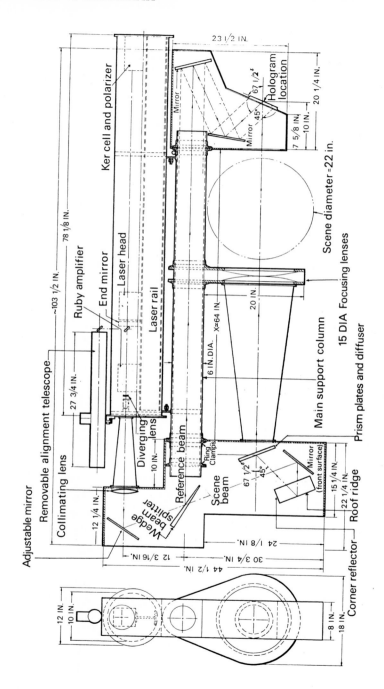

FIG. 17. Schematic of pulsed laser transmission holocamera (after Wuerker and Heflinger, 1968).

have designed and built a variety of " holocamera's " for particle size analysis, particularly for rocket engine studies. Again a pulsed ruby laser beam was used for the illumination for the same reasons that they were used in the hologram cameras discussed earlier. Here we will describe one of the systems and follow quite closely the description of it given by Wuerker and Heflinger (1968) in a recent review paper on pulsed laser holography. These authors point out quite clearly the need for taking considerable trouble with the ruby laser to increase the temporal and spatial coherence of the beam. Furthermore, because they used a separate reference beam, it is necessary then to match the paths of the diffracted and reference beams quite carefully.

A schematic diagram of the holocamera is shown in Fig. 17 designed for use with a 25,000 lb thrust 18 in. diameter engine. The laser beam is expanded and collimated by a Galilean telescope. A beam splitter provides the illumination and reference beams. The illumination beam passes through the beam splitter and is reflected by a front surface mirror and a 90° roof reflector into a prism plate and ground glass diffuser. The prism plate directs the illumination beam parallel to the axis of the two focusing lenses which form the scattered

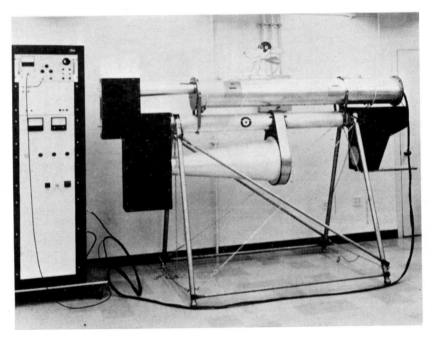

FIG. 18. Photograph of the holocamera system of Fig. 17 (after Wuerker and Heflinger, 1968).

light from the diffuser into the hologram plane. The reference beam is reflected from the beam splitter, passes through the 6 in. diameter pipe and is reflected by two mirrors into the holographic plane. The two beams are at 45° to each and were determined by the properties of the Agfa 10E75 emulsion. Two shutters are used in the system—an electric capping shutter and a window shade shutter which triggers the laser when it is in the open position. Wavelength discrimination techniques removed the majority of the self-luminosity of the flame and sunlight. The apparatus is shown in Fig. 18. The holograms produced by this system are illuminated with light from a helium–neon laser, and images of the field can be seen with a resolution of better than 100 μ.

D. PHOTOGRAPHY

1. *Pulsed Laser Photography*

An advantage can be gained by using holographic methods to photograph transient or high speed events especially when it is not certain where in a given volume the event may occur. Hence, the techniques used in particle sizing can be applied to macrophotography. Brooks *et al.* (1965) realized this and used the ruby laser in both the conventional and Q-switched modes. These workers recognized the importance of designing the system so that the path of the reference beam carefully matched that of the illuminating beam. Figure 19 shows a schematic of apparatus used in this original experimentation. The output from the laser is diverged slightly and split in two by the beam splitter. The scene was diffusely illuminated. By careful positioning of the mirrors the optical paths were matched and the angle between the two beams was 20°. Photographs were obtained of a 22-caliber bullet cutting a wire while moving at 375 meter/sec. The image was formed by the conventional method of illuminating the hologram with a He–Ne laser. Photography of slower phenomena such as water jets were accomplished without Q-switching the laser. Resolution obtained by this process was about 20 lines per millimeter. These results are interesting but similar records can be obtained with conventional high-speed photographic techniques. However, the holographic method has a greater depth of field.

Tanner (1966) has pointed out how these techniques might be used in fluid mechanics and illustrated the principles using a gas flame. Of particular importance was Tanner's observation and illustration that once the hologram was made the image could be recorded and seen as if it had been photographed in a conventional Schlieren or shadow system.

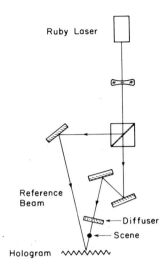

FIG. 19. Schematic diagram of holographic photographic system using equalization of optical path (after Brooks *et al.*, 1965).

For successful application of holographic methods to photography it is necessary to have good control of the laser output parameters particularly the temporal coherence. With good temporal coherence considerable path differences can be tolerated between the object and reference beams. Ansley and Siebert (1968) have obtained laser output in a single transverse and axial frequency mode resulting in coherence lengths of greater than 1 meter. The typical pulse lengths are 30 nsec and the energy 250 mJ. Figure 20 shows the experimental arrangement used by these authors. The reflecting mirrors are external to the ruby rod and a cryptocyanide *Q*-switch is employed which

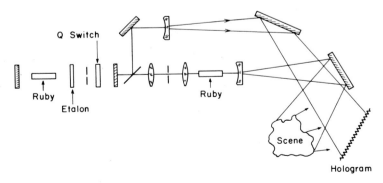

FIG. 20. Schematic design of highly coherent pulsed laser holographic system (after Ansley and Siebert, 1968).

suppresses the lower axial modes. An amplifier rod is used to provide a factor of five gain per pass through the rod. Excellent portrait photographs have been taken as well as more scientific subjects with this method.

2. Microcircuit Manufacture

One of the problems in microcircuit manufacture is purely optical. Each silicon disk of approximately 2.5 cm in diameter contains tens or often hundreds of microcircuits requiring a resolution of a few microns. The master for producing the contact exposure on the photoresist coating on the silicon disk is made by a step and repeat technique after a two-step reduction from the original art work. The masters can only be used a limited number of times for contact printing before they have to be discarded. Dust particles are disastrous in this process. Projection printing techniques cannot be used because of the high resolution required over a large format. In principle holography can help since it is conceptually possible to produce a hologram of a single high resolution element and then use the hologram to form an image of the required resolution (Beesley, 1968); the format could be greater than that available with a lens. The possible application to microcircuit manufacture is discussed in two recent papers (Kiemle, 1968; Beesley, 1968).

A combination of this idea plus that of image replication (Parrent and Thompson, 1964b) could be of value. The principle of image replication involves coherently illuminating the single object of interest and allowing the diffracted light to fall on a periodic structure. The periodic structure is chosen so that in the final image plane a set of delta functions are produced at which locations the image of the object is positioned. Originally this was achieved by the use of grating structures. However, the process can be significantly improved by making the periodic structure a hologram of the required array of delta functions. This was recognized by a number of workers as well as the ones referenced above (Groh, 1967; Lu, 1968; Grosso et al., 1968; Lowenthal et al., 1968).

A related approach discussed by Kiemle (1968) is to illuminate the hologram of a single element with an array of beams.

All these approaches are interesting but as yet have not been used in the microcircuit manufacture in production.

E. DATA STORAGE AND RETRIEVAL

As early as 1964 Leith and Upatnieks demonstrated the possibility of storing more than one image on a holographic plate. In this example the two objects were placed at different distances from the hologram so that neither obscured the other when viewed from the position of the hologram. Storage of several images can be achieved by rotating the hologram between exposures (Van Ligten and Lawton, 1967). This type of arrangement is similar to earlier nonholographic multiplexing techniques. There are a number of advantages to be gained in storing information as a hologram rather than a microimage. The hologram is not greatly affected by the presence of scratches, dust, pinholes in the emulsion and other localized defects. These same defects in a microimage could completely eliminate the stored information or a significant portion of it. Hence there is a built-in advantageous redundancy in the holographically stored information.

1. *Holographic Memories*

These advantages have led to very serious considerations of holographic memories by a number of companies notably RCA, Bell Telephone Laboratories, and IBM. A holographic memory based on a page organization could have a capacity of 2×10^7 bits at a data rate of 50×10^6 bps and an access time of 3×10^{-6} sec (LaMacchia, 1969, 1970).

A typical example of a random access memory is that under development by Bell Telephone Laboratories. The light from an argon laser is deflected acoustooptically by a pair of lead molybdate cells into the holographic memory (see Fig. 21). The image produced by the illuminated hologram is formed on an

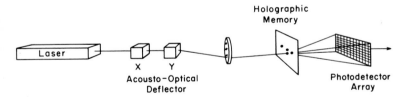

FIG. 21. Holographic memory with random access under development by Bell Telephone Laboratories.

array of photodetectors. The data bits appear as bright and dark areas and are converted into electrical impulses by the photodetector. The memory is produced by a step and repeat process (LaMacchia, 1969) each hologram being put down separately as a Fourier-transform hologram formed between the Fourier transform of the data mask produced by an $f/1.3$ system and the reference waves. This hologram is actually recorded in a localized area of the recording medium. A typical array may consist of 32×32 holograms, each hologram containing 4096 bits: the holograms have a center to center spacing of 2 mm. Hence some of the advantages of the holographic recording are negated by the very small area that each hologram occupies. In the image formed the bit has a diameter of 1.5 mm. With a $f/0.7$ system the capacity can be increased to 16×10^7 bits by using a 64×64 array of holograms.

One suggested application of an optical memory is in the printing industry for typesetting (Meyerhofer, 1970). The memory consists of a set of holograms of characters of one or more fonts. A pulsed argon laser beam is deflected by two galvanometer mirrors to the correct location, and a real image of the required character is produced at a fixed location on the face plate of a camera tube. This image is then scanned with an electron beam to produce a video signal. Subsequent processing then determines the exact size and shape of the character before it is displayed on a cathode-ray tube. Finally the character is positioned optically. Clearly this technique will have to compete technologically and economically with current systems available to the industry.

The viability of holographic memories will probably depend upon the developments in recording materials. Initially the prime candidate is, of course, silver halide emulsion. However, increased diffraction efficiency can be obtained with dichromated-gelatin which produces a phase record. The major drawback to these recording materials is that they are irreversible. A significant technological improvement can be obtained if the material can be erased so that the memory can be updated locally. Hence a variety of photochromic materials have been considered (Bosomworth and Gerritson, 1968). A typical photochromic material is written on with blue light and erased with red. For readout an intermediate wavelength is used. It must be remembered, of course, that this material is much slower than silver halide emulsions, which may not be a problem since relatively high energy densities are available with laser beams.

Thermoplastic materials have also been evaluated (Urbach and Meier, 1966) which again provide a sensitive reversible material that shows little sign of fatigue after many cycles.

Recent work on materials has included the so-called Curie point writing in thin films of ferromagnetic materials. Manganese bismuth has been used (Chen et al., 1968; Mezrich, 1969). The thermal effect of the light is to change the magnetization in the film. The readout from this magnetic record is accomplished by illuminating the record with a lower power laser beam and detecting the phase modulation produced by the Faraday effect. The record is erased by raising the temperature to a point above the Curie temperature which for manganese–bismuth is 150° C.

Finally we may note that index changes produced in some of the ferroelectric crystalline material have been examined as phase recording materials. The most interesting materials at the moment are probably lithium niobate (Chen et al., 1968) and barium titanate (Townsend and LaMacchia, 1969).

Clearly a considerable amount of effort has yet to be expended in the area before holographic memories can become part of the everyday technology.

2. *Television Tape Player*

Very recently RCA introduced a new concept for a color videotape that consists of a holographic record embossed into a vinyl tape.[1] Here again we have the use of a new holographic material that uses a phase image in a relatively cheap material. The holograms are recorded as Fourier transform holograms that have the advantage of producing an image that is not subject to lateral motion of the hologram. The overall system is currently under development, and it is intended that SelectaVision will be introduced into the home entertainment market in 1973. This development could be the first truly commercial application of holography. The specific implementation of the principles of holography are quite interesting. The required hologram is initially recorded using a helium–cadmium laser at 4416 Å in photoresist coated onto a cronar tape. When the photoresist has been developed, it is plated with nickel. The resulting nickel master is then used to produce holograms on a vinyl tape by heat and pressure. Hence a large number of vinyl replicas can be produced rapidly from a single master, each tape being ½ inch

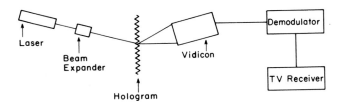

FIG. 22. RCA's holographic videotape play back system.

wide film containing 10-mm wide holograms. The image is produced from the hologram by transilluminating with a 2 mW helium–neon laser onto the vidicon (Fig. 22). The color is encoded in a set of superimposed modulated areas for the blue and red images and the green information is recovered by subtracting the red and blue signals from the total luminance signal.

F. IMAGE FORMATION THROUGH AN IRREGULAR MEDIUM

The fact that the hologram records the actual wavefront information present in that plane offers the possibility of compensating for errors introduced by the medium between the object and the hologram recording plane

---

[1] This discussion is based on press releases and semitechnical reports in trade journals (e.g., see Scott, 1969) since no literature exists in the normal scientific journals.

through which the light passes. Leith and Upatnieks (1966) and (Upatnieks *et al.* (1966) showed how this idea could be applied to the defects caused by the spherical aberration present in a lens. A hologram is made of the aberrated wavefront by using a point source. This hologram is then used as a corrector plate to minimize the effect of the aberration on an image. In a sense this technique is perhaps more closely related to the optical processing schemes to be discussed in a later section.

A more important application of this principle is the production of an image when the light has to pass through an irregular medium, such as a turbulent atmosphere or a diffuser. Several workers have exploited this technique (Goodman *et al.*, 1966; Stroke, 1969; Kogelnik, 1965). Figure 23 shows the principle quite clearly; the hologram is the interference pattern formed between light from the object that passes through the aberrating medium and light from a point source that also passes through the same medium. Hence when an image is formed from this record the effect of the aberration is effectively cancelled out. Figure 24 shows the normal image formed through an aberrating medium of a photograph of a Gemini spacecraft! Figure 25 shows the image formed by the holographic method—a clearly recognizable image is formed, that is still somewhat degraded by the presence of noise. Nevertheless the result is dramatic. Goodman has also conducted experiments over a long optical path to attempt to remove the effects of the atmosphere. Positive results were obtained but not nearly as dramatic as the laboratory result shown above. It must be stressed that the reference beam must "see" the same turbulence or distortion that the object beam is subjected to.

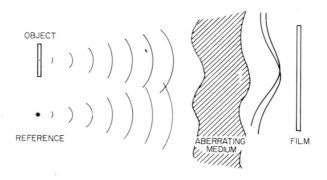

OBJECT

REFERENCE

ABERRATING
MEDIUM

FILM

FIG. 23. Recording a hologram in the presence of an aberrating medium (after Goodman *et al.*, 1969).

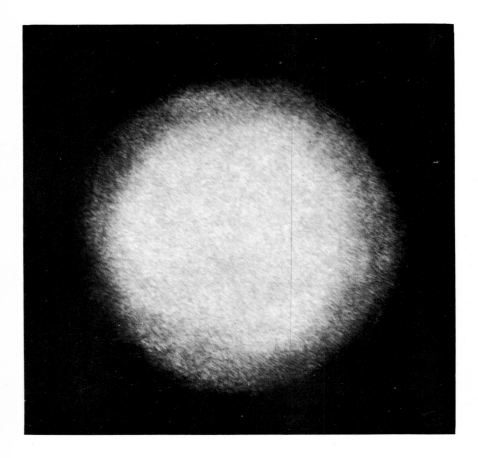

FIG. 24. Conventionally formed image of a photograph of a Gemini spacecraft with the aberrating medium present. (Photograph provided by Goodman *et al.*, 1969.)

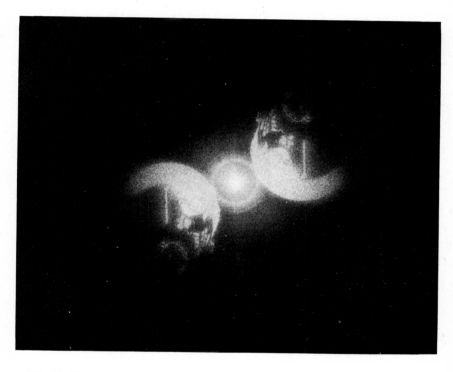

FIG. 25. Holographically formed image of a photograph of a Gemini spacecraft with the aberrating medium present. (Photograph provided by Goodman *et al.*, 1969.)

G. Nonoptical Holography

The majority of the realized and suggested applications of holography have involved visible light in both the recording and reconstruction of the wavefronts. The original applications, however, involved forming the hologram with a nonoptical beam. The second step in the image forming process was to form the required image optically. This we discussed earlier as examples of electron and X-ray holography.

Considerable attention has been given to acoustic holography during the last few years, and two conferences have now been devoted to the subject (Metherell *et al.*, 1969, 1970). In addition, a good popular article has appeared (Metherell, 1969) as well as useful review papers (Korpel, 1968; El Sum, 1968).

The hologram is produced by the interference of two sound fields produced when two sources are tuned for the same frequency and one is used to irradiate the object and the other is used to provide the reference wave. The resulting sound interferogram has then to be detected to record the required hologram. Mueller and Sheridan (1966) described the original scheme shown in Fig. 26; the quartz transducers were fed from the same 7 MHz rf generator and beam divergence obtained with acoustic lenses. The interference between the two sound waves produces a standing wave pattern on the surface of the

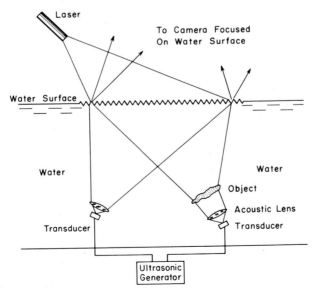

Fig. 26. One of the techniques for producing acoustic holograms.

water whose amplitude is proportional to the acoustic intensity of the surface. This pattern is recorded by illuminating it with a helium–neon laser—the photographic record is now the required hologram. The wavelength change inherent in the process produces a distortion in the final image because the longitudinal magnification is proportion to the ratio of wavelengths, whereas the lateral magnification is not. Mueller and Sheridan also pointed out the principle of using the surface deformation directly as a phase hologram. Improvements in the basic technique can be obtained by placing a membrane on the water surface and covering the membrane with a thin film of oil. The required wave pattern is now formed on the surface of the oil. Thus motion picture records have been made by photographing a TV tube using such subjects as goldfish swimming in a tank of water which shows the internal organs of the fish since the soft tissue is transparent to the sound beam.

A scanning technique can also be used to scan the field produced on or in the liquid surface with piezoelectric transducers. At longer wavelengths the scanning method can be used directly in air. Unfortunately these techniques are slow, but could possibly be improved by using large arrays of detectors.

The electrical output from a microphone that is detecting a sound field has the same frequency and phase as the sound field. Hence the required hologram can be made electronically by mixing the microphone output with a suitable electrical reference signal. A flexibility exists now to produce complex amplitude records or phase-only holograms.

Application for acoustic holography could occur in a number of fields including nondestructive testing, medical diagnostics that would not have a detrimental effect upon the subject, and oceanography. It appears that further effort is still required to determine the applicability of acoustic holography in the various fields mentioned above.

There is another aspect of nonoptical holography that has also received a passing attention. A hologram can be made at microwave frequencies and then an image formed optically (Dooley, 1965; Stockman and Zarwyn, 1968). At present there seems little application in this area.

Synthetic aperture radar was developed and used successfully without anyone's consciously thinking of it as a holographic process, but in retrospect it certainly resembles holographic image formation. In a recent article Leith (1970) stated

the synthetic antenna concept is credited independently to C. Wiley of the Goodyear Aircraft Corp. (about 1950) and to the group of C. Sherwin at the University of Illinois (about 1951). Various synthetic antenna systems were constructed and tested in the 1950s, including a highly sophisticated system at the University of Michigan by a group headed by L. J. Cutrona.

The similarity of synthetic aperture radar to holography is clearly seen since Doppler frequencies are generated when the radar is moved with respect to the ground. As the airborne system moves the Doppler frequency is changed, and hence a single point object produces an electrical signal that has the same form as the classical zone plate. Other related radar systems such as pulse-compression radar and phased-array antennas can have holographic interpretations.

It is not appropriate to dwell on this subject here since it cannot be considered in the main stream of holographic applications. However, a summary can be found in the literature (Goodman, 1968; Leith and Ingalls, 1968).

IV. Nonimage-Forming Applications

It was natural that the initial applications of holography made use of its special image-forming properties. The real gain, however, came when the techniques involved in holographic recording was used for some nonimaging applications that at first sight could be easily overlooked. In this section the nonimage-forming applications are discussed with special reference to interferometry. Of all the applications that have been described thus far in the literature on holography, this is certainly the most exciting with the largest diversity of technological impact.

A. INTERFEROMETRY

The discovery and development of holographic interferometry was a natural and simultaneous reaction by a number of groups working in holography and related laser technologies. In 1965, therefore, at least six separate and independent efforts lead to essentially the same general result. It is impossible to say who was first and so they are listed alphabetically here (Brooks et al., 1965; Burch, 1965a,b[2]; Collier et al., 1965; Haines and Hildebrand, 1965; Horman, 1965; Powell and Stetson, 1965). Since 1965 the literature has contained a large number of papers devoted to the ideas outlined by these authors and as expected many of the significant results were obtained by the originators themselves and their co-workers (Stetson and Powell, 1965, 1966; Haines and Hildebrand, 1966a,b; Burch et al., 1966; Archbold et al., 1967; Heflinger et al., 1966).

---

[2] In Burch's paper he also gives credit to C. Reid and N. R. Wall of AWRE Aldermaston, England for simultaneous and independent discovery.

Basically there are three interrelated methods which can be considered: single-exposure, double-exposure, and multiple-exposure holographic interferometry.

1. Single-Exposure Holographic Interferometry

This is the method to which Haines and Hildebrand devoted much of their time. The principle involved recording a hologram of a given object. The developed hologram was then placed again in exactly the same position so that the image formed fell exactly on the original object. The object was then moved or deformed and the object and the image interfere, the inter-ference fringes being related to the change that has taken place. Consider a hologram made by the light reflected by the object $a_1(x) \exp [i\phi(x)]$ and a plane wave $a_2 \exp (ikx \sin \alpha)$, incident at an angle α. From Eq. (10) the intensity of the resultant hologram field is

$$I(x) = a_1{}^2(x) + a_2{}^2 + a_2 a_1(x)\{\exp [i\phi(x) - kx \sin \alpha]$$
$$+ \exp [-i(\phi(x) - kx \sin \alpha)]\} \tag{14}$$

The hologram is then replaced and is illuminated with the wave formed by the addition of the light from the object and the same reference wave. If the object has been changed slightly then the amplitude will be essentially the same but the phase will have changed, hence the new object wave is $a_1(x) \exp [i\theta(x)]$. The resultant wave $\psi(x)$ transmitted by the hologram is thus,

$$\psi(x) = a_1{}^3(x) \exp [i\theta(x)] + a_1(x)a_2{}^2 \exp [i\theta(x)]$$
$$+ a_2 a_1{}^2(x) \exp [i(\phi(x) - \theta(x) - kx \sin \alpha)]$$
$$+ a_2 a_1{}^2(x) \exp [-i(\phi(x) - \theta(x) - kx \sin \alpha)]$$
$$+ a_1{}^2(x)a_2 \exp (ikx \sin \alpha)$$
$$+ a_2{}^3 \exp (ikx \sin \alpha) + a_2{}^2 a_1(x) \exp [i\phi(x)]$$
$$+ a_2{}^2 a_1(x) \exp [-i(\phi(x) - 2kx \sin \alpha)] \tag{15}$$

The various terms represent waves propagating in different directions. The first, second, and seventh terms are in the direction of the original wave. Collecting these three terms gives:

$$\psi_0(x) = a_1(x)\{[a_1{}^2(x) + a_2{}^2] \exp [i\theta(x)] + a_2{}^2 \exp [i\phi(x)]\} \tag{16}$$

Hence the resultant intensity distribution in this "image" is

$$|\psi_0(x)|^2 = a_1{}^2(x)\{[a_1{}^2(x) + a_2{}^2]^2 + a_2{}^4$$
$$+ 2a_2{}^2[a_1{}^2(x) + a_2{}^2] \cos [\theta(x) - \phi(x)] \tag{17}$$

Hence fringes are formed as determined by the value of the phase difference of the cosine term, and a dark fringe will occur when

$$\theta(x) - \phi(x) = (2n + 1)\pi/2, \qquad n = 0, 1, 2 \tag{18}$$

Haines and Hildebrand (1966a,b) have shown how this method may be used for a variety of problems; their results include structures subjected to strain and translation and target mesh deformation in an image orthicon. These workers analyzed in some detail the effects on the fringe patterns of various deformations, rotations, and translations.

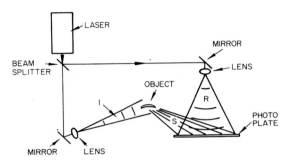

FIG. 27. A typical method of producing the hologram for holographic interferometry. This particular arrangement is that used by Alwang *et al.* (1969). (*R* is the reference beam, *I* the illuminating beam, and *S* the signal beam.) Courtesy of United Aircraft Corporation (Pratt and Whitney Aircraft Division).

Figure 27 shows a typical arrangement for recording the hologram for holographic interferometry. This particular system is that used by Alwang *et al.* (1969) for the study of turbine blades. Figure 28 shows a result obtained with this system for a mechanically deformed turbine blade.

One of the major problems that exists is the correct and accurate interpretation of the fringe pattern. A number of theoretical treatments have been made which give a partial picture of the interpretation (Haines and Hildebrand, 1966a,b; Brown *et al.*, 1969). This comment is true of all the holographic interferometric systems.

2. Double-Exposure Holographic Interferometry

An equivalent process to the one discussed above would be to record the holograms of the same object at different times. This method has some advantages over the previous technique particularly for studying transient phenomena. Hence double-exposure pulsed laser holograms have been studied extensively (Heflinger *et al.*, 1966). The analysis is, of course, not significantly different from the analysis given for the single exposure system, and the resulting fringe pattern is determined by the phase difference between

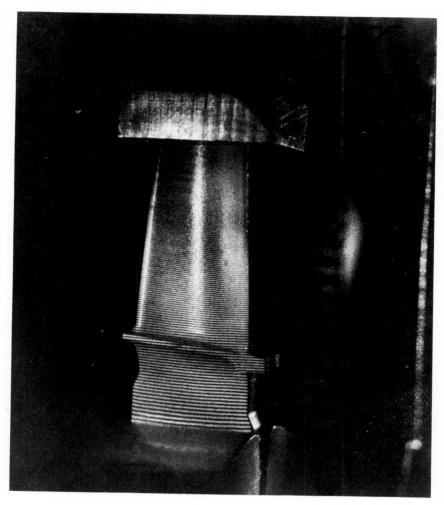

FIG. 28. Interference fringes in a mechanically deformed turbine blade (after Alwang *et al.*, 1969). Courtesy of United Aircraft Corporation (Pratt and Whitney Aircraft Divion).

the object wave in its first position and the object wave in its second position. Likewise, the experimental arrangements used are similar to that shown in Figure 27.

A range of interesting examples have been studied by a number of groups. For example, Jeffers (1969) has used the method for the investigation of diaphragm-type pressure transducers. The motion in this situation is perpendicular to the plane of the hologram; the first hologram is made in the unpressured state and the second with pressure applied. Figure 29 shows an interferogram of a poorly bonded pressure transducer of diameter 2.5 cm. The fringe spacing is approximately 0.16 cm.

The problem of debonds has also been studied by a group at G. C. O., Inc. Debonds in a rubber-to-aluminum laminate have been detected.

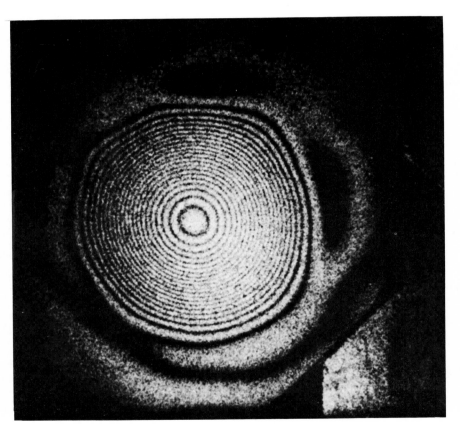

Fig. 29. Interferogram of a poorly bonded diaphragm-type pressure transducer (after Jeffers, 1969).

A uniform vacuum is applied to the test panel and then returned to atmospheric pressure. Figure 30 shows a typical result from a double-exposure hologram. The debonded regions are seen as concentric interference fringes. This same company has devised and used an apparatus for the simultaneous testing of both the side walls and tread of motor vehicle tires. Figure 31 shows a holographic interferogram of a 8.25 × 14 four-ply tire. The first hologram was recorded when the tire was not inflated and the second after inflation to 50

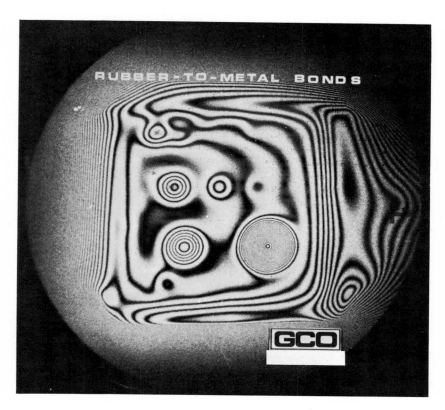

FIG. 30. Double-exposure holographic interferometric study of a rubber-to-aluminum laminate (courtesy of G. C. O., Inc. Ann Arbor, Michigan.)

pounds per square inch. The creep of the material brings out a flaw that exists between the liner and the first ply on the shoulder (top left-hand corner of photograph); the fringe pattern on the tread is apparently indicative of a separation between the first and second plies. The broad widely spaced fringes contain the overall change in dimensions caused by the pressure change.

3. Multiple-Exposure Holography

Powell and Stetson's independent discovery of the principle of holographic microscopy lead them to investigate very thoroughly the properties of multiple-exposure holographic interferometry (or equivalently, time-averaged holographic interferometry). This method has particular applicability to the study of vibrating objects (Powell and Stetson 1965; Stetson

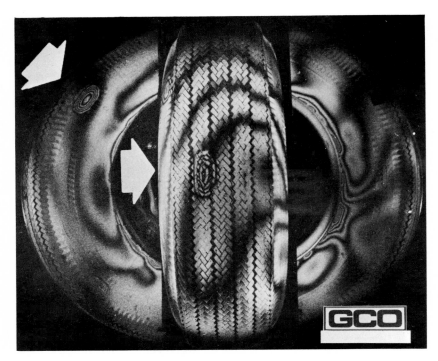

FIG. 31. Double exposure holographic interferogram of two views of a car tire showing clearly the local separation that has occurred between various plies (courtesy of G. C. O., Inc., Ann Arbor, Michigan.)

and Powell, 1965, 1966; Powell, 1968; Stetson, 1968). The technique involved is to record a hologram continuously while the object is vibrating. This composite hologram can be thought of as a superposition of a large number of holograms or as a single time-averaged hologram. Following these authors fairly closely and after an excellent brief description given by Leith and Upatnieks (1967) we will consider the image formed from the time-averaged hologram produced by an off-axis reference beam and the object wave. The virtual image in this case is essentially $a_2{}^*\langle a_1 \rangle$, where the angular brackets denotes a time average.[3] Hence the virtual image I_v is given by

$$I_v = \frac{K}{t} \int_0^t \iint 0(x_0 + x', y_0 + y', z')$$

$$\exp\{ikr(t)\}\, d(x_0 + x')\, d(y_0 + y')\, dt \qquad (19)$$

[3] The total record is, of course, a time average but a_2 does not vary with time while a_1 does.

where K is a constant including the constant $a_2{}^*$, t is the exposure time, and the double integral represents the object field a_1 in the recording plane in terms of the object itself; x_0, y_0, 0 are some average coordinates of the object, and x', y', and z' are the time dependent variations about that position $(x_0, y_0, 0)$; $r(t)$ is the distance from the point $(x_0 + x', y_0 + y', z')$ and a point in the hologram plane (x, y, z). Thus

$$[r(t)]^2 = (x - x_0 + x')^2 + (y - y_0 + y')^2 + (z - z')^2 \qquad (20)$$

since $z \gg z'$ Eq. (20) can be expanded binomially and

$$r(t) \approx z - z' + (z'^2/2z) + [(x - x_0 - x')^2/2z] + [(y - y_0 - y')^2/2z] + \cdots \quad (21)$$

Hence Eq. (19) becomes

$$I_v = K \exp (ikz) \int_0^t \exp (-ikz')(1 - z'/z) \iint O(x_0 + x', y_0 + y', z')$$

$$\times \exp \{ik(x - x_0 - x')^2/2z\}$$

$$\times \exp \{ik(y - y_0 - y)^2/2z\} \, d(x_0 + x') \, d(y_0 + y') \, dt \qquad (22)$$

For a general vibration, Eq. (22) must be evaluated, however, as a useful example the case of $x' = y' = 0$ can be considered. The vibration then is the z direction only. Furthermore we will consider small vibrations so that terms in $(z')^2$ can be neglected. Then

$$I_v = C \int_0^t \iint O(x_0, y_0, z') \exp (ikz') \exp [ik(x - x_0)^2]/2$$

$$\times \exp [ik(y - y_0)^2]/2 \, dx_0 \, dy_0 \, dt \qquad (23)$$

and the image finally may be written approximately as

$$I_v = CO(x_0, y_0) \int_0^t \exp [ikz'(t)] \, dt \qquad (24)$$

Thus the image can be considered to be the original object multiplied by a time averaged function determined by the motion $z'(t)$. For an object that is vibrating sinusoidally

$$z'(t) = 2a(x_0, y_0) \cos \omega t \qquad (25)$$

The integral part of Eq. (24) then yields a zero-order Bessel function $J_0[2ka(x_0, y_0)]$. Thus fringes will be seen that relate to constant amplitudes of vibration of the object. Figure 32 shows a photograph of virtual image

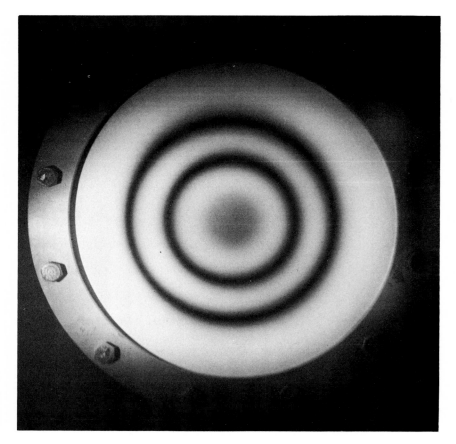

FIG. 32. Contours of equal amplitude of vibration resulting from a multiple exposure (time average) hologram of an acoustic transducer (after Monahan and Bromley, 1968).

produced by an acoustic transducer vibrating in its fundamental mode with an applied signal of 490 · 1 Hz and a driving voltage of 10 V (Monahan and Bromley, 1968). Figure 33 shows one of the original results of Powell and Stetson (1965) that illustrates the vibration amplitude of the second resonance of a can bottom. As the amplitude of vibration is increased the number of fringes seen also increases.

The implication of the interferometric techniques discussed above does not really do justice to the impact that this technology could have in the area of nondestructive testing. Hence many applications are being pursued with particular reference to the testing of engineering components (Waddell and

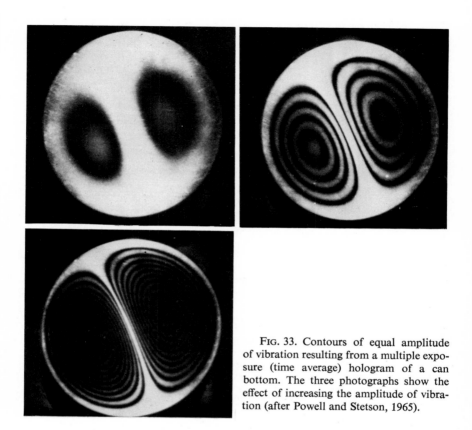

FIG. 33. Contours of equal amplitude of vibration resulting from a multiple exposure (time average) hologram of a can bottom. The three photographs show the effect of increasing the amplitude of vibration (after Powell and Stetson, 1965).

Kennedy, 1968; Archbold and Ennos, 1967, 1968; Alwang *et al.*, 1969). Finally mention should be made of the possible application to experimental photoelasticity measurements (Rogers, 1966; Fourney, 1967; Hovanesian *et al.*, 1967).

B. CONTOUR GENERATION

Several methods have been proposed for producing a set of fringes that provide an accurate contour mapping of the object under test. The first method (Haines and Hildebrand, 1967) uses two sources which produce two holograms either sequentially or simultaneously. Hence two images are produced that have a phase difference between them. The resulting cosine fringes formed are localized at the object and represent a family of hyperboloids. When the two sources are at infinity and the line passing through the object perpendicular to the line of sight bisects the angle, β, between the propagation directions from the sources, then contour fringes are produced that have a separation d given by

$$d = \lambda/2 \sin (\beta/2) \tag{26}$$

Some problems exist with the method since some areas are in shadow.

A second method (Haines and Hildebrand, 1967) again forms two holograms, but this time with different wavelengths from an argon–ion laser. The fringes observed in the image again are contours where the separation is now

$$d = \lambda_1\lambda_2/2(\lambda_1 - \lambda_2) \tag{27}$$

where λ_1 and λ_2 are the two wavelengths used. It is interesting to note that both these methods could be generalized to obtain multiple beam fringes by using multiple sources or wavelengths (Haines and Hildebrand, 1967; Zelenka and Varner, 1968).

A third technique has been suggested by Tsurata et al. (1967) and investigated by Zelenka and Varner (1969). Two holograms are made: the first with a medium of index n_1 surrounding the object and the second with a medium of index n_2 surrounding the object. The distance between the resulting contours for normal illumination of the object is now given by

$$d = \lambda_v/2(n_2 - n_1) \tag{28}$$

where λ_v is the wavelength of the coherent beam. Wuerker et al. (1968) show some excellent results using this method and report that using air and CO_2 for the two media gives contours separated by 1.4 mm, whereas air and sulfur hexafluoride produce a spacing of 0.6 mm.

C. INTERFERENCE MICROSCOPY

In Section III,A the principles of holographic microscopy were described. A related development is the application of holography to interference microscopy (Snow and Vandewarker, 1968). These workers modified a conventional microscope so that a hologram is used to generate one of the beams in a two-beam interference method. For transmitted light a system is used similar to that illustrated in Fig. 8. A hologram is made of a microscope slide in its normal position on the stage. The slide of interest is now inserted, and the processed hologram returned to its original position. Interference then results from the image formed by the hologram and the image of the object. This process eliminates the need for matched optics that are required in conventional systems. In reflected light a hologram is made of a reference flat placed on the stage: the interferogram is then made by replacing the processed hologram and inserting the specimen of interest. Various forms of interferograms can be produced by these methods, e.g., horizontal and oblique sections or differential and totally doubled interferograms.

V. The Hologram as an Optical Element

In the holographic image forming process, the hologram has built into it a structure that acts like a lens. In fact, the hologram of a point object is a zone lens (or a sine-wave zone plate). This property was recognized early in the history of the subject (Rogers, 1950). It is not unreasonable, then, to ask how a hologram may be used as an optical element in its own right. Two areas will be discussed briefly here—holographic lenses and gratings and holographic filters for coherent optical processing systems.

A. HOLOGRAPHIC LENSES AND GRATINGS

Zone lenses with large apertures could be fabricated, and it has been suggested Kock (1966) that they could be manufactured, rolled-up, launched in a satellite rocket, and unfurled in space, thus achieving a high resolution system of minimum cost and weight. This still remains only an idea; the problem of achromatizing the zone lenses has received some attention by Snow and Givens (1968).

Holography is being very seriously considered as a method of producing diffraction gratings that could give better performance than the machine-ruled gratings (Labeyrie and Flamand, 1969a,b; Cordelle et al., 1969). It has been reported that gratings 15 × 11 cm with 3000 lines per millimeter have been made. The method of production consists of recording the required interference pattern in a photosensitive layer which is then treated to get the correct profile. The surface is finally metallized to give approximately 40% efficiency in the wavelength range 2500 Å to 10,000 Å. Plane and concave gratings have been fabricated and a Schmidt plate has been designed to be used with a cadadioptric system.

B. FILTERS FOR OPTICAL DATA PROCESSING

Coherent optical data processing is a subject that is almost as broad as holography in its diversified literature and number of suggested (and perhaps unfulfilled) applications. It would be impossible to do any justice to the subject here; another review article would be needed to cover this topic.

However, some comments are certainly appropriate. It is interesting to note that optical processing is about the same age as holography as a serious scientific and technological endeavor. It existed quite independently of holography until a few years ago. One of the major problems in optical processing is the fabrication of the required filter, particularly when complex filters are necessary.

The impact that holography has had on optical spatial filtering is in the use of holographic filters. This idea was first introduced by Vander Lugt (1964) in a paper on signal detection by complex spatial filtering. A filter was constructed that produced a delta function in the image plane at the location of the object for which the filter was designed. The principles can be illustrated in the following way. The desired form of the required response of the system (impulse reponse) $f(x, y)$ is Fourier transformed by a lens to give $F(\xi/\lambda f, \eta/\lambda f)$, and a plane reference wave is added of the form $a_0 \exp (2\pi i\, \alpha\xi)$. The resulting interference pattern is

$$I(\xi, \eta) = a_0{}^2 + F(\xi/\lambda f, \eta/\lambda f)^2 + a_0 F(\xi/\lambda f, \eta/\lambda f) \exp 2\pi i\alpha\xi$$
$$+ a_0 F^*(\xi/\lambda f, \eta/\lambda f) \exp -2\pi i\alpha\xi \qquad (29)$$

where x, y, and ξ, η are coordinates in the appropriate plane and the asterisk denotes a complex conjugate. $I(\xi, \eta)$ is recorded and becomes the filter that is used in the optical processer. If the input to the usual coherent optical chain is $a(x, y)$ which is Fourier transformed and operated upon by the filter, then the transmittance through the filter is

$$U(\xi, \eta) = a_0{}^2 A(p, q) + |F(p, q)|^2 A(p, q)$$
$$+ a_0 F(p, q)A(p, q) \exp 2\pi i\alpha\xi$$
$$+ a_0 F^*(p, q)A(p, q) \exp -2\pi i\alpha\xi \qquad (30)$$

where p and q are written for $\xi/\lambda f$ and $\eta/\lambda f$, respectively. This optical field is then retransformed by the second lens in the coherent optical system to give a distribution $\psi(x'\, y')$ given by

$$\psi(x', y') \propto a_0{}^2 a(x', y') + f(x', y') \circledast f^*(x', y') \circledast a(x', y')$$
$$+ a_0 f(x', y') \circledast a(x', y') \circledast \delta(x' + \alpha\lambda f, y')$$
$$+ a_0 f^*(x', y') \circledast a(x', y') \circledast \delta(x' - \alpha\lambda f, y') \qquad (31)$$

The first two terms in Eq. (31) continue along the axis, whereas the third and fourth terms are displaced upwards and downwards from the axis. The third term is the convolution denoted by $\circledast$, of $f(x', y')$ with $a(x', y')$, and the fourth term is the cross-correlation of $f(x', y')$ with $a(x', y')$. For the filter to select a given object we make $f(x', y') = a(x', y')$. This process clearly lends itself to the detection process of specific objects in a scene or specific characters on a page.

One of the original ideas in optical processing was the correction of aberrated images—an idea introduced by Maréchal and Croce (1953) (a valuable summary can be found in a review paper by Tsujiuchi, 1963). The concept of using a holographic correction plate (or filter) was introduced by Leith *et al.* (1965b) and Upatnieks *et al.* (1966). A hologram is made of the wavefront emerging from the aberrated lens. This hologram is then used together with the lens to correct the aberration.

Stroke and Zech (1967) have used a related method to correct photographic images that have image motion blurr. Figure 34 shows one of their

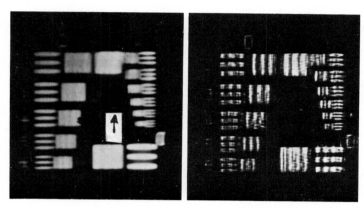

Photo
blurred
by motion

Holographically
deblurred photo

Fig. 34. Image deblurring using a holographic Fourier-transform filter (after Stroke *et al.*, 1969).

results. The required filter is made from the known point-spread function (indicated by the arrow).

As mentioned earlier a full discussion of the topic of optical data processing is not possible here. However, the above example should give some brief introduction to the role to be played by holographic filters.

VI. Conclusions

This review of applications of holography is an attempt to discuss the applications to date. Clearly many ideas for applications have been omitted and a complete bibliography of those applications discussed is not possible. Holography has proved to be an exciting science for the many people working in the field; unfortunately, the application of holographic ideas and principles to solving problems in science and technology has been slow forthcoming. However, interest is high and work continues and those deeply involved have a healthy optimism for the future of holography.

REFERENCES

Alwang, W. G., Cavanaugh, L. A., Burr, R., and Sammartino, E. (1969). *Proc. Electro-Optical System Design Conf.*, p. 79.

Anonymous (1968). "Holography Index." Andersonian Library, Univ. of Strathclyde, Glasgow (and Supplements).

Ansley, D. A., and Siebert, L. D. (1968). *Holography, Proc. Seminar-in-Depth, Soc. Photo-Opt. Instrum. Eng.*, p. 127.

Archbold, E., and Ennos, A. E. (1968). *Nature (London)* **217**, 942.

Archbold, E., Burch, J. M., and Ennos, A. E. (1967). *J. Sci. Instrum.* **44**, 489.

Armstrong, J. A. (1965). *IBM J. Res. Develop.* **9**, 171.

Baez, A. V. (1952). *J. Opt. Soc. Amer.* **42**, 756.

Baez, A. V., and El Sum, H. M. A. (1957). "X-Ray Microscopy and Microradiography, Proceedings" (V. E. Cosslett, A. Engstrom, and H. H. Patte, Jr., eds.), p. 347. Academic Press, New York.

Beesley, M. J. (1968). *Proc. Symp. Engineering Applications of Holography, Univ. of Strathclyde, Glasgow*, p. 503.

Bosomworth, D. R., and Gerritson, H. J. (1968). *Appl. Opt.* **7**, 95.

Bragg, W. L., and Rogers, G. L. (1951). *Nature (London)* **167**, 190.

Brooks, R. E., Heflinger, L. O., Wuerker, R. F., and Briones, R. A. (1965). *Appl. Phys. Lett.* **7**, 92.

Brooks, R. E., Heflinger, L. O., and Wuerker, R. F. (1966). *IEEE J. Quantum Electron.* **2**, 275.

Brown, G. M., Grant, R. M., and Stroke, G. W. (1969). *J. Acoust. Soc. Amer.* **45**, 1166.

Buerger, M. J. (1950). *J. Appl. Phys.* **21**, 909.

Burch, J. M. (1965a). "The 1965 Viscount Nuffield Memorial Paper." Prod. Eng., **44**, 431

Burch, J. M. (1965b). *Z. Angew. Math Phys.* **16**, 111.

Burch, J. M., Ennos, A. E., and Wilton, R. J. (1966). *Nature (London)* **209**, 1015.

Carter, W. H. (1969). Private communication.

Carter, W. H., and Dougal, A. A. (1966). *IEEE J. Quantum Electron.* **2**, lxiv.

Carter, W. H., Engeling, P. D., and Dougal, A. A. (1966). *IEEE J. Quantum Electron.* **2**, 44.

Chambers, R. P., and Courtney-Pratt, J. S. (1966a). *J. SMPTE (Soc. Motion Pict. Telev. Eng.)* **75**, 373.

Chambers, R. P., and Courtney-Pratt, J. S. (1966b). *J. SMPTE (Soc. Motion Pict. Telev. Eng.)* **75**, 359.

Chen, F. S., LaMacchia, J. T., and Frazer, D. B. (1968). *Appl. Phys. Lett.* **13**, 223.

Collier, R., Doherty, E., and Pennington, K. S. (1965). *Appl. Phys. Lett.* **7**, 223.

Cordelle, J., Flamand, J., Pieuchard, G., and Labeyrie, A. (1969). *Proc. 8th Congr. of ICO, Reading, England*, p. 117.

DeVelis, J., and Reynolds, G. O. (1967). "Introduction to Holography," Addison-Wesley, Reading, Massachusetts.

DeVelis, J., Parrent, G. B., and Thompson, B. J. (1966). *J. Opt. Soc. Amer.* **56**, 423.

Dooley, R. P. (1965). *Proc. IEEE* **53**, 1733.

El Sum, H. M. A. (1952). Reconstructed Wavefront Microscopy. Ph.D. Thesis, Stanford Univ., Palo Alto, California.

El Sum, H. M. A. (1968). *Holography, Proc. Seminar-in-Depth, Soc. Photo-Opt. Instrum. Eng.*, p. 137.

Ennos, A. E., and Robertson, E. R., eds. (1968). *Proc. Symp. Engineering Applications of Holography, Univ. of Strathclyde, Glasgow.*

Fourney, R. E. (1967). *Proc. 12th Ann. Tech. Symp. of Soc. Photo-Opt. Instrum. Eng.*, SPIE Publications, Redondo Beach, California.

Gabor, D. (1948). *Nature (London)* **161**, 777.

Gabor, D. (1949). *Proc. Roy. Soc. Ser.*, *A* **197**, 454.

Gabor, D. (1951). *Proc. Phys. Soc. London, Sect. B* **64**, 221.

Goodman, J. W. (1968). "Introduction to Fourier Optics." McGraw-Hill, New York.

Goodman, J. W., Jackson, D. W., Lehmann, M., and Knotts, J. (1969). *Appl. Opt.* **8**, 1581.

Goodman, J. W., Huntley, W. H., Jackson, D. W., and Lehmann, M. (1966). *Appl. Phys. Lett.* **8**, 311.

Groh, G. (1967). Holographic Arbeitstagung, Frankfurt.

Grosso, R. P., Kishner, S. J., and Vesper, R. M. (1968) *In* "Applications of Lasers to Photography and Information Handling," *Proc. SPSE Semin.* (R. Murray, ed.), p. 131. SPSE Publications, New York.

Haine, M. E., and Dyson, J. (1950). *Nature (London)* **166**, 315.

Haine, M. E., and Mulvey, T. (1952a). *J. Opt. Soc. Amer.* **42**, 763.

Haine, M. E., and Mulvey, T. (1952b). *Nature (London)* **170**, 202.

Haines, K. A., and Hildebrand, B. P. (1965). *Phys. Lett.* **19**, 106.

Haines, K. A., and Hildebrand, B. P. (1966a). *Appl. Opt.* **5**, 595.

Haines, K. A., and Hildebrand, B. P. (1966b). *IEEE Trans. Instrum. Meas.* **15**, 149.

Haines, K. A., and Hilbebrand, B. P. (1967). *J. Opt. Soc. Amer.* **57**, 155.

Hanson, A. W. (1952). *Nature (London)* **170**, 580.

Harburn, G., and Taylor, C. A. (1962). *Proc. Roy. Soc., Ser. A* **264**, 339.

Heflinger, L. O., Brooks, R. E., and Wuerker, R. F. (1966). *J. Appl. Phys.* **37**, 642.

Hickling, R. (1968). *J. Opt. Soc. Amer.* **58**, 275.

Horman, M. H. (1965). *Appl. Opt.* **4**, 333.

Hovanesian, J. D., Bricic, V., and Powell, R. L. (1967). *Can. Congr. Appl. Mech. Proc.* **1**, 104.

Jeffers, L. A. (1969). *Proc. Electro-Optical System Design Conf.*, p. 115.

Kallard, T. (1969). "Holography—State of the Art Review," Optosonic Press, New York.

Kiemle, H. (1968). *Proc. Symp. Engineering Applications of Holography, Univ. of Strathclyde, Glasgow*, p. 233.

Kock, W. (1966). *IEEE Proc.* **54**, 1610.

Kock, W. (1969). "Lasers and Holography," Doubleday, New York.

Kogelnik, M. (1965). *Bell Syst. Tech. J.* **44**, 2451.

Korpel, A. (1968). *IEEE Spectrum* **5** (10), 45.

Kozma, A. (1966). *J. Opt. Soc. Amer.* **56**, 428.

Labeyrie, A., and Flamand, J. (1969a). *Opt. Commun.* **1**, 1.

Labeyrie, A., and Flamand, J. (1969b). *Optical Spectra* Nov/Dec, p. 50.

LaMacchia, J. T. (1969). *IEEE Int. Conv. Rec.* p. 238.

LaMacchia, J. T. (1970). *Laser Focus* **6** (6), 35.

LaMacchia, J. T., Lin, J. H., and Burckhardt, C. B. (1969). *J. Opt. Soc. Amer.* **59**, 490A.

Latta, J. N. (1968). *J. SMPTE (Soc. Motion Pict. Telev. Eng.)* **77**, 540.

Leith, E. N (1970). *Laser Focus* **6**, 2, 29.

Leith, E. N., and Ingalls, A. L. (1968). *Appl. Opt.* **7**, 539.

Leith, E. N., and Upatnieks, J. (1962). *J. Opt. Soc. Amer.* **52**, 1123.

Leith, E. N., and Upatnieks, J. (1963). *J. Opt. Soc. Amer.* **53**, 1377.
Leith, E. N., and Upatnieks, J. (1964). *J. Opt. Soc. Amer.* **54**, 1295.
Leith, E. N., and Upatnieks, J. (1965). *J. Opt. Soc. Amer.* **55**, 569.
Leith, E. N., and Upatnieks, J. (1966). *J. Opt. Soc. Amer.* **56**, 523.
Leith, E. N., and Upatnieks, J. (1967). *Progr. Opt.* **6**, 3.
Leith, E. N., Upatnieks, J., and Haines, K. A. (1965a). *J. Opt. Soc. Amer.* **55**, 981.
Leith, E. N., Upatnieks, J., and Vander Lugt, A. (1965b). *J. Opt. Soc. Amer.* **55**, 595.
Lomas, G. M. (1969). *Appl. Opt.* **8**, 2037.
Lowenthal, S., Werts, A., and Rembault, M. (1968). *C. R. Acad. Sci.* **267**, 120.
Lu, S. (1968). *Proc. IEEE* **56**, 116.
Lu, S. (1969). *J. Opt. Soc. Amer.* **59**, 1544A.
Maréchal, A., and Croce, P. (1953). *C. R. Acad. Sci.* **237**, 607.
Meier, R. W. (1965). *J. Opt. Soc. Amer.* **55**, 987.
Metherell, A. T. (1969). *Sci. Amer.* **221** (4), 36.
Metherell, A. T., El Sum, H. M. A., and Larmore, L., eds. (1969). "Acoustical Holography,"
    Vol. 1. Plenum Press, New York.
Metherell, A. T., El Sum, H. M. A., and Larmore, L., eds. (1970). "Acoustical
    Holography," Vol. 2. Plenum Press, New York.
Meyerhofer, D. (1970). *Laser Focus* **6** (2), 40.
Mezrich, R. S. (1969). *Appl. Phys, Lett.* **14**, 132.
Michelson, A. A. (1927). "Studies in Optics," p. 60. Univ. of Chicago Press, Chicago,
    Illinois.
Monahan, M. A., and Bromley, K. (1968). *J. Acoust. Soc. Amer.* **44**, 1225.
Mueller, R. K., and Sheridan, N. K. (1966). *Appl. Phys. Lett.* **9**, 328.
Murata, K., Fujiwara, H., and Asakura, T. (1968). *Proc. Symp. Engineering Applications
    of Holography, Univ. of Strathclyde, Glasgow*, p. 289.
Parrent, G. B., and Thompson, B. J. (1964a). *Opt. Acta* **11**, 183.
Parrent, G. B., and Thompson, B. J. (1964b). U.S. Patent No. 3,320,852.
Powell, R. L. (1968). *Proc. Symp. Engineering Applications of Holography, Univ. of Strath-
    clyde, Glasgow*, p. 333.
Powell, R. L. (1969). *Ind. Res.* **11**, 50.
Powell, R. L., and Stetson, K. A. (1965). *J. Opt. Soc. Amer.* **55**, 1593.
Reick, M. (1968). *Proc. Symp. Engineering Applications of Holography, Univ. of Strath-
    clyde, Glasgow*, p. 261.
Rogers, G. L. (1950). *Nature (London)* **166**, 237.
Rogers, G. L. (1952). *Proc. Roy. Soc. Edinburgh, Sect. A* **63**, 313.
Rogers, G. L. (1966). *J. Opt. Soc. Amer.* **56**, 831.
Rose, H. W. (1965). *J. Opt. Soc. Amer.* **55**, 1565 (A).
Scott, J. B. (1969) *Microwaves* Dec., p. 19.
Silverman, B. A., Thompson, B. J., and Ward, J. (1964). *J. Appl. Meteorol.* **3**, 792.
Smith, H. M. (1969). "Principles of Holography," Wiley, New York.
Snow, K. A., and Givens, M. P. (1968), *J. Opt. Soc. Amer.* **58**, 871.
Snow, K. A., and Vandewarker, R. (1968). *Appl. Opt.* **7**, 549.
Stetson, K. A. (1968). *Proc. Symp. Engineering Applications of Holography, Univ. of Strath-
    clyde, Glasgow*, p. 123.
Stetson, K. A., and Powell, R. L. (1965). *J. Opt. Soc. Amer.* **55**, 1694.
Stetson, K. A., and Powell, R. L. (1966). *J. Opt. Soc. Amer.* **56**, 1161.
Stockman, H. E., and Zarwyn, B. (1968). *Proc. IEEE* **56**, 763.
Stroke, G. W. (1966). "An Introduction to Coherent Optics and Holography," Academic
    Press, New York.

Stroke, G. W. (1969). *Opt. Acta* **16**, 401.
Stroke, G. W., and Falconer, D. G. (1964). *Phys. Lett.* **13**, 306.
Stroke, G. W., and Zech, G. (1967). *Phys. Lett. A* **25**, 89.
Stroke, G. W., Brumm, D., and Funkhouser, F. (1965). *J. Opt. Soc. Amer.* **55**, 1327.
Stroke, G. W., Furrer, F., and Lamberty, D. R. (1969). *Opt. Commun.* **1**, 141.
Tanner, L. H. (1966). *J. Sci. Instrum.* **43**, 81.
Thompson, B. J. (1963). *Soc. Photo-Opt. Instrum. Eng., 8th Annu. Tech. Symp., Los Angeles.*
Thompson, B. J. (1964a). *J. Soc. Photo-Opt. Instrum. Eng.* **2**, 43.
Thompson, B. J. (1964b). *J. Opt. Soc. Amer.* **54**, 1406A.
Thompson, B. J. (1967). *Proc. IEEE 9th Annu. Symp. on Electron, Ion, and Laser Beam Technology* (R. I .W. Pease, ed.), p. 295.
Thompson, B. J. (ed.) (1968a). *Holography, Proc. Seminar-in-Depth, Soc. Photo-Opt. Instrum. Eng.*
Thompson, B. J. (1968b). *Holography, Proc. Seminar-in-Depth, Soc. Photo-Opt. Instrum. Eng.,* p. 25.
Thompson, B. J. (1969a). *Physics-in-Depth, a seminar sponsored by AIP and NASW. Image* **1** (1). Inst. of Opt., Rochester, New York.
Thompson, B. J. (1969b). *In* "Technological Forecast 1980," Proc. of Polytechnic Inst. of Brooklyn Symp. (A. E. Schillinger, ed.). In press.
Thompson, B. J. (1970). *Electro-Optical Systems Design Magazine* p. 32.
Thompson, B. J., and Ward, J. (1967). *J. Opt. Soc. Amer.* **57**, 275.
Thompson, B. J., and Zinky, W. (1969). *Appl. Opt.* **7**, 2426.
Thompson, B. J., Parrent, G. B., Ward, J., and Justh, B. (1966). *J. Appl. Meteorol.* **5**, 343.
Thompson, B. J., Ward, J., and Zinky, W. (1967). *Appl. Opt.* **6**, 519.
Thompson, J. F., Ward, J., and Zinky, W. (1965). *J. Opt. Soc. Amer.* **55**, 1506A.
Tollin, P., Main, P., Rossman, M., Stroke, G. W., and Restrick, R. C. (1966). *Nature (London)* **209**, 603.
Tonomura, A., Funkumara, A., Watawabe, M., and Komoda, T. (1968). *Jap. J. Appl. Phys.* **7**, 295.
Townsend, R. L., and LaMacchia, J. T. (1969). *J. Opt. Soc. Amer.* **59**, 1530A.
Tsujiuchi, J. (1963). *Progr. Opt.* **2**, 133.
Tsurata, T., Shiotake, N., Tsujiuchi, J., and Matsuda, K. (1967). *Jap. J. Appl. Phys.* **6**, 661.
Upatnieks, J. (1967). *Appl. Opt.* **6**, 1905.
Upatnieks, J. (1969). *J. Opt. Soc. Amer.* **59**, 1539A.
Upatnieks, J., Vander Lugt, A., and Leith, E. N. (1966). *Appl. Opt.* **5**, 589.
Urbach, J. C., and Meier, R. W. (1966). *Appl. Opt.* **5**, 666.
Vander Lugt, A. (1964). *IEEE Trans. Inform. Theory* **1T-10**, 12.
Van Ligten, R. F. (1967). *J. Opt. Soc. Amer.* **57**, 564A.
Van Ligten, R. F. (1968). *Holography, Proc. Seminar-in-Depth, Soc. Photo-Opt. Instrum. Eng.,* p. 75.
Van Ligten, R. F., and Lawton, K. C. (1967). *J. Appl. Phys.* **36**, 1996.
Van Ligten, R. F., and Osterberg, H. (1966). *Nature (London)* **211**, 282, 5046.
Waddell, P., and Kennedy, W. (1968). *Proc. Symp. Engineering Applications of Holography, Univ. of Strathclyde, Glasgow,* p. 347.
Ward, J., and Thompson, B. J. (1967). *Proc. Brooklyn Polytech. Symp. on Modern Optics,* p. 649.
Welford, W. T. (1966). *Appl. Opt.* **5**, 872.
Winthrop, J. T., and Worthington, C. R. (1965). *Phys. Lett.* **15**, 124.
Wuerker, R. F., and Heflinger, L. O. (1968). *Proc. Symp. Engineering Applications of Holography, Univ. of Strathclyde, Glasgow,* p. 99.

Wuerker, R. F., Heflinger, L. O., and Zivi, S. M. (1968). *Holography, Proc. Seminar-in-Depth, Soc. Photo-Opt. Instrum. Eng.*, p. 97.
Zelenka, J. S., and Varner, J. R. (1968). *Appl. Opt.* **7**, 2107.
Zelenka, J. S., and Varner, J. R. (1969). *Appl. Opt.* **8**, 1431.

LASER APPLICATIONS
IN METROLOGY AND GEODESY

James C. Owens[1]

Research Laboratories, Eastman Kodak Company
Rochester, New York

[1] Formerly with the Environmental Science Services Agency (ESSA) Research Laboratories, Boulder, Colorado, where much of the work described here was carried out.

I. Introduction

Optical methods of distance and angle measurement are well known in industrial metrology and geodetic surveying, but their use has generally been restricted by the light sources available to telescopic methods of alignment and angle measurement and to rather specialized interferometric comparisons of nearly equal optical path lengths as in gage block calibration, refractometry, and lens and mirror testing. Outdoor distance measurements using modulated light have been limited to ranges of a few kilometers.

The introduction of lasers, and especially visible-light gas lasers, has dramatically expanded the utility of these optical methods and has in some cases simplified their use. The spatial coherence of laser light permits the collimation of beams to diffraction-limited directivity while retaining a useful level of irradiance. In such cases of maximal collimation (or, equivalently, focusing) the total uniphase power of the laser can be used, whereas with an incoherent source only the power radiated from a surface area less than one square wavelength is available. It can be shown by straightforward physical optics that the advantage of the laser is four to five orders of magnitude over the most intense unfiltered incoherent sources. Hence alignment can be performed by projecting a light beam in the direction of interest, interferometry can be carried out in normally lighted rooms and even outdoors, and optical ranging can be done over much longer paths than before. The great temporal coherence of gas laser light permits direct fringe-counting interferometry to be carried out over far larger optical path length differences than have previously been possible.

In this article we shall consider some practical ways to make use of this unique spectral radiance of lasers. Most of the discussion is restricted to linear measurements (which can sometimes be cascaded), but some comments on direct three-dimensional surface figure problems are included. No attempt is made to give comprehensive summaries of optical theory or conventional practice; good texts on interferometry (Steel, 1967; Baird and Hanes, 1967) and alignment (van Heel, 1965), as well as more specialized treatments (Mollet, 1960) are available. Instead, the chapter is intended as a systematic collection of ideas on how to align structures and how to measure short and long distances, fluid velocities and turbulence, and surface vibration patterns, suggesting the methods which seem to me the most reasonable for each problem. Analyses are included of several topics which may be helpful but which are not easily found in the metrological literature: atmospheric refraction and dispersion, projected fringe patterns with compensated and uncompensated interferometers, the outputs and errors of the two most satisfactory fringe-counting interferometers, the use of Jones matrices in analyzing electro-optical distance measuring instruments, and the operation of phase-locked transponder systems in long-distance measurement.

II. Alignment

A. BEAM DIRECTIONALITY

A collimated light beam in vacuum or in a homogeneous medium travels in a straight line, spreading slightly because of diffraction. The output from a single-mode laser has a Gaussian irradiance distribution, given by

$$I(r) = (2P/\pi R^2) \exp [-2r^2/R^2] \qquad (1)$$

where r is the radial distance from the beam center, P is the laser power, and R is the radius at which the irradiance falls to e^{-2} times its central value. If the full beam is transmitted the irradiance remains Gaussian at any distance, and the full divergence angle in the far field to the e^{-2} irradiance points is given by

$$\varphi = 2\lambda/\pi R \qquad (2)$$

where λ is the wavelength of the light. A plot of spot diameter versus distance for various beam sizes and a wavelength of 632.8 nm is shown in Fig. 1,

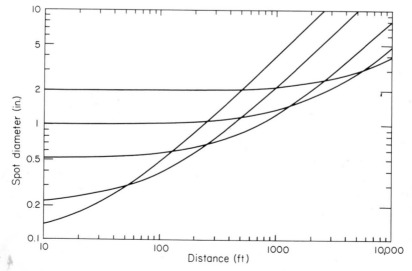

FIG. 1. Spot diameter to the e^{-2} irradiance points versus distance for collimated Gaussian beams of wavelength 632.8 nm.

from which it can be seen that there is an optimum collimated beam size giving the smallest possible spot at any given distance. Focusing further reduces the spot size in the near field (roughly speaking, at distances less than that at which the collimated beam would double its original diameter) at the expense of far-field divergence.

In practice, of course, the beam will be truncated by the transmitting optics and the received spot will not be exactly Gaussian. The minimum spot size on a distant target is achieved if the beam greatly overfills the objective lens of the beam expanding telescope, giving approximately uniform illumination of the aperture, but this wastes laser power. It can be shown either analytically or numerically (Buck, 1967) that the largest irradiance results at the center of the received spot if the transmitted beam is truncated at the radius where its irradiance has dropped to 8.1 % of the maximum value.

The utility of such an optical " piano wire " is obvious; a single man can set up the laser and then walk along the beam aligning various components with it. More accurate settings can be made if a simple detector array, such as the quadrant detector indicated in Fig. 2, is used. Currently available commercial instruments give an angular precision of 1 μrad over working distances as large as several hundred feet, and the method does not require the operator judgment needed with transits and autocollimators. Servo-control can be added to maintain the alignment. Furthermore, the output of a gas laser is normally linearly polarized, and hence a polarization measurement can be used to give roll angles.

This straightforward technique is gaining widespread use in the building of large structures, such as the assembly of the jigs and fixtures around which

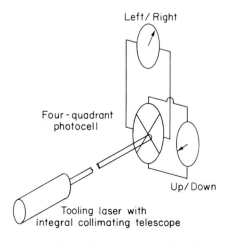

FIG. 2. Use of simple detector array in alignment.

an airplane or a ship will be framed and assembled. Special tooling lasers designed for stable pointing and good single-mode operation are used. With larger, less precise detector arrays, the method is used in grading, trenching, and tunnel boring. In the laboratory, the alignment of multielement optical systems is simplified by using a laser beam. For a linear system such as a telescope, the optical axis is first defined by apertures and crosshairs and then the optical components are inserted one by one and adjusted until the transmitted and reflected beams coincide with the axis.

B. USE OF DIFFRACTION

For alignment over distances of several hundred feet or more, the spot size will be rather large and it may not be possible to determine the position of a collimated beam's center to the required accuracy with a simple detector array. Rather than using an inverted telescope to focus successively at each distance of interest, which may cause changes in beam direction, the beam can be made divergent and lenses or equivalent symmetrical diffracting screens (Fresnel zone plates) inserted at each alignment location in turn as is done at the Stanford 2-mile linear accelerator (Herrmannsfeldt *et al.*, 1968). There, the accelerating tube is mounted on top of a large support pipe, 60 cm in diameter and 3 km long, which must be maintained straight to within ± 0.25 mm over its length. As indicated in Fig. 3, each 12 meter section of pipe carries a

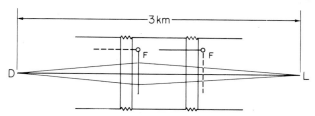

FIG. 3. Schematic illustration of the Stanford accelerator alignment system. A typical Fresnel lens F focuses light from laser L to an image at the detector plane D.

rectangular Fresnel zone plate which can be pivoted down into the laser beam. In addition to the 294 plates fastened to the pipe, there are three plates attached to pillars going down to bedrock. Each plate is designed to focus the incident light on the detector plane. The image is a pair of crossed lines, the width of the intersection point corresponding to the diffraction limit of the Fresnel zone plate. Alignment is carried out by first checking the optical axis defined by the three pillar plates and the detector pillar, taken in pairs. The alignment targets are then inserted into the beam, one at a time, and each section of pipe is moved until the image falls on the same place at the detector plane. The minimum sensitivity of the system, occurring for the plates near the center of the accelerator, is about ten times better than the required ± 0.25 mm. The support pipe is evacuated to a pressure of about 1×10^{-5} atm to prevent refraction effects from deflecting or distorting the image.

A variant of the diffraction method convenient for applications where alignment is to be done continuously rather than at fixed points along a line has been suggested by Betz (1969), who noted that a line of zero irradiance would cross the beam if a suitable phase-shifting plate were inserted near the laser. If the upper half of the beam, for example, is retarded in phase by π radians relative to the lower half, the diffraction pattern at any distance will show a symmetrical minimum along a horizontal line passing through the center of the beam. If the phase plate is divided into quadrants of alternating phase shift, the pattern will show both a horizontal and a vertical dark line. The width of the line increases with distance, of course, the full width at approximately half the irradiance of the adjacent maxima being given by

$$\Gamma = \{\lambda s[(r + s)/r]\}^{1/2} \tag{3}$$

where r is the effective distance between the laser point source and the phase plate, and s is the distance from the plate to the observation plane. The fact that the beam "carries its own crosshairs" is convenient for preliminary alignment. For higher accuracy, an aperture can be placed in the plane of interest and the doubly diffracted light observed on a screen behind this aperture as indicated in Fig. 4. If the aperture is exactly centered, this second

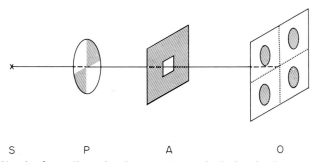

FIG. 4. Sketch of two-dimensional asymmetry method, showing laser source S, phase plate P, detecting aperture A, and observing screen O with irradiance maxima.

diffraction pattern is exactly symmetrical, but a displacement between the aperture and the optical axis causes asymmetry in the diffraction pattern. Betz shows that this asymmetry is quite sensitive to displacement and that for a reasonable divergence of the laser beam the accuracy achievable with the double-diffraction method is considerably better than that given by using a detector array to locate the center of the original Gaussian beam.

C. REFRACTION EFFECTS

In alignment and vertical angle measurement with long paths, the curvature of the beam due to atmospheric refraction may not be negligible. Air density and hence refractive index decrease with increasing height above the earth, and therefore light rays curve downward. An analysis of these effects in radio propagation, along with relevant climatological data, has been given by Bean and Dutton (1966). The geometry of point-to-point measurements over horizontal paths, the case of most interest here, is shown in Fig. 5. The

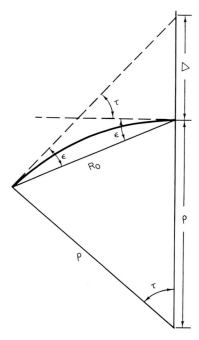

FIG. 5. Geometry of refraction over approximately horizontal paths. The diagram is distorted for clarity; for the cases considered here, $\Delta \ll R_0 \ll \rho$ and all angles are very small.

radius of curvature of the ray at any point is given by

$$\rho = -1/(dn/dh) \tag{4}$$

where (dn/dh) is the derivative of refractive index n with respect to height h. In general, this quantity varies along the path, but for approximately horizontal line-of-sight paths it can normally be considered constant. The refraction angle ε at either end of the path, half the "total bending" τ, can easily be shown to be

$$\varepsilon = -(R_0/2)(dn/dh) \tag{5}$$

where R_0 is the true distance, while the displacement of the spot on the receiving plane is given by $\Delta = R_0\,\varepsilon$.

To find (dn/dh), it is adequate to use

$$n - 1 = K(P/T) \tag{6}$$

where P is total pressure, T is temperature in $°K$, and K is a parameter depending only on wavelength. Hence we find

$$dn/dh = (n-1)[(1/P)(dP/dh) - (1/T)(dT/dh)] \tag{7}$$

Pressure is determined from the hydrostatic equation (Valley, 1965) and is given by

$$P = P_0 \exp\left(-\frac{gM}{R}\int_0^h \frac{dz}{T}\right) \tag{8}$$

where P_0 is the pressure at sea level, g is the acceleration of gravity, M is the molecular weight of air, and R is the gas constant. It we assume a constant temperature lapse rate so that $T = T_0 - \alpha z$, we readily find the well-known exponential result

$$P = P_0 \exp(-h/H) \tag{9}$$

where the pressure scale height, $H = RT_0/gM$, is typically about 8.3 km. Hence Eq. (7) becomes

$$dn/dh = -(n-1)[1/H + (1/T)(dT/dh)] \tag{10}$$

Combining Eqs. (5) and (10) and evaluating the result for 632.8 nm, 15° C, sea level pressure (hence $n - 1 = 276 \times 10^{-6}$) and $R_0 = 10$ km, we find

$$\varepsilon = 166 + 4.8(dT/dh) \qquad \mu\text{rad} \tag{11}$$

For a typical gradient of $-6.5°$ C/km, $(dn/dh) = -27 \times 10^{-6}$/km and $\varepsilon = 135\ \mu\text{rad}$, so that the spot displacement Δ is 135 cm.

On the average, the refractive index varies approximately exponentially with height as does pressure, but with a scale height of about 9.8 km. Hence for a path high above the ground, refraction can be estimated from surface meteorological measurements. Surveyors working under good conditions normally need not do even this; first-order leveling is carried out by measuring from a central position to stations approximately equidistant from the measuring point so that the relative elevation of the stations can be determined without knowing the actual (assumed uniform) refraction. Another method is to use a theodolite at each end of the path, each sighting at the other, and to measure vertical angles simultaneously. In the absence of lateral refraction or other errors, any difference between the sum of the angles and 180° must be due to refraction, which can then be corrected.

Although Eq. (5) shows that refraction is normally dominated by the pressure gradient, which generally changes slowly along with gross weather conditions, diurnal and more rapid variations in refraction are caused by changes in the temperature gradient. In clear weather, it can be several times as large in the first few meters above the ground as the typical $-6.5°$ C/km value, negative in daytime, and positive during a nighttime inversion. Measurements of laser beam refraction over outdoor paths 5.5, 15, and 45 km long have been reported by Ochs and Lawrence (1969), who found diurnal variations as large as 40 μrad/km.

Small-scale refractive index inhomogeneities caused by local temperature variations can give rise to significant problems of beam spreading and scintillation in outdoor work. Information can be found in two good review papers (Strohbehn, 1968; Lawrence and Strohbehn, 1970).

III. Interferometry

A. PRINCIPLES

After alignment, the most straightforward and reasonable application of lasers is to the measurement of length, using direct optical interferometry for short distances and modulated light for long ones. Although Babinet proposed in 1827 that the meter be defined in terms of the wavelength of light, it was not until 1895 that Michelson and Benoit actually measured a standard meter bar using the cadmium line at 643.8 nm, and not until the Eleventh General Conference on Weights and Measures in 1960 was the meter formally defined in terms of the 606.0 nm line of ^{86}Kr. Before lasers became available, the low coherence and brightness of available light sources made the interferometric measurement of length a difficult task, used only for the high-precision comparison of end standards and similar applications. A discussion of incoherent-source interferometer design and fringe interpretation has been given by Candler (1951). In length measurement with laser sources we can ignore several of the compensation problems which were formerly important.

The basic principles may be understood with the aid of Fig. 6, a diagram of the Twyman–Green (collimated light) version of the Michelson interferometer, and Fig. 7, its simplified optical equivalent. Light from the laser is collimated and incident on a partially reflecting, partially transmitting beamsplitter. The reflected fraction is again reflected by a fixed reference

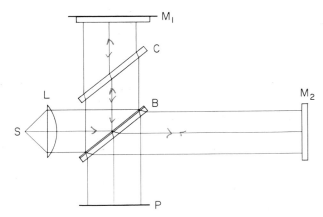

FIG. 6. Diagram of Twyman–Green interferometer, showing laser source S, collimating lens L, beamsplitter B, compensating plate C, fixed mirror M_1, moving mirror M_2, and observing plane P.

mirror and returns to the beamsplitter, where part is reflected back to the laser and part is transmitted to the observing plane. We call this latter part the reference beam. The light originally transmitted by the beamsplitter is reflected by a moving mirror that traverses the distance to be measured. This light also returns to the beamsplitter, where part is transmitted to the laser and part (the signal beam) is reflected to the observing plane and super-imposed on the reference beam. The compensating plate, identical to the beamsplitter except for the partially reflecting coating and parallel to it, makes the two arms optically identical. For this simple interferometer with plane-wave illumination, the viewing screen will be illuminated with a simple truncated Gaussian spot if the virtual image of the fixed mirror is parallel to the moving mirror. An output lens can be added, of course, to focus the light onto a photodetector. Constructive interference will occur, giving maximum irradiance on the viewing screen, whenever the difference in optical path of the two arms is an integral number of wavelengths:

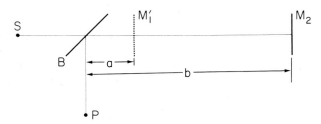

FIG. 7. Optical equivalent of Fig. 6, showing position of virtual image M_1' of fixed mirror. Effective source position is at a finite distance if interferometer illumination is divergent, and at infinity for full collimation.

$$2 |b - a| = N\lambda, \qquad N \text{ an integer} \tag{12}$$

The irradiance on the screen is given by

$$I = I_0 \cos^2 [2\pi |b - a|/\lambda] \tag{13}$$

where I_0 is the irradiance which the screen would have if the light from the collimator fell directly on it, and all of the other components, assumed lossless, were absent. If the mirrors are not quite parallel, the Gaussian spot will be traversed by bright and dark fringes, the form of which we will describe in the next section. With severe misalignment, the reference and signal beam spots will not overlap.

The maximum difference in optical path length $2|b - a|$ over which fringes may be observed depends on the temporal coherence of the light source, as may be seen from a simple argument. Consider a lamp emitting two distinct and sharply defined spectral lines whose separation $\Delta\lambda$ is small compared to the mean wavelength $\bar{\lambda}$ of the two. Each will give rise to interference, but the shorter-wavelength one will give a pattern which varies more rapidly as the moving mirror is displaced. At certain distances, constructive interference will occur simultaneously for both wavelengths, the local fringe visibility $V = (I_{max} - I_{min})/(I_{max} + I_{min})$ will be maximum, and the irradiance will reach an absolute maximum; at distances halfway between, a bright fringe for one wavelength will occur simultaneously with a dark one for the other, and the net fringe visibility will be minimum. It is straightforward to show that the visibility, which is the envelope of the fringe pattern, is periodic with period $\lambda^2/\Delta\lambda$, to extend the analysis to the case of a laser source emitting several equally spaced lines, and to show that for a single spectral line of Gaussian profile the variation of fringe visibility with optical path length difference is also Gaussian. In general, the range of distances over which fringes can be observed with a single spectral line is inversely proportional to the width of the line, and hence a narrow line will permit fringes to be observed while the moving mirror traverses a long distance. Michelson, using the 643.8 nm line of Cd, was able to observe fringes for mirror movements of only a few millimeters, and hence the meter bar measurement required many steps. The ^{86}Kr lamp (Engelhard and Vieweg, 1961) has a considerably greater coherence length, permitting fringe observation over a few decimeters, but the lamp is rather inconvenient to use and is low in intensity because of the 60° K operating temperature required for small Doppler linewidth. A well-designed single-frequency laser can give acceptable fringes at essentially any distance; the practical limits are set by acoustical disturbances perturbing the laser wavelength, modulation required by some stabilization methods, or atmospheric distortion, rather than by the fundamental coherence length of the laser. This same coherence, which permits direct fringe counting while one mirror traverses long distances, also causes some problems: undesired reflections from other surfaces, such as the air–glass interface on the back side of the beamsplitter, give rise to spurious interference patterns on the viewing screen. Laser interferometers are therefore designed with a minimum number of surfaces, and where possible the optical elements are thick and wedged so that the spurious beams are thrown to the side and do not reach the detector. A related problem arises because the laser is a resonant structure, and if any light is reflected back from the interferometer into the laser, as would happen in Fig. 6, the laser output amplitude and wavelength will, in general, be unstable and vary with the position and alignment of the moving mirror. The total system of laser plus interferometer must then be analyzed as a single multiply resonant system. Such an approach has been used for the supression of unwanted laser modes, but in general the final output must not be reflected back into the laser. The simplest and least desirable way to provide isolation is simply to attenuate the beam between laser and interferometer by inserting a filter of some kind. If the interferometer can operate with circularly polarized light, a better isolator consisting of a polarizer and quarter-wave plate can be used; if linear polarization is required, a Faraday rotation isolator would be needed. A better solution in many cases is to use a geometrical design for which no light is reflected back to the laser.

The basic unit of length measurement, $\lambda/2$, gives sufficient precision for most applications. At 632.8 nm, about 30,000 fringes must be counted as the moving mirror traverses one centimeter. We will find in Section III,C that it is convenient to reflect the light back and forth once more in the test leg, thus doubling its sensitivity, and another factor of four can be gained in the electronics. Hence the least count in a simple digital system not using phase measurement can be $\lambda/16$ or about 1.5 μin. In environments where vibration is present this precision may be awkwardly high, and it may be desirable to use infrared rather than visible-light lasers. On the other hand, higher precision can be achieved by using multiple-beam Fabry–Perot interferometers rather than the simple Michelson type (Herriott, 1967). Spherical rather than plane mirrors are normally used to reduce diffraction losses. Although the basic fringe spacing, $\lambda/2$, is unchanged, the fringes are no longer sinusoidal and can be two orders of magnitude narrower. For a given precision of setting on a fringe, the precision is increased proportionately. Alignment is critical, and hence these interferometers are not typically used for direct fringe counting but instead to measure small changes in length. Of particular interest is the 30 meter instrument of Boyne et al. (1970), built in an unused gold mine for measuring the velocity of light.

B. INTERFERENCE PATTERNS

With imperfect collimation or alignment, the output plane will not show the simple truncated Gaussian spot but will carry a superimposed pattern of interference fringes. Normally a fringe-counting interferometer is set up to show as few fringes as possible, but this is not necessarily the case in other applications. We now derive the shape of the patterns which can be observed.

1. Compensated Interferometer

An interferometer is said to be compensated if it is designed to be insensitive to changes in some parameter or adjustment. For example, it may be compensated for tilt. Historically, the phrase "compensated interferometer" without specification of a particular parameter means an instrument in which the light paths are identical except for length. One of the conditions of such identity is that each pair of rays generated by the beamsplitter traverse equivalent paths in glass. This has normally been done by making a single plane-parallel glass plate, cutting it in two, and using one half as the beamsplitter and the other as the compensating plate as shown in Fig. 6. Symmetrical beamsplitters such as the ones shown in Fig. 8 can also be used. For

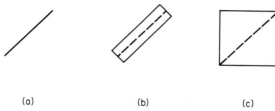

(a)   (b)   (c)

FIG. 8. Three types of symmetrical beamsplitter: (a) thin plastic pellicle; (b) cemented plates of equal thickness with a partially reflective coating between them; (c) cube form of type (b).

small-diameter beams the cube form is convenient because it can serve as a part of the mechanical structure of the interferometer, with other elements evaporated onto it or cemented to it. For beams of larger diameter, the plane-parallel plate is normally chosen because of its lower cost. For single-wavelength laser use spectral compensation is not required, and the choice of beamsplitter type is usually determined by mechanical considerations, spurious beam suppression, or cost. We will show in Section III,B,2 that there are characteristic asymmetries in the interference patterns of uncompensated interferometers, though, and for some uses, therefore, it will be desirable to have one of the compensated forms.

We first analyze the compensated case, in which we can consider the beamsplitter to be a single surface of negligible thickness, finding the interference pattern projected on a screen for either diverging or collimated light from a perfect point source. The coordinate system and basic lengths are shown in Fig. 9. The origin is at the position of source S, the z axis coincides with the optical axis from S to the center of moving mirror M_2, and the y axis lies in the plane determined by this axis and the second optical axis defined by

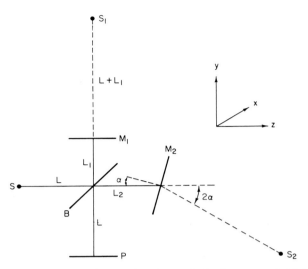

FIG. 9. Distances and coordinate system for analysis of compensated interferometer.

the center of the beamsplitter B and the center of fixed mirror M_1. We assume that mirror M_1 is normal to its optical axis and that mirror M_2 is tilted by a small angle α; we can take this angle to be in the yz plane at no loss of generality. Source S is at distance L from the center of B, while the corresponding distances for M_1 and M_2 are L_1 and L_2, respectively. For the beams reflected by the two mirrors, we wish to find the locus of points of constant phase difference on an observing screen P normal to the optical axis and at distance L from the beamsplitter.

Behind each mirror is an image of source S, as indicated in Fig. 9. The optical equivalent of the system is shown in Fig. 10, and we see that our problem is merely to calculate the interference pattern for two point sources, S_1 at position $2(L + L_1)[0, 0, 1]$ and S_2 at $(L + L_2)[0, \sin 2\alpha, 1 + \cos 2\alpha]$. It is straightforward trigonometry to find the distance from either to a general point $[x, y, 0]$ on the observing plane. We set the difference in distances equal to $N\lambda$, finding the equation defining the fringes to be

$$(N\lambda)^2 x^2 + [(N\lambda)^2 - (L' + \Delta L)^2 \sin^2 2\alpha] y^2$$
$$+ (L' + \Delta)(\sin 2\alpha)[4(L' + \Delta L)^2 \cos^2 \alpha - (N\lambda)^2 - 4(L')^2] y$$
$$= 2(L' + \Delta L)^2 (\cos^2 \alpha)[2(L' + \Delta L)^2 \cos^2 \alpha - (N\lambda)^2 - 4(L')^2]$$
$$+ \tfrac{1}{4}[(N\lambda)^2 - 4(L')^2]^2 \tag{14}$$

where L' and ΔL are given by

$$L' = L + L_1$$
$$\Delta L = L_2 - L_1 \tag{15}$$

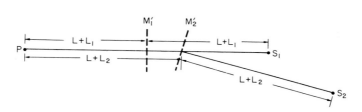

FIG. 10. Optical equivalent of system shown in Fig. 9.

The physical interpretation of this result is simple. The loci of points of equal phase difference are hyperboloids of revolution about the straight line S_1S_2 passing through the sources. In the case $\alpha = 0$, so that S_1S_2 is normal to plane P, the fringes will be circles. If $\alpha \neq 0$ but $\Delta L = 0$, so that S_1S_2 is nearly parallel to P, the fringes will be hyperbolas. If S_1S_2 intersects P at an angle which is not too large, elliptical fringes will be observed near the point of intersection. We now consider these cases in somewhat more detail. Note that the maximum path length difference is just the separation of S_1 and S_2, which for small α is given by

$$(N\lambda)_{max} = 2[L'\alpha^2(L' + 2\Delta L) + (\Delta L)^2(1 + \alpha^2)]^{1/2} \tag{16}$$

which reduces, of course, to $(N\lambda)_{max} = 2\Delta L$ for $\alpha = 0$.

(a) $\alpha = 0$. Circular fringes are observed. For $\Delta L = 0$, the illumination is just the Gaussian spot; if ΔL, $N\lambda \ll L'$, the circles have radius

$$r = 2L'[(2\Delta L/N\lambda)^2 - 1]^{1/2} \tag{17}$$

(b) $\Delta L = 0$. For $\alpha \ll 1$ and $N\lambda \ll L'$, we find simple hyperbolas shifted downward along the y axis:

$$x^2 + [1 - (2L'\alpha/N\lambda)^2]y^2 - 2L'\alpha y + 4(L')^2 = 0 \tag{18}$$

(c) $N\lambda < (L' + \Delta L) \sin 2\alpha$. In this case, the sources are nearly side by side so that S_1S_2 is roughly parallel to P, and the fringes are hyperbolic. We start by assuming $\alpha \ll 1$, $\Delta L \ll L'$, and $N\lambda \ll L'$, finding that the general result, Eq. (14), reduces to

$$(N\lambda)^2 x^2 + [(N\lambda)^2 - (2L'\alpha)^2]y^2 + 16(L')\alpha(\Delta L)y$$
$$= 4(L')^2[4(\Delta L)^2 - (N\lambda)^2] \tag{19}$$

This can be rewritten in the standard form

$$[(y - k)^2/b^2] - (x^2/a^2) = 1 \tag{20}$$

where the parameters a, b, and k are given by

$$a^2 = 4(L')^2[4(L')^2\alpha^2 + 4(\Delta L)^2 - (N\lambda)^2]/[(2L'\alpha)^2 - (N\lambda)^2]$$

$$b^2 = a^2\{(N\lambda)^2/[(2L'\alpha)^2 - (N\lambda)^2]\} \qquad (21)$$

$$k = [8(L')^2\alpha(\Delta L)]/[(2L'\alpha)^2 - (N\lambda)^2]$$

This is the equation of a two-branch hyperbola with center at $(0, k)$ and transverse axis of length $2b$ along the y axis.

(d) $N\lambda > (L' + \Delta L) \sin 2\alpha$. This occurs when α is very small but $\Delta L \neq 0$, so that some of the hyperboloids fully intersect the screen and give closed figures, although the axis $S_1 S_2$ is not normal to the screen. The ellipses can be described by Eq. (19), although strictly speaking Eq. (14) should be used because within the assumptions of the simplified equation the maximum value of $N\lambda$ is only $2L'\alpha$.

(e) $N\lambda = (L' + \Delta L) \sin 2\alpha$. For this intermediate case the fringes are parabolic. If $\Delta L = 0$ and $N\lambda \ll L'$, the equation is simply

$$x^2 - (N\lambda)y + 4(L')^2 = 0 \qquad (22)$$

(f) Collimated illumination. The results for fully collimated illumination can be obtained by simply allowing L' to approach infinity. The fringes are those for the interference of two plane waves, straight lines given by

$$y = (2\Delta L \pm N\lambda)/\alpha \qquad (23)$$

and hence of spacing λ/α.

2. Uncompensated Interferometer

The uncompensated case, in which we have a plane-parallel glass slab in one arm but not in the other, is somewhat more complicated because of the astigmatism of the slab. We again consider the basic interferometer of Fig. 6, but now without plate C. The variation of phase retardation with angle of incidence on the beamsplitter is different in different planes, and hence the patterns predicted in the preceding section for a diverging source will be distorted. We begin by considering the change in optical path length and the beam offset occurring when a ray traverses a plane-parallel plate. Consider a ray incident at angle I on a plate of thickness d and refractive index n, as indicated in Fig. 11. We find using Snell's law and simple geometry that the extra optical path length due to the presence of the plate is

$$\Delta(nL) = n(QB) + BC - QA$$
$$= [(n^2 - \sin^2 I)^{1/2} - \cos I]d \qquad (24)$$

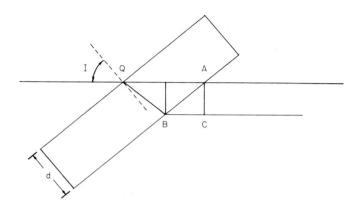

FIG. 11. Refraction by a plane-parallel plate.

With actual components, tilts are normally made around fixed axes, so that an angle of incidence is most easily specified by giving two angles of tilt around orthogonal axes rather than as a single angle I in a varying plane of incidence. We can rewrite Eq. (24) in terms of an angle I_y measured around a vertical axis and an angle I_x measured around a horizontal one, finding the necessary trigonometric relations from Fig. 12. The result is

$$\Delta(nL) = \left\{ \frac{[n^2 + (n^2 - 1)(\tan^2 I_x + \tan^2 I_y)]^{1/2} - 1}{[1 + \tan^2 I_x + \tan^2 I_y]^{1/2}} \right\} d \qquad (25)$$

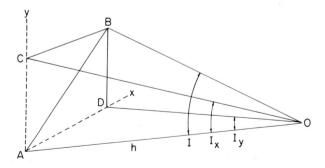

FIG. 12. Diagram used in finding the relation between a general angle of incidence I and its components I_x and I_y, measured in orthogonal planes. Line OA is the optical axis, normal to the reference plane ACD; line OB is the normal to the glass plate at O.

We expand this result for small tilts around a basic angle of 45°. For an angle $I_x = 45° + \theta_x$ around the horizontal axis and θ_y around the vertical one, the difference between the actual optical path length and that at 45° is

$$\delta(nL) = \frac{d}{\sqrt{2}} \left\{ \left[1 - \frac{1}{(2n^2 - 1)^{1/2}} \right] \left(\theta_x + \frac{1}{4} \theta_y{}^2 \right) + \frac{1}{2} \left[1 - \frac{1}{(2n^2 - 1)^{3/2}} \right] \theta_x{}^2 \right\}$$

(26)

We choose to put the uncompensated plate in the reference arm for convenience, which can be done by having the partially reflecting surface on the side of the beamsplitter away from the source. The first step in forming an equivalent system without mirrors is indicated in Fig. 13, where the images of

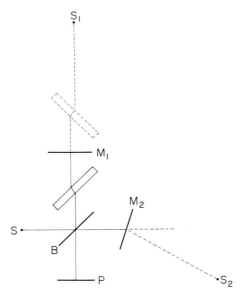

FIG. 13. First step in finding the equivalent system for an uncompensated interferometer, showing the image of the uncompensated plate.

the plate and of the source are shown, and we see that the light from S_1 will pass through two plates, each at 45° to the optical axis and therefore perpendicular to each other, before interfering with the light from S_2. For rays lying in the plane of the interferometer (the yz plane), for which $\theta_y = 0$, the angle of incidence on one plate will be $(45° + \theta_x)$ and on the other it will be $(-45° + \theta_x)$. Because only the form $\tan^2 I_x$ appears in Eq. (25), we can use $(45° - \theta_x)$ for the second plate and need not reexpand around $-45°$.

For rays lying in the perpendicular (xz) plane, the angle of incidence θ_y is the same for both plates. We see from the linearity of Eq. (26) in θ_x that there is no net change in optical thickness to first order in either plane; the additional optical path in the yz plane due to one plate is canceled by that of the second. The terms quadratic in θ_x and θ_y represent increases in wavefront curvature. The plate acts like a weak negative lens having different focal lengths in the two planes, so that source S_1 appears to be moved closer to the beamsplitter, but by different amounts for the rays lying in the two planes. It is straightforward to show that the change in radius of curvature is four times the coefficient of the quadratic term in Eq. (26), one factor of two arising from the effective presence of two plates and another from the geometry. Hence in the fully simplified diagram analogous to Fig. 10, source S_1 appears to be not at z coordinate $2L'$ but at $(2L' - h)$, where the shift h is given by

$$h_{yz} = \sqrt{2}\, d\{1 - [1/(2n^2 - 1)^{3/2}]\} \tag{27}$$

in the yz plane and by

$$h_{xz} = (d/\sqrt{2})\{1 - [1/(2n^2 - 1)^{1/2}]\} \tag{28}$$

in the xz plane.

Another astigmatic effect is the offset of all rays but the axial one. As sketched in Fig. 14, a given ray lying in the yz plane and passing through the

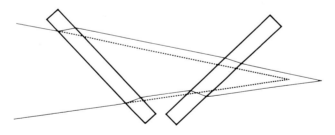

FIG. 14. Sketch indicating the source displacement effect of the uncompensated plate and its image.

two plates exits parallel to the incident ray but with an offset depending on θ_x. Again using Fig. 11, we can show that the beam offset AC for a single plate is given by

$$D = d(\sin I)\left\{1 - \frac{(1 - \sin^2 I)^{1/2}}{n[1 - (1/n^2)\sin^2 I]^{1/2}}\right\} \tag{29}$$

Rewriting in terms of $I_x = 45° + \theta_x$ and $I_y = \theta_y$, we find

$$D = \frac{d}{\sqrt{2}} \left\{ \left[1 - \frac{1}{(2n^2 - 1)^{1/2}} \right] + \left[1 - \frac{1}{(2n^2 - 1)^{3/2}} \right] \theta_x + \left[1 - \frac{n^2}{(2n^2 - 1)^{3/2}} \right] \frac{\theta_y^2}{2} \right\}$$

(30)

Noting that Eq. (29) changes sign when expanded around $-45°$, we find the total deviation by both plates to be, in lowest order,

$$D_{tot} = \sqrt{2} \, d\{1 - [1/(2n^2 - 1)^{3/2}]\}\theta_x \tag{31}$$

Because this offset is linear in θ_x, we see that all rays again appear to come from a point source that is closer to the beamsplitter than is the actual source. The apparent source position for rays in the yz plane is the same as given by Eq. (27). To find the effect in the xz plane we must resolve the total offset D, measured in the plane of incidence, into its components D_x and D_y, corresponding respectively to θ_x and θ_y. It is obvious that D_y will vary linearly with θ_y, again giving an apparent source shift.

Although the presence of the plate makes the source appear closer, it also adds an extra optical path which is the same as that for a single plate of thickness $2d$ at $45°$. Measured by optical path length, source S_1 appears to be farther away rather than closer with the glass present. It can quite easily be shown that the pair of tilted plates is equivalent, except for the fixed phase shift, to a single thicker plate inserted normal to the optical axis, although the plate thickness must be different in the xz and yz planes. The thickness

$$d' = \frac{\sqrt{2} \, d\{1 - [1/(2n^2 - 1)^{3/2}]\}}{(1 - 1/n)} \tag{32}$$

gives the same apparent source position in the yz plane as the actual tilted ones, although the extra axial optical path added is too large. Hence it is impossible to have the two sources S_1 and S_2 appear to be superimposed, even in one plane, and also to have the optical path lengths equal so that $N\lambda = 0$. If the true optical path lengths are equal at some point, the sources do not appear to coincide; if the wavefront curvatures are matched, the optical paths differ. The fact that these two conditions cannot be simultaneously satisfied was a significant drawback of uncompensated interferometers when only thermal light sources were available, although with laser sources the unmatched fixed path causes no difficulty. The astigmatism of the plate, however, distorts the fringe patterns; for example, fringes which would have been circular in the compensated case will now be elliptical. The patterns can be predicted by including Eq. (26) in the earlier trigonometric analysis.

C. Limiting the Degrees of Freedom

A simple Twyman–Green interferometer has many degrees of freedom, linear and angular, and is awkwardly sensitive to misalignment. It is possible to use cube-corner or cat's-eye retroreflectors instead of plane mirrors, replacing the two angular degrees of freedom of each mirror by two lateral ones. The interferometer will still operate as long as any part of the beam is reflected back on itself, and hence the sensitivity to lateral misalignment is very low compared to the original angular sensitivity. If the cube corners are offset as shown in Fig. 15, the additional advantage is gained that there is

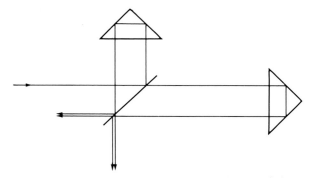

Fig. 15. Interferometer with offset retroreflectors. No light is reflected back into the laser, and both output patterns can be observed.

no feedback into the laser. A simpler version of the same design is shown in Fig. 16. Another design, currently in use, is sketched in Fig. 17. At the expense of returning light to the laser and hence requiring the use of an absorber or isolator, this version is insensitive to both rotation and lateral translation of the moving retroreflector. It thus achieves the minimum number of effective degrees of freedom along with double sensitivity because of the folded path. As in the other good designs, all of the optical elements can be cemented together into a single rugged package. Further discussion and references to aberration analyses can be found in the thesis by Foster (1965).

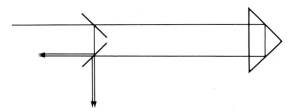

Fig. 16. Simpler version of the same design as Fig. 15.

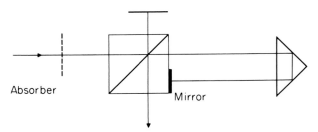

FIG. 17. Folded-path instrument sensitive only to longitudinal displacement.

D. REVERSIBLE COUNTING

A practical instrument must be capable of reversible fringe counting so that measurements can be made with the mirror moving both out and back and, more important, so that no fringes are miscounted in the presence of vibration. In order to do this, resolving the ambiguity of the circular functions, the interferometer must provide two outputs in quadrature. The two signals, one varying sinusoidally and one cosinusoidally with path length, are first converted to square waves. Successive pulses in one channel are tallied by the counter, the phase relation of the two signals controlling whether the count is recorded as positive or negative. The basic technique, including circuit details, has been described by Cook and Marzetta (1961). Reversible electronic counters suitable for direct connection to photodetectors and capable of counting rates of 1 MHz or greater are now commercially available.

The simplest method of generating quadrature signals is simply to tilt the reference mirror as indicated in Fig. 18. A tilt of 32 μrad gives a fringe spacing of 1 cm. Two detectors, properly spaced, then give the desired signals. If these are applied to the X and Y deflection terminals of an oscilloscope, the beam will be deflected in a circle, the sense of rotation giving the direction of motion of the moving mirror. A length measurement could be made by tallying the integral number of revolutions on a counter and measuring the fractional rotation of the spot to interpolate between fringes.

This method of generating the quadrature signals is a poor one, however, because slight misalignments will change the fringe spacing and therefore the phase relation of the outputs, possibly causing count errors. A better system is shown in Fig. 19, where a $\lambda/8$ step in the fixed mirror divides the illuminated field into two parts having irradiances in quadrature.

For reliable operation in the presence of vibrational misalignment or wavefront distortion due to atmospheric turbulence, it is necessary to generate the two signals by division of amplitude rather than by spatial division of wavefront. A good method for doing so was suggested by Peck and Obetz

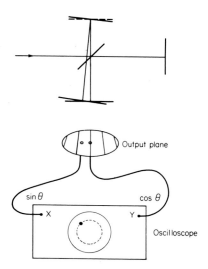

FIG. 18. Simplest method of generating quadrature signals. Tilting the reference beam gives straight fringes, and properly spaced detectors give the desired outputs.

(1953), who used the offset interferometer of Fig. 15 and placed one detector at the center of each of the two output patterns. If the beamsplitter is a lossless dielectric one, the two outputs are required to be complementary by conservation of energy. If the beamsplitter is a lossy metallic one, however, the outputs need not be in antiphase; the actual phase shift between the two

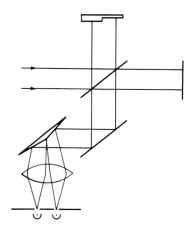

FIG. 19. Quadrature signal generation by division of wavefront, using $\lambda/8$ step in fixed mirror.

outputs depends sensitively on the thickness and composition of the beam-splitter coating. This method has recently been utilized by Rowley (1966), who has found that certain alloys of gold and silver provide satisfactory shifts. It is a good approach because there is no feedback to the laser, no division of wavefront, and all of the light except that absorbed by the beam-splitter (typically about 40%) is used, although we have found that making good beamsplitters is something of a problem.

A variety of polarization methods have also been proposed. A good one is shown in Fig. 20. The input light is polarized linearly at 45° to the plane of the interferometer. After reflection from the moving mirror and beam-splitter, the output light in the signal beam is still polarized linearly at 45°, so that its vertical and horizontal components are in phase. In the reference arm, however, a quarter-wave plate makes the reference beam circularly polarized, so that its vertical and horizontal components are in quadrature. After the beams recombine, a Wollaston prism separates the vertical and horizontal components, giving two interference patterns which are also in quadrature and thus the desired outputs. If the horizontally polarized components are in phase, for example, one of the vertically polarized ones will be shifted by 90° with respect to the other.

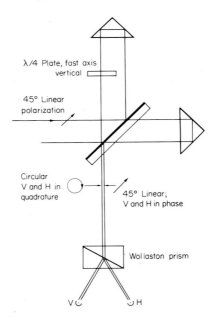

FIG. 20. Polarization method for obtaining quadrature outputs. A linearly polarized signal beam interferes with a circularly polarized reference one. A Wollaston prism separates the interference patterns of the vertically and horizontally polarized components.

Several problems of polarization compensation arise. In general, polarization is altered by any reflection not occurring at normal incidence, and hence the use of beamsplitters mounted at 45° and of retroreflectors other than cat's eyes of long focal length will cause deviations from simple quadrature phase relationships and equal amplitudes. In addition, an unsymmetrical beamsplitter may give a different depolarization in reflection from the air-coating interface than from the glass-coating one. Compensation can be achieved by replacing the simple wave plate by an adjustable Babinet–Soleil compensator, but a better solution if cube corners must be used is to make the system fully symmetrical by orienting the retroreflectors identically and using a beamsplitter which is both symmetrical and nonpolarizing. The output beams will be elliptically polarized, but the vertical and horizontal components will have the desired quadrature relation. For use with offset beams, an effectively symmetrical beamsplitter can be made by cutting an unsymmetrical one in half and reversing one part, or by applying the coating to the top half of one side and to the bottom half of the other; now the reflections giving the normal output beams will both occur at air-coating interfaces or at glass-coating ones. The next step, making the beamsplitter nonpolarizing, can be accomplished simply by mounting it at a small angle of incidence (10° to 15°) rather than at 45°. Finally, adjusting the angle of linear polarization of the input light does not change the relative phase shift of the outputs but does change their intensity. If a second beamsplitter and two separate polarizers are used instead of the Wollaston prism, the relative phase shift of the outputs can be varied.

The polarization method has the disadvantage that half the output light is not used unless a second pair of detectors is employed, but it has the real advantage that the outputs can be adjusted in phase and amplitude. Variants of Fig. 20 can also be used, of course, such as the ones suggested in Figs. 16 and 21. In the latter design, polarization compensation makes use of the fact that for linearly polarized light there exists an angular roll position which

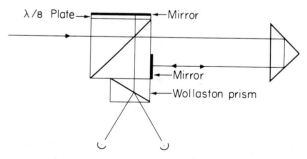

FIG. 21. Folded-path version of polarization interferometer.

exactly preserves the polarization after a double transit through the cube corner (Peck, 1962).

A different method of reversible counting has recently been developed in which the light source is a helium–neon laser placed in an axial magnetic field so that it oscillates simultaneously at two different optical frequencies separated by about 2 MHz. The superimposed output beams have opposite circular polarizations. They are separated by a beamsplitter and two filters, each consisting of a quarter-wave plate and a linear polarizer, so that one provides the reference beam and the other the signal beam. If the signal-beam mirror is moving, the beat frequency observed at the detector will be different from the fundamental 2 MHz beat (which can be observed using a second beamsplitter and detector at the laser output), and this difference in frequency can be used to measure the mirror motion. The system is attractive because this ac mode of operation is considerably less sensitive to signal-beam attenuation than are the dc methods. Because a special laser is required, however, we shall not analyze the system further here; details are available elsewhere (Dukes and Gordon, 1970).

E. ANALYSIS OF OUTPUTS

For simple fringe counting over short paths, either the lossy-beamsplitter method or the more complicated but adjustable polarization method will be satisfactory. For operation over longer paths, especially where air turbulence may cause scintillation and pattern distortion, and for subfringe measurements in vibration and propagation studies, the actual outputs and sources of error must be considered in more detail. We start with the simpler method, showing how fractional-fringe data reduction can be carried out, and then analyze the polarization interferometer.

1. *Lossy-Beamsplitter Method*

The interferometer to be analyzed is shown in Fig. 22. We assume that the input light is linearly polarized in the p or s plane of the beamsplitter (the plane of the diagram or the perpendicular plane passing through the optical axis, respectively) and that the retroreflectors are either cat's eyes or dihedral mirrors with intersection lines normal to the plane of the diagram, so that polarization effects can be neglected. The laser output can be taken to be a plane wave of uniform irradiance I_0 over the area of interest and described by $[A \cos \omega t]$, where A is the light amplitude, ω is the optical frequency, and t is the time. Hence the average irradiance is $I_0 = \frac{1}{2}A^2$. The reference

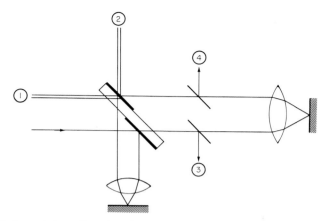

FIG. 22. Lossy-beamsplitter interferometer. Detectors 1 and 2 are located at equivalent points of the interference patterns, while 3 and 4 monitor the transmitted and received signal beams, respectively, using the light reflected by uncoated glass plates. The retroreflectors shown are one form of cat's eyes, and the beamsplitter is effectively symmetrical.

beam reaching detector 1, twice reflected by the beamsplitter of reflectivity r, is given by $[r^2 A \cos \omega t]$. We need not include the reflectivity of the retroreflector because it affects outputs 1 and 2 symmetrically. The reference beam reaching detector 2 is given by $[rtA \cos (\omega t + \theta/2)]$, where t is the magnitude of the beamsplitter transmissivity and $\theta/2$ is its associated phase. The existence of this phase shift between reflected and transmitted beams is the crux of the method. The signal beam at detector 1 is given by $[t^2 t_p A \cos (\omega t + \theta - \varphi)]$, where t_p is the magnitude of the transmissivity of the measuring path and $\varphi = 2\pi/\Delta L$ is the phase shift associated with the difference in optical path ΔL between the signal and reference beams. The signal beam at detector 2 is given by $[rtt_p A \cos (\omega t + \theta/2 - \varphi)]$. The outputs from detectors 1 and 2, found by adding the reference and signal beams at each detector, squaring and time-averaging, are given by

$$I_1 = C_1 A^2 RT \sqrt{T_p}\{[(R/T)^2 + T_p]/2(R/T)\sqrt{T_p} + \cos (\theta - \varphi)\}$$
$$I_2 = C_2 A^2 RT \sqrt{T_p}[(1 + T_p)/2\sqrt{T_p} + \cos \varphi]$$

(33)

where $R = r^2$, $T = t^2$, and $T_p = t_p{}^2$ are power reflection and transmission coefficients, and C_1 and C_2 are parameters describing the photomultiplier gain setting and other adjustments. One of the output currents varies as $\cos \varphi$ and the other as $\cos (\theta - \varphi)$, but neither fringe pattern will, in general, have unit visibility. In the absence of scintillation (time varying T_p), it is possible to operate by merely blocking the dc components and amplifying the ac signals to equal amplitude. These are digitized and recorded, and it is straightforward to estimate θ and to find φ using a computer. Let us denote the normalized ac parts of I_1 and I_2 by primes, so that we have

$$I_1' = \cos(\theta - \varphi)$$
$$I_2' = \cos\varphi$$
(34)

From these we can easily find the signal in quadrature with I_2', $I_3' = \sin\varphi$:

$$I_3' = [I_1' - I_2' \cos\theta]/\sin\theta \tag{35}$$

Making use of the identity $\sin^2\varphi + \cos^2\varphi = 1$, we can solve for θ:

$$\cos\theta = I_1'I_2' \pm [(I_1'I_2')^2 - (I_1')^2 - (I_2')^2 + 1]^{1/2} \tag{36}$$

From one pair of values (I_1', I_2') we obtain θ. For each succeeding pair, Eqs. (34) and (35) give the desired signals, and φ is simply found by computing arccos I_2' and using the relative signs of I_2' and I_3' to determine the quadrant. We have found in practice that phase shifts as small as a few degrees give quite acceptable results, and that the results are quite insensitive to errors in θ.

They are more sensitive, however, to amplitude changes, and in the presence of scintillation or laser variation it may be necessary to monitor the laser output and the returning light level. Unless the interferometer is symmetrical and perfectly aligned, θ will vary as well, and we must consider all four variables A, T_p, θ, and φ. The outputs of detectors 3 and 4 are given by

$$I_3 = \tfrac{1}{2}C_3 A^2 T$$
$$I_4 = \tfrac{1}{2}C_4 A^2 T T_p$$
(37)

where C_3 and C_4 are adjustable parameters as before. The outputs of all four detectors are recorded and digitized, and the normalized signals I_1' and I_2' computed from them. For the special case of $R = T$ and $C_1 = C_2 = C_3 = C_4$, they are given by

$$I_1' = \tfrac{1}{2}(I_3/I_4)^{1/2}[(I_1/RI_3) - (I_4/I_3) - 1]$$
$$I_2' = \tfrac{1}{2}(I_3/I_4)^{1/2}[(I_2/RI_3) - (I_4/I_3) - 1]$$
(38)

After the normalized signals have been found, the computation of φ proceeds as before.

2. Polarization Method

Even in interferometers not specifically designed to measure or make use of polarization, changes in polarization may affect fringe visibility and, as in the lossy-beamsplitter method, the relative irradiance of the two outputs.

We now outline how to analyze these effects, finding, as an example, the outputs for one polarization method of obtaining quadrature signals.

For fully polarized light it is most convenient to use the Jones calculus, which has been well described by Shurcliff and Ballard (1964). We consider light propagating in the positive direction along the z axis of a right-handed Cartesian coordinate system. The Jones vector is the two-element column vector defined by

$$J = \begin{pmatrix} E_x \\ E_y \end{pmatrix} \tag{39}$$

where E_x and E_y are the complex amplitudes of the electric field components in the x and y planes, respectively. Angles are measured in the usual way, from the $+x$ axis toward the $+y$ axis, and the handedness of rotation of polarization vectors is defined for an observer looking back along the $+z$ axis toward the source, rather than for one looking in the direction of propagation of the light. Hence linear polarization at 45° is described by the vector $E_0\begin{pmatrix} 1 \\ 1 \end{pmatrix}$, and right circular polarization by $E_0\begin{pmatrix} -i \\ 1 \end{pmatrix}$. Jones vectors are usually normalized by discarding amplitude or phase factors common to both elements, but if two coherent beams are to be superimposed the full vectors must be retained so that the relative amplitudes and phases of the beams are preserved. The irradiance of a beam is found by adding the irradiances of the orthogonal components, that is, by finding the time average of the sum of the squares of the magnitudes of the elements,

$$I = \tfrac{1}{2}\langle E_x^* E_x + E_y^* E_y \rangle \tag{40}$$

The effect of any optical component is found by multiplying the Jones vector of the incident light by a matrix characterizing the component. A birefringent plate of retardation γ with fast axis at 0°, for example, acts as if it were thicker for y-polarized than for x-polarized light. The emerging y component is retarded by γ, and hence multiplied by a phase factor exp $(-i\gamma)$, relative to the x component. To within a constant phase factor, the plate is represented by the matrix

$$R(\gamma) = \begin{pmatrix} e^{i(\gamma/2)} & 0 \\ 0 & e^{-i(\gamma/2)} \end{pmatrix} \tag{41}$$

If the fast axis of the retarder is at angle θ, its effect may be found by rotating the coordinates of the incident light to match the retarder axes, multiplying by $R(\gamma)$, and then rotating back to the original axes. The output polarization is given by

$$J' = S(-\theta)R(\gamma)S(\theta)J \tag{42}$$

where the rotation matrices have the well-known form

$$S(\theta) = \begin{pmatrix} \cos\theta & \sin\theta \\ -\sin\theta & \cos\theta \end{pmatrix} \tag{43}$$

For a reflecting surface with its normal lying in the xz plane, the matrix may be written

$$M = \begin{pmatrix} r_p & 0 \\ 0 & r_s \end{pmatrix} \tag{44}$$

where r_p and r_s, the amplitude reflection coefficients for light polarized parallel to the plane of incidence or perpendicular to it, may differ in both magnitude and phase. Note that reflection in a mirror inverts the coordinate system, changing the sense of the z axis but not the others. After a non-polarizing reflection, light which was initially linearly polarized at angle φ remains linearly polarized, but at angle $-\varphi$.

We now consider a simple example, the polarization interferometer of Fig. 20. We assume that the beamsplitter is unsymmetrical, coated on the laser side, and mounted at a large angle. The reference arm lies in the xz plane. The two polarization components will, in general, be reflected with differing reflectivities and a phase shift, and these parameters may differ for incidence on the coated and uncoated sides. The matrix for reflection from the coated side is written

$$\begin{pmatrix} R_p e^{i(\Gamma/2)} & 0 \\ 0 & R_s e^{-i(\Gamma/2)} \end{pmatrix}$$

and from the uncoated ones,

$$\begin{pmatrix} R_p{}' e^{i(\Gamma'/2)} & 0 \\ 0 & R_s{}' e^{-i(\Gamma'/2)} \end{pmatrix}$$

We assume there is no phase shift in transmission. For incidence on the coated side we have

$$\begin{pmatrix} T_p & 0 \\ 0 & T_s \end{pmatrix}$$

for the uncoated,

$$\begin{pmatrix} T_p{}' & 0 \\ 0 & T_s{}' \end{pmatrix}$$

For simplicity we choose the mirrors to be dihedrals mounted with all mirror normals lying in the xz plane so that the matrix for each reflection is diagonal,

$$\begin{pmatrix} r_p e^{i(\gamma/2)} & 0 \\ 0 & r_s e^{-i(\gamma/2)} \end{pmatrix}$$

and the double reflection restores the original coordinate system. Finally, we describe the effect of the extra optical path in the signal arm by an isotropic attenuation t and phase shift η.

The sequence of operations for the signal arm is indicated in Fig. 23. The

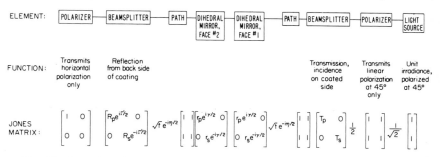

FIG. 23. Sequence of optical elements and associated Jones matrices for the signal arm of the interferometer in Fig. 20. Only the output linearly polarized at 0° is indicated.

diagram is to be read from right to left, in the order of matrix multiplication. For a source linearly polarized at 45° and the output polarizer set at 0°, the output amplitude is

$$(1/\sqrt{2})te^{-i\eta}R_p'e^{i(\Gamma'/2)}r_p^2 e^{i\gamma}T_p\begin{pmatrix} 1 \\ 0 \end{pmatrix} \tag{45}$$

We can find the output of the reference arm analogously, add the signal and reference amplitudes, and calculate the irradiance of the resulting fringes by Eq. (40). The resultant irradiances of the outputs at 0° and 90° are, respectively,

$$\tfrac{1}{2}r_p^4 T_p^2\{(tR_p')^2 + R_p^2 + 2tR_p'R_p \cos[\eta + (\Gamma - \Gamma')/2 + \pi/4]\}$$
$$\tfrac{1}{2}r_s^4 T_s^2\{(tR_s')^2 + R_s^2 + 2tR_s'R_s \cos[\eta - (\Gamma - \Gamma')/2 - \pi/4]\} \tag{46}$$

If the source is linearly polarized at 0° and the fast axis of the quarter-wave plate is at 45°, the output irradiance in the 45° channel is given by

$$\tfrac{1}{2}r_p^4\{(tR_p'T_p)^2 + \tfrac{1}{2}(T_p^2 + T_s^2)R_p^2$$
$$+ \sqrt{2}\,tR_p'T_pR_p(T_p^2 + T_s^2)^{1/2}\cos[\eta + (\Gamma - \Gamma'/2) + \varphi]\} \tag{47}$$

where

$$\tan \varphi = T_s/T_p \tag{48}$$

The fringe irradiance of the other output, with polarizer at $-45°$, is identical except for the sign of φ; unlike the case of a source at $45°$, the sign of $(\Gamma - \Gamma')/2$ is identical in the two outputs.

From these results we see that if the source is linearly polarized at $45°$, the fringe visibilities of the two outputs will, in general, be nearly equal, will be identical if the beamsplitter is symmetrical even if polarizing, and will be low only if the path loss is high. The irradiances of the outputs may differ significantly if the beamsplitter or dihedral mirrors have reflection coefficients of unequal magnitude; for this reason roof prisms utilizing total internal reflection would be preferable to metallized mirrors. If the quarter-wave plate is accurate, the only source of quadrature error is lack of beamsplitter symmetry through $(\Gamma - \Gamma')$.

For a source polarized at $0°$, the fringe visibilities will be equal and, in general, nearly unity for low transmission loss. The output irradiances are equal. Deviations from quadrature do not depend on asymmetry but vary quite strongly with transmission polarization as indicated by Eq. (48).

The same approach can be used, of course, to analyze other systems. Often much can be learned about the polarization properties of an interferometer by simple inspection of its matrices. An interferometer cannot be compensated for polarization, for example, unless the overall matrices for the signal and reference arms are identical except for isotropic factors. If cube corners are used, for which the matrices are not diagonal, the individual matrices cannot be commuted and the overall matrices will not be identical unless the beamsplitter is symmetrical and nonpolarizing. Information on the detailed polarization properties of cube corners has been given by Peck (1962) and by Walsh and Krause (1966).

F. Wavelength Stabilization

The ^{86}Kr standard lamp gives 3×10^5 fringes in 10 cm; if a resolution of 1/300 fringe is achieved, a precision of 1 part in 10^8 is possible in the length measurement. The spectral line is slightly asymmetrical, but the ultimate precision of length measurement with this light source is probably limited by coherence length rather than by inherent wavelength instability. Gas lasers, on the other hand, provide much greater coherence lengths, but they normally use lighter atoms and operate at much higher temperatures than the krypton lamp, and hence their emission lines are strongly Doppler broadened. The instantaneous linewidth of a single-mode He–Ne laser can be extremely narrow and its short-term stability very good because the resonator Q is high. A serious defect, however, is that this laser will continue to operate while the resonator length, and hence the operating wavelength, are changed over a range of about 3 parts in 10^6. Mielenz et al. (1966) have shown that the operating wavelength of a free-running He–Ne laser can be manually set to the line center with a reproducibility of a few parts in 10^8, although the wavelength then normally drifts by about 3 parts in 10^8 per minute. This sensitivity to thermal, acoustical, and atmospheric perturbations of the resonator, as well as sensitivity to the composition and pressure of the operating gas mixture, have prevented the free-running gas laser from replacing the krypton lamp as a wavelength standard.

The long-term stability of He–Ne lasers has been improved not only by thermal compensation of the resonator structure but also through the use of several ingenious servomechanism methods that continuously reset the cavity resonance to some given point on the atomic emission profile or to some external atomic or resonator standard. A good review describing a number of these methods has been given by Birnbaum (1967), and a briefer, more recent one by Hall (1968). The best known of these methods and the one used in commercially available lasers makes use of the Lamb dip, the minimum in the output power occurring at the center of the emission line of a laser containing only one isotope of neon. One of the laser mirrors is mounted on a piezoelectric crystal, and a sinusoidal voltage applied to this crystal causes the operating wavelength to scan back and forth over a small range. The laser output is monitored and a servo system maintains the average wavelength at the intensity minimum, where the first derivative of the line profile is zero and the second derivative is positive. The width of the Lamb dip is about 1 part in 10^7 of the operating wavelength, more than an order of magnitude less than the atomic linewidth, and a good servo system can maintain the operating wavelength within 1% of the center of the dip. Unfortunately the resulting resettability of 1 part in 10^9 is not representative of the laser's long-term stability because of the rather large pressure shifts of the entire spectral line. A recent comparison by three national standards laboratories in which the wavelength of a single commercial self-stabilized laser was measured against ^{86}Kr gave results agreeing with ±5 parts in 10^9, but a similar laser of different manufacture was found to have a center wavelength differing from the others by more than 1 part in 10^7. To make a primary standard it is necessary to servo-control a laser using as the reference an external absorption cell containing a gas at low temperature and pressure having a narrow absorption line that is only weakly affected by external perturbations and that falls within the laser's operating range. The most promising system at this time appears to be stabilization of the He–Ne laser by using the coincidence of its emission at 3.39 μm with a saturable absorption line of methane. Barger and Hall (1969) have built two independent systems and have shown that their wavelengths coincide within 1 part of 10^{11}. The pressure shifts and other perturbations of the methane line are small enough that the long-term stability may be comparable to the reproducibility.

G. REFRACTIVE INDEX CORRECTION

In any interferometric measurement, the length corresponding to a given fringe count obviously depends on the wavelength of the light used. For a given source the wavelength in air λ_a is slightly smaller than the wavelength in vacuum λ_v and their ratio defines the refractive index:

$$n \equiv \lambda_v / \lambda_a \tag{49}$$

The refractive index of air is a function of pressure, temperature, composition, and wavelength. Under normal conditions it differs only slightly from unity, varying from about 1.000283 at 400 nm to about 1.000276 at 700 nm for dry air under standard conditions, at a pressure ot 1013.25 mbar and a temperature of 15° C. For most purposes the refractive index at the He–Ne wavelength $\lambda_v = 632.991$ nm is predicted adequately by the simple expression

$$(n - 1) \times 10^6 = (78.64/T)P_t - (12/T)P_w \tag{50}$$

where P_t is the total pressure and P_w is the partial pressure of water vapor, both in millibars, and T is the temperature in °K. More accurate expressions will be given in Section IV,C.

Near standard conditions, a change of 1 part in 10^6 in wavelength (and hence in the conversion of fringe count to length) is caused by a change in temperature of 1° C, by a change in pressure of 3.7 mbar, or by a change in the partial pressure of water vapor of 23 mbar. In practice, variations of temperature and relative humidity are relatively unimportant in reasonably controlled environments. A change in relative humidity from 10% to 90% at 70° F, for example, changes P_w by only 20 mbar. Atmospheric pressure, however, cannot be controlled and must be monitored for accurate work. In an unpublished study described by Foster (1965), pressure variations were measured in New York during the month of December for the period 1957–1962. It was found that the typical errors would be as follows: If the pressure were measured at 8.00 A.M. each day and the wavelength corresponding to this pressure used all day, the error would be less than ±4.8 parts in 10^6; if the pressure were measured once during each 24-hour day and the corresponding wavelength used for that period, the error would be less than ±10.9 parts in 10^6; and if the pressure were measured once each month and

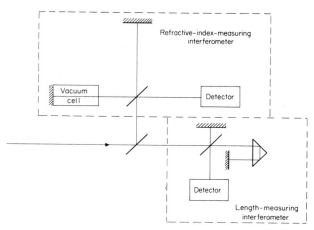

Fig. 24. Double interferometer, one section for monitoring refractive index and the other for measuring length.

used all month, the error would be less than ± 15.1 parts in 10^6. Commercially available interferometers usually include pressure, temperature, and humidity sensors, the outputs of which are automatically included in the conversion of fringe count to distance. An alternative approach used in metrology laboratories is indicated in Fig. 24. Two interferometers are used, one having fixed mirrors and one arm in vacuum so that its output monitors changes in refractive index, while the other is used for the actual length measurement.

H. THREE-DIMENSIONAL APPLICATIONS

In addition to the linear methods described so far, which can be cascaded as in x, y tables for two- and three-dimensional measurement, interferometric methods have long been used for checking the surface figures of mirrors and flats as well as the quality of lenses and other transmission elements. The limited spatial and temporal coherence of available light sources has required the use of a number of sophisticated interferometers, especially of the shearing type, and interpreting the resulting fringe patterns is not always simple. Laser methods, in spite of the problem of spurious fringes, have significantly simplified and broadened these techniques. In the production of large optics, for example, the laser provides the first light of sufficient coherence to permit the inspection and evaluation of thick lenses and prisms with precision interferometers. Fringe scanning and computer analysis permits this work to be done on a reasonably routine basis.

A particularly significant development has been that of holographic interferometry, which considerably expands the domain of interferometric measurement. Its applications include nondestructive testing, surface contouring, and vibration studies on surfaces which are not optically finished, and the testing of aspheric optical surfaces for which no master surface actually exists by using a computer-generated hologram to provide the reference wavefront. A general introduction to holography has been given by Smith (1969), while details of these and other applications may be found in another article in this book (see Thompson, page 1, this volume).

IV. Modulated-Light Methods

A. PRINCIPLES

For measuring distances of several kilometers or more in the open air, direct optical interferometry is precluded by atmospheric turbulence. Geodetic distance measurements of high accuracy are now usually made by measuring the time required for an electromagnetic wave to travel from a transmitter to a distant retroreflector or transponder and back. The observed transit time is multiplied by the appropriate propagation velocity to give the distance. Both transit time and propagation velocity, therefore, must be determined for the path being measured. An accuracy of 10 ppm (parts per million) in distance is normally considered adequate for "first-order" work, but 1 ppm is often required for specialized geodetic applications, and significantly higher accuracies would be desirable for geophysical measurements of earth strain.

Simple microwave or optical pulse techniques are useful in military ranging and other coarse measurements, but they do not, at present, provide satisfactory precision for geodetic applications. For a round-trip path length of 10 km, for example, the transit time is about 33 μsec, and hence the time measurement must be accurate to 3 psec if the distance measurement is to have a precision of 1 ppm. The transit time may be found by measuring the phase delay of a cw radio or microwave signal traversing the path. This signal may be either transmitted directly or used to modulate a microwave or optical carrier wave. The accuracy of the transit time measurement depends on both the accuracy with which phase can be measured and the signal frequency, and for a given accuracy of phase measurement the transit time can be measured more accurately at higher frequencies. Although it appears that the optimum frequency for distance measurement lies in the microwave region, the use of microwaves propagating directly through the

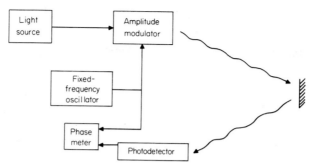

FIG. 25. Phase-meter method of measuring transit time.

atmosphere suffers from multipath errors and high sensitivity to atmospheric water vapor. These disadvantages can be largely overcome by using a light beam modulated at the microwave frequency rather than transmitting the microwave signal itself.

There are two basic methods of measuring transit time with such a signal; these are shown in Figs. 25 and 26. In Fig. 25 the optical carrier wave is sinusoidally amplitude modulated at frequency v, and the modulation of the returning light, detected by a photomultiplier, is measured with a phase meter. This phase shift is related to the path length by

$$\varphi = 2\pi(2\langle n^G\rangle L/\lambda) \tag{51}$$

where L is the one-way path length, λ is the modulation wavelength in vacuum, and $\langle n^G\rangle$ is the group refractive index averaged over the path. The use of modulation phase requires that the group index, defined by

$$n^G = c/U \tag{52}$$

where U is the group velocity and c is the velocity of light in vacuum, be used instead of the ordinary phase refractive index. In the second method, used by Fizeau in the first terrestrial measurement of the velocity of light, the light returns through the modulator after reflection from the distant mirror:

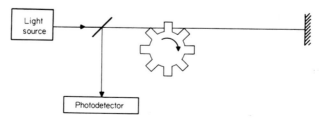

FIG. 26. Fizeau method of measuring transit time. The chopper would now be replaced by an amplitude modulator driven by a variable-frequency oscillator.

It will pass through and reach the detector only if the modulator is transmitting when the light returns; a maximum occurs in the average irradiance at the detector if the transit time is an integral number N of modulation periods τ:

$$2\langle n^G \rangle L/c = N\tau \tag{53}$$

In this method the photomultiplier is normally used as a null detector, and the modulation frequency $v = 1/\tau$ is adjusted until the output is maximized or minimized.

For general surveying use, the phasemeter method is probably preferable because of its simplicity and linear readout. It is used almost exclusively in present commercial instruments. The precision is limited, however, because the modulation frequency is generally restricted to 50 MHz or less by the frequency response of the photomultiplier. It is possible to use one of the microwave-frequency detectors described by Anderson and McMurty (1966), by Kerr (1967), and by Ross in the chapter on laser communications, this volume, page 239, although problems of reliability and limited gain have so far prevented their wide use. For measurements of highest accuracy, the two-pass Fizeau method is probably better because it permits high modulation frequencies to be used while retaining a sensitive photomultiplier of limited frequency response, and because the method avoids certain systematic errors. We will, therefore, analyze the operation of a system using this method in some detail, commenting only at the end, in Section IV,F, on a more complicated instrument utilizing phase measurement.

One disadvantage of a high modulation frequency is that the ambiguity resolution problem becomes more difficult. Both types of instrument effectively determine only the last fractional wavelength, and if the path length being measured is greater than half a modulation wavelength it is necessary to determine the integral number N as well.

With a frequency of 3 GHz and a distance of 10 km, for example, we have $N = 2 \times 10^5$. The normal procedure with a phasemeter instrument is to measure the fractional wavelength using three or more different modulation frequencies and to apply the well-known method of exact fractions. If the modulation frequency is continuously variable it is possible instead to measure the difference in frequency of successive integral-wavelength points. This is explained more fully in Section IV,D.

The first modern optical instrument was the "Geodimeter," originally developed by Bergstrand (1950) for a measurement of the velocity of light. Although the range of the first instrument was only a few kilometers, its convenience and accuracy were recognized as important for geodetic work and it soon became available commercially. Information on current instruments and their geodetic use can be found in a comprehensive book (Rinner and Benz, 1966) and in two volumes of conference proceedings (International Association of Geodesy, 1967; Angus-Leppan, 1968), while a review of interferometric and modulated-light methods for geophysical measurement has been given by Bender (1967).

B. LIGHT MODULATION AND SYSTEM OPERATION

We now describe briefly the operation of electrooptic light modulators and their use in a basic Fizeau-type system. Although the light finally reaching the photomultiplier must be amplitude modulated, other forms of modulation are satisfactory if they can be converted to amplitude modulation before reaching the detector. Polarization modulation, for example, can be used because transmission through a simple fixed polarizer provides the necessary conversion; phase or frequency modulation can be used by superimposing a coherent reference beam on the signal beam at the detector surface. All known modulators giving a reasonably large modulation index at high frequencies are of the nonabsorbing, variable retardation type. Polarization modulation is the easiest to use and the normal choice.

Although Bergstrand used Kerr cells, the liquids having the largest Kerr constants, such as nitrobenzene, are lossy at microwave frequencies, and the most satisfactory modulators utilize the linear electrooptic effect, called the Pockels effect. When an electric field is applied to a crystal lacking a center of inversion symmetry, the birefringence of the crystal is altered linearly. The basic effect is electronic, and hence very fast, although there is an additional contribution from ionic motion at frequencies below a few megahertz. The change in birefringence causes the crystal to act as an electrically variable wave plate and to modulate the polarization of light transmitted appropriately through it. The actual comparison of various electrooptic materials and the choice of a crystal and a modulator configuration are rather complicated, for the relationship between an external electric field applied in any direction and the resulting changes in shape and orientation of the index ellipsoid are given by an 18-element tensor. Fortunately, it can be shown by symmetry arguments that for any given crystal class a number of the elements will be zero. A good elementary introduction to crystal optics has been given by Wood (1964). Kaminow and Turner (1966) have described the best materials available, tabulated their important parameters, and discussed modulator design. Unfortunately, although many papers describing individual modulators have been published, a complete tabulation of the tensors for all crystal classes and a step-by-step outline of modulator design seem to exist only in unpublished reports.

Potassium dihydrogen phosphate (commonly called KDP) is the most commonly used crystal because of its ready availability in good optical quality. In the simplest configuration for microwave use, with the direction of light propagation and of the applied field along the c axis of the crystal and the incident light polarized linearly along the a or b axis, there is no residual birefringence. Ten times as much retardation for a given voltage can be achieved if the electric field is applied transverse to the direction of propagation and the ratio of crystal length (the direction of propagation) to thickness (the field direction) is twenty, a reasonable number. Because there is a large and temperature-dependent residual birefringence in this transverse configuration, it is necessary to have very good temperature control or to use a pair of crystals in series, mounted so that the modulations add but the birefringences cancel. Lithium niobate and lithium tantalate are about an order of magnitude better in modulation at the same voltage and ratio of length to thickness, giving an induced differential retardation of π radians (acting as a half-wave plate) for an applied voltage of about 140 V. They suffer from the same residual birefringence problem as KDP, but the effect is small in lithium tantalate. Kaminow and Sharpless (1967) have successfully operated 4 GHz modulators using both of these materials.

We can analyze the operation of a Fizeau-type system using polarization modulation by again applying the Jones calculus. Consider a simple system in which the light is emitted by a source, polarized linearly in the vertical direction, passed through a modulator having (time-dependent) retardation Γ_1 with the fast axis at $45°$, transmitted over a path to a retroreflector and back, passed through the modulator a second time to receive the additional retardation Γ_2 (which is in general different from Γ_1 because the electric field in the modulator changes during the transit time of the light), and finally passed through a polarizer crossed with the first one to reach a detector. This system is equivalent to the one shown in Fig. 27, in which we represent the second pass through the modulator by passage through a physically separated modulator. The Jones matrices describing the operations of each element

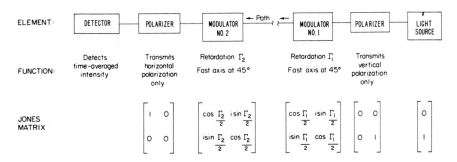

FIG. 27. Effective sequence of elements in simple Fizeau-type system with associated Jones matrices.

are also given. In general, an odd number of reflections followed by passage back through a retarder is equivalent to passage through a half-wave plate having its fast axis at $0°$ or $90°$ and rotation of the axes of the retarder from θ to $-\theta$, but the horizontal setting of the output polarizer gives identical results with the system of the figure. The output reaching the photodetector is found by matrix multiplication to be

$$\begin{pmatrix} \sin \tfrac{1}{2}(\Gamma_1 + \Gamma_2) \\ 0 \end{pmatrix}$$

The two retardations have the same amplitude and frequency, but Γ_2 is advanced relative to Γ_1 by the phase shift φ of Eq. (51), which is just the optical path length between the modulators expressed in radians:

$$\Gamma_1 = \Gamma e^{i\omega t}$$
$$\Gamma_2 = \Gamma e^{i(\omega t + \varphi)} \tag{54}$$

The output amplitude is thus

$$\left[\begin{array}{c} \sin[(\Gamma \cos \varphi/2)e^{i(\omega t + \varphi/2)}] \\ 0 \end{array} \right]$$

Note that the output irradiance varies at twice the modulation frequency. The photomultiplier cannot follow the modulation, and we average over a modulation period. The resulting average irradiance can be written, as is well known, in terms of the Bessel function $J_0(x)$,

$$\bar{I}/I_0 = \tfrac{1}{2}[1 - J_0(2\Gamma \cos \varphi/2)] \tag{55}$$

If the retardation amplitude Γ is small, we can expand this result and retain only the term of lowest order, obtaining

$$\bar{I}/I_0 = (\Gamma^2/4)(1 + \cos \varphi) \tag{56}$$

The average irradiance depends consinusoidally on path length, and hence distance measurements can be made exactly as with Fizeau's toothed-wheel modulator. We remember that the retardation amplitude is proportional to the electric field amplitude, and in the absence of a net residual birefringence, therefore, the average irradiance at the detector is proportional to the microwave power fed to the modulator.

It is straightforward to analyze possible variants of this system in the same way. If the modulator were followed by a horizontal polarizer, for example, so that the light transmitted over the path was amplitude modulated, and if the final output polarizer were vertical, the irradiance would be

$$\bar{I}/I_0 = (\Gamma^4/64)[\tfrac{1}{2} + \cos^2 \varphi] \tag{57}$$

For an ordinary KDP microwave modulator giving about $\Gamma = 0.1$ radian, it is clear that such a system is undesirable.

C. Atmospheric Limitations and the Dispersion Method

Before describing an actual instrument using the Fizeau method, we consider the accuracy that can be expected if measurements are made at only a single optical wavelength, as well as a method of obtaining significantly better results.

The principal limitation to the ultimate accuracy of electromagnetic distance measurements through the atmosphere is uncertainty in the average propagation velocity of the radiation, for inhomogeneity and turbulence in the lower atmosphere cause the refractive index to vary along the path. If the velocity assumed is c, the distance determined is the optical path length $L' = \langle n^G \rangle L$, where $\langle n^G \rangle$ is the average group refractive index and L is the true geometrical distance along the ray path. For very long paths it is necessary to estimate not only the value of $\langle n^G \rangle$ but also the average vertical gradient of the phase refractive index n, for refraction causes L to be larger than the true straight-line distance L_0. The uncertainty in this correction is normally much smaller than the uncertainty due to n^G for ground-to-ground paths, however; for a distance of 25 km and a typical gradient $(dn/dh) = -30 \times 10^{-6}/\text{km}$, the ratio $(L - L_0)/L_0$ is 3×10^{-8}.

The group refractive index is related to the phase index by (Brillouin, 1960)

$$n^G = n + \sigma \, dn/d\sigma \tag{58}$$

where $\sigma = 1/\lambda_v$ is the vacuum wavenumber in μm^{-1}. Expressions for the phase and group indices useful over broad ranges of pressure, temperature, composition, and wavelength have recently been given (Owens, 1967). A simplified formula for the group index that gives results in agreement with those of the best expression within 1 part in 10^8 except under conditions of extreme temperature and humidity is

$$(n^G - 1) \times 10^8 = \left[2371.34 + 683939.7 \frac{(130 + \sigma^2)}{(130 - \sigma^2)^2} + 4547.3 \frac{(38.9 + \sigma^2)}{(38.9 - \sigma^2)^2} \right] D_s$$

$$+ [6487.31 + 174.174\sigma^2 - 3.55750\sigma^4 + 0.61957\sigma^6] D_\omega \tag{59}$$

where the density factors D_s and D_w for dry air and for water vapor are given by

$$D_s = (P_s/T)\{1 + P_s[57.90 \times 10^{-8} - (9.3250 \times 10^{-4}/T) + 0.25844/T^2]\} \tag{60}$$

and

$$D_w = (P_w/T)\{1 + P_w[1 + (3.7 \times 10^{-4})P_w][-2.37321 \times 10^{-3}$$
$$+ 2.23366/T - 710.792/T^2 + (7.75141 \times 10^4/T^3)]\} \tag{61}$$

in which P_s and P_w are the partial pressures in millibars of dry air containing 0.03% carbon dioxide and of water vapor, respectively, and T is the temperature in °K. The variation of $(n^G - 1)$ with wavelength is shown in Fig. 28.

Near sea level the refractivity $(n^G - 1)$ and hence the ratio $(L' - L)/L$ are approximately 300×10^{-6}. In order to determine L with an accuracy of 1 ppm, assuming that L' has been measured sufficiently well, it is necessary to estimate the average refractivity to 1 part in 300. The density factors are the same for group as for phase index, and hence the sensitivity to atmospheric conditions is the same. This uncertainty of 1 in 300 corresponds to an uncertainty in average temperature of 1° C, in average pressure of 3.7 mbar, or in average partial pressure of water vapor of 23 mbar. For a microwave rather than optical carrier the temperature and pressure uncertainties allowable would be very nearly the same, but that for water vapor would be only 0.2 mbar. The saturation vapor pressure of water at 15° C is 17 mbar, and hence we see that the uncertainty in refractivity due to water vapor, which is a highly variable constituent of the atmosphere, is relatively unimportant when an optical carrier is used but is a serious source of error for microwave systems.

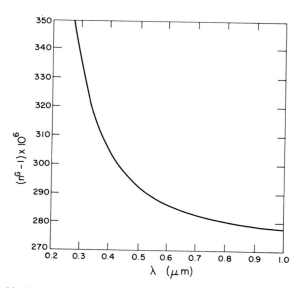

FIG. 28. Group refractive index of dry air at 15° C and 1013.25 mbar.

Even for optical systems, for which temperature variations are the most important source of error, it can be difficult to estimate the average atmospheric refractive index well enough to achieve 1 ppm accuracy in a distance measurement by the usual procedure of measuring pressure, temperature, and humidity at one or both ends of the path. Good results can be achieved when the terrain is uniform, meteorological conditions along the path are reasonably uniform and slowly varying in time, averaging times are sufficiently long that short-period fluctuations tend to cancel, and, if possible, several sets of sensors are used. Under nonuniform conditions, such as in mountainous terrain, systematic errors of many parts per million may occur because the center of the path remains at a temperature quite different from those of the end points. Surveyors have learned that the most reliable operation is achieved when the path is high above the ground, the wind velocity is greater than 1 meter/sec, and measurements are made at night or during an overcast day. The precision attainable with microwave measurements over both uniform and nonuniform terrain has been discussed by Thompson and Janes (1967). They used meteorological data from one or both ends to correct distance measurements over a series of paths, calculating the standard deviation of the mean corrected distance as a function of averaging time. For their best path, a 17.1 km line along the coast of Florida, averaging times of 7 hours or more were required to reduce the standard deviation of the mean to 1 ppm.

A direct optical method for measuring not only transit time, but also the group refractive index averaged over the path, has been suggested repeatedly, but not until recently did it appear feasible. A brief history of the idea and summary of recent work may be found elsewhere (Owens, 1968). The method may be qualitatively understood as follows: The refractive index of air is dispersive, as shown in Fig. 28, and hence light of two different wavelengths propagating over the same path will travel at slightly different velocities. Because the refractivity at a given wavelength is proportional to air density, the difference in refractivity, and hence the difference in transit time for the two wavelengths, will be proportional to the average air density over the path. A measurement of the difference in transit time, therefore, can be used with the total transit time for either wavelength to find the average density over the path and hence the average refractive index for either wavelength.

To be more explicit, we consider a geometrical path length L between light source and reflector. The one-way optical path length can be written $\langle n^G \rangle L = L + S$, where the additional contribution due to the air is denoted by S. This quantity is given by

$$S = \int_0^L (n^G - 1)\, dx \qquad (62)$$

For a 10 km path at sea level, S is about 300 cm. If the He–Ne laser line of vacuum wavelength 632.99 nm and the 368.36 nm line from a mercury arc lamp are used, the extra optical paths S_B and S_R for the blue and red light, respectively, will differ by about 10%, giving a difference $\Delta S = S_B - S_R$ of about 30 cm. This difference in path may be written

$$\Delta S = \int_0^L (1/A_R)(n_R{}^G - 1)\, dx \tag{63}$$

where

$$A_R = (n_R{}^G - 1)/(n_B{}^G - n_R{}^G) \tag{64}$$

Because A_R is independent of atmospheric density, as can be seen from Eq. (59), and is only weakly dependent on atmospheric composition, we can replace it by its average value $\langle A_R \rangle$ and take it outside the integral sign. We now have

$$S_R = \langle A_R \rangle (\Delta S) \tag{65}$$

If the difference in optical path length is measured to 1 part in 300 (to 1 mm in this example), the correction S_R can be found to approximately the same fractional precision and therefore the true distance to about 1 ppm.

The most serious noninstrumental source of error is uncertainty in average humidity, which changes the dispersion parameter A_R. It can be shown from Eq. (59) that an error of about 9 mbar in the estimated average water vapor pressure leads to an error of 1 ppm in corrected distance, nearly independent of temperature. For most purposes, therefore, a rough estimate of the average humidity will suffice. A thorough analysis of the errors due to humidity estimation and to refraction has been given by Thayer (1967), who concluded that for ground-to-ground paths, none of the geometrical errors would be as important as the 5% uncertainty in relative humidity which seems to be about the minimum that can be achieved with measurements at both ends of the path. He concluded that the dual-wavelength method could give an accuracy of about 0.1 ppm except for paths more than 25 km long or in tropical weather conditions of high humidity with temperatures over 25°C.

The radio refractive index is about 100 times as sensitive to water vapor as the optical one (Bean and Dutton, 1966); a partial pressure of 10 mbar at 15° C increases the radio index by 45×10^{-6} relative to that for the same total pressure of dry air, while it decreases the optical group index for red light by about 0.4×10^{-6}. By simply extending the dispersion idea and adding a third wavelength in the microwave region to the two optical ones, the microwave-optical dispersion could be measured and used to find the average water vapor density over the path. Thayer analyzed this technique in the same report, concluding that an accuracy of 0.03 ppm or better should be possible for path lengths up to 50 km and temperatures as high as 30° C under reasonably normal refractive conditions.

Uncertainty in the vacuum velocity of light is not a source of error in the same sense as those described above. No geometrical inconsistencies such as triangle nonclosures will result from this uncertainty; its only effect is to give a slight uncertainty in the overall scale factor of the geodetic network.

D. A Prototype Geodetic Instrument

A dual-wavelength instrument of the Fizeau type has been built in the Environmental Science Services Agency (ESSA) Research Laboratories with the goal of providing measurements of at least 1 ppm accuracy over distances of 10 km or more. A block diagram of the instrument is shown in Fig. 29. Its operation for either wavelength is exactly as described in Section IV,B. Two separate light sources are simultaneously used, a helium–neon gas laser and a high-pressure mercury arc lamp filtered to emit a narrow spectral band centered near 368 nm. The light beams from the two sources are superimposed, vertically polarized, passed through a KDP modulator that varies their polarization between right-handed and left-handed elliptical

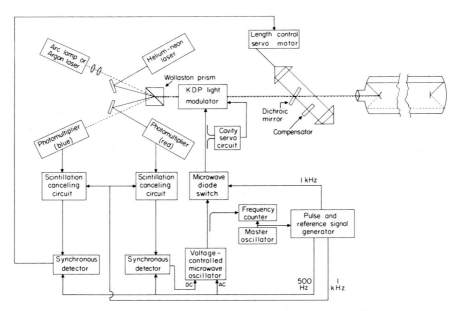

FIG. 29. Block diagram of the ESSA dual-wavelength, Fizeau-type instrument.

at a 3 GHz rate, and transmitted by a 20 cm Cassegrainian telescope. The light traverses the path to be measured and is returned by a cat's-eye retro-reflector, a second 20 cm telescope with a plane mirror at its focal point. It passes through the modulator a second time, where the modulation is doubled or canceled when the modulation phase of the returning light is, respectively, in or out of phase with the modulator excitation, through a horizontal polarizer, and is separated into two beams reaching separate photomulti-pliers. Because the polarization rather than the amplitude of the light is modulated, a Wollaston prism can be used to perform the combined functions of polarizing and analyzing the light as well as joining and separating the two colors. The dispersion of the prism permits the beams to be superimposed without using a dichroic mirror, simply by using the correct angle of incidence for each color. The quartz lens used as a telescope eyepiece has longitudinal chromatic aberration, but this can be compensated by slightly adjusting the divergence of the blue beam with a pair of lenses near the arc lamp so that both red and blue emerge from the telescope well collimated.

The arrangement shown for measuring the difference in optical path ΔS is very simple. The blue light is transmitted directly from the modulator to the telescope, but the red light is diverted by a dichroic mirror and two prism reflectors around an adjustable supplementary path. A polarization compensator corrects for the effects of the prisms. With the modulation frequency set to give an irradiance maximum for blue light, one of the prisms is moved to give a simultaneous maximum for red. Hence the optical paths for both colors are made equal (aside from an integral number of modulation wavelengths) and the difference in optical path length can be simply read out in terms of the distance the prism is moved from a reference position.

The microwave system must provide enough power to give a reasonable modulation index at a stable, accurately measured frequency. Thermal distortion of the KDP crystal limits the power dissipation of the modulator to about 1 W, and when operated continuously at this level a peak retarda-tion of only about 0.1 rad results. It is convenient instead to operate with high power pulses at a low duty cycle. The modulation pulses must be long compared to the time required for light to traverse the measured path, while the pulse repetition rate should be high compared to the rate of atmospheric density fluctuation. The system is designed to deliver 10 W at a 10% duty cycle at pulse repetition frequencies of 1 kHz (for distances up to 8 km) or 500 Hz (for distances up to 16 km). In order to ensure frequency stability the microwave oscillator is operated continuously and phase-locked to a crystal oscillator, while the pulses are gated by a microwave diode switch. Because the modulator cavity has a Q of several hundred, it is continuously tuned to resonance at the driving frequency by a servo-control circuit. The error signal for this servo loop is generated by a balanced mixer which compares the phase of the microwaves incident on the cavity with those reflected back from it. In order to track changes in atmospheric conditions, a second servo loop locks the modulation frequency to the optical path length so that the path for one color always remains an integral number of modulation wavelengths. A third servo loop can be used to control the length of the supplementary path, maintaining the other color at an integral number also. The effects of scintillation are largely cancelled by automatic normalizing circuits. Further details are available elsewhere (Earnshaw and Owens, 1967).

In making an actual distance measurement the first step is ambiguity resolution, which requires determining the optical path length to within a quarter of a modulation wavelength. For red light the integral number N_R of modulation wavelengths along the two-way path is related to the modulation frequency v by

$$N_R = (\langle n_R{}^G\rangle L + k_R + \Delta)(2v/c) \tag{66}$$

and hence we can write

$$\Delta N_R/\Delta v = (2/c)(\langle n_R{}^G\rangle L + k_R + \Delta) \tag{67}$$

where L is the total one-way geometrical path length between modulator and retroreflector, Δ is the supplementary path, and k_R is the apparent increase in one-way path length due to the optical components. In practice it is not possible to determine the right-hand side of Eq. (67), and hence N_R, with sufficient accuracy by measuring the frequency at two adjacent lock-in points, but once such a measurement of $\Delta N_R/\Delta v$ is made, successively more accurate values can be found by changing the frequency in larger increments. The frequency need not be swept continuously because the value of ΔN_R for each step can be determined from the approximate value of $\Delta N_R/\Delta v$ obtained in each preceding one. The process is continued until the uncertainty in N_R due to uncertainty in the frequency measurement is less than 1.

Next, the frequency is set close to one of the values for which N_R is known and the servo-control circuits for frequency and supplementary path are turned on, maintaining both red and blue path lengths at integral values. The apparent distances are obtained from the two relations

$$\begin{aligned}\langle n_R{}^G\rangle L &= (N_R c/2v) - k_R - \Delta\\ \langle n_B{}^G\rangle L &= (N_B c/2v) - k_B\end{aligned} \tag{68}$$

where the subscripts R and B refer to red and blue light, respectively. The corrected distance is given by

$$L = \langle n_R{}^G\rangle L - \langle A_R\rangle[\langle n_B{}^G\rangle L - \langle n_R{}^G\rangle L] \tag{69}$$

where the appropriate value of $\langle A_R \rangle$, defined in Eq. (64), is determined by using measurements of pressure, temperature, and humidity made at one end of the path.

Several field tests were carried out during the development of the instrument. During August 1966, measurements were made over a 1.6 km path across Lake Hefner, near Oklahoma City. The precision of the instrument in detecting optical path length changes was found to be about 3 parts in 10^8 for an averaging time of 10 sec. This was checked by randomly moving the retroreflector; a motion of about 5×10^{-3} cm could be detected. For 177 measurements of corrected length made over a 4-day period, the standard deviation was 1.55 mm, slightly better than 1 ppm. In this work it was necessary to measure red and blue sequentially rather than simultaneously, which can cause a significant loss of accuracy. After rebuilding the instrument, further tests were made during the summer of 1967 using a 5.3 km path between two hills north of Boulder, Colorado. The precision of the instrument, given by the root-mean-square fluctuations of 1 sec averages relative to a 30 sec moving average, was 3 parts in 10^9 during a relatively quiet period at night and about ten times worse immediately after a storm. The reproducibility of corrected length was found to be about 3 parts in 10^7. Because the numerical value of A_R is about 10, we would expect that the reproducibility of corrected length would be about ten times poorer than the instrumental precision; the additional order of magnitude actually found indicated that other errors were present. The most serious source of systematic error was probably uncertainty in the mean wavelength of the blue light, which gives an error in corrected length of 3 ppm/nm. The mercury arc lamp was replaced in 1968 with a pulsed argon laser operating at a wavelength of 351.1 nm, reducing this uncertainty and providing much greater spectral radiance. In addition, it has proven difficult to maintain alignment while changing the supplementary path, and so the "line stretcher" was replaced by another of improved design. At Christmas, 1968, the instrument was tested using one mile of the support pipe of the Stanford Linear Accelerator. This approach, measuring the reproducibility of corrected length through a pipe while varying the pressure and, if possible, the humidity over wide ranges, is the most direct way of testing the dispersion method. A reproducibility of 1 part in 10^7 was found over a range of pressure from 20 to 256 mmHg, consistent with the earlier outdoor results. Refraction prevented operation at higher pressures. It is believed that significantly better results should be obtained when several remaining sources of systematic error are corrected.

Development of this instrument is continuing (Hernandez, 1970) and several changes have recently been made. The voltage-tunable magnetron used as a microwave source has been replaced by a voltage-controlled crystal oscillator driving a high-power multiplier chain. The troublesome line

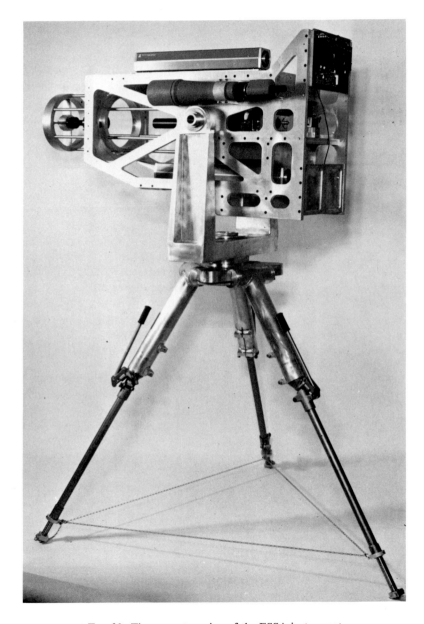

FIG. 30. The current version of the ESSA instrument.

stretcher has been eliminated and now the red and blue path lengths are measured alternately at a 500 Hz rate. The pulsed argon–ion laser has been replaced with a more reliable helium–cadmium one operating at 441.6 nm. Finally, the mechanical layout of the instrument has been improved. The present version is shown in Fig. 30.

Although this dual-wavelength instrument is the only one of Fizeau type known to the author, development programs for at least two other dual-wavelength instruments of the phase-meter type have recently been under way. In addition, several instruments for the measurement of average water vapor density over a path by using microwave or microwave-optical dispersion have been built or are currently under consideration. Information about these efforts can be found in the references cited by Owens (1968), while more recent microwave-optical work has been described by Wood and Thompson (1968).

E. Optical Power Required

The laser power required as a function of distance for measurements of a given precision can be calculated in a straightforward way. We outline the factors to be considered and give results for the instrument described in the preceding section, assuming that the light sources and modulator are all operated continuously. We then comment on the improvements gained by pulsing the lasers and modulator even if their average powers are held constant and by using systems of "one-way" measurement in which a transponder replaces the retroreflector.

1. Geometrical Attenuation

Ochs and Lawrence (1969) have found that laser beam spreading angles for paths 5–45 km long are typically 15–60 μrad at night and average about 60 μrad during the day, although angles over 100 μrad are not uncommon in daytime. If this spreading caused by atmospheric turbulence is large compared to the intrinsic divergence due to the optics, the total beam divergence is essentially independent of the transmitter and reflector apertures. Consider a transmitted beam of power P_0 spreading at angle α, part of which is intercepted by the retroreflector of radius R_r at distance L. This fraction is returned, again in a cone of angle α, and is collected by the receiver of radius R_t. The ratio of received to transmitted power is

$$P_r/P_0 = [16(R_r)^2(R_t)^2/(\alpha L)^4] \tag{70}$$

Evaluating this expression for 20 cm optics, an angle of 50 μrad, and a distance of 15 km, we find that only 0.54 % of the power is collected.

2. *Instrumental Attenuation*

A significant amount of light is lost by absorption and reflection in the optics even though antireflection coatings having minima at both wavelengths are used. Assuming that the laser outputs are vertically linearly polarized and that the modulator gives a fixed two-pass retardation of π radians so that the Wollaston prism has no effect, the overall transmittance from laser to photomultiplier is typically 12% for the red light and 4% for the blue.

3. *Modulator Efficiency*

The ratio of average irradiance at the photodetector to incident irradiance at the modulator input is given in Eq. (56). The maximum value of this ratio, which we shall call the modulator efficiency, is $\Gamma^2/2$. The KDP modulator of this instrument, operated continuously, gives a peak retardation Γ of 0.106 rad for red light and 0.15 rad for blue. Hence the efficiency is 0.56% for red and 1.12% for blue. The use of lithium tantalate or niobate, of which quite good crystals are now available, will improve these figures considerably.

4. *Attenuation Caused by Scattering*

Elterman (1968) has found that aerosol scattering is normally dominant over Rayleigh scattering for altitudes up to 3 km above sea level. His tables predict a total sea-level attenuation coefficient K of 0.62 dB/km at 633 nm and 1.1 dB/km at 350 nm. This reduction in irradiance for the round-trip path can be written

$$I/I_0 = 10^{-(2 \times 10^{-6})KL} \tag{71}$$

where L is the one-way distance in centimeters.

5. *Attenuation by Absorption in Atmospheric Gases*

Absorption by spectral lines in the visible region is not ordinarily a problem, although the coincidence of one of the wavelengths with a weak line might change the dispersion parameter A_R significantly. An extensive study covering the wavelength range from 0.6 to 20 μm has been given by Long (1963), while Curcio *et al.* (1964) have discussed absorption at shorter wavelengths.

6. *Signal-to-Noise Requirement*

For a fixed modulation frequency the number of modulation wavelengths is proportional to path length. Hence for a given relative accuracy in distance measurement, the absolute precision (in wavelengths) with which the modulation wavelength must be locked to the optical path length decreases as the distance increases, and hence a lower signal-to-noise ratio (SNR) can be tolerated. In terms of phase measurement, we would say that the absolute precision (in radians) required in the modulation phase measurement decreases as the distance increases. This effect can be described by including a "negative attenuation" factor,

$$P/P_0 = (L \times 10^{-5})/500 \tag{72}$$

where L is again to be expressed in centimeters. For a distance of 500 km, when the precision of 0.1 ppm required to give corrected distance to 1 ppm demands that the round-trip path length be determined only to a precision of 10 cm (one modulation wavelength), the SNR can be unity. For shorter distances better determinations, and hence greater signal-to-noise ratios, are required.

When measurements are made in daylight the noise level is much higher because of increased turbulence resulting in scintillation, and also because some scattered sunlight reached the detectors even when narrowband filters are used. Experience indicates that for the same accuracy the average received power in daytime may have to be as much as 100 times greater than that required at night. We therefore include a parameter A that is taken to be 1 for night measurements and 100 for daytime ones.

7. Required Laser Power

The ratio of received power at the photomultiplier to overall laser power is found by multiplying the various factors. Taking the received power P to be the minimum detectable, we find the required laser power for red light to be

$$(P_L)_R = \frac{P_R \alpha_R{}^4 L^3 [10^{(2 \times 10^{-6})K_R L}](4.65 \times 10^9)A}{R_r{}^2 R_t{}^2} \tag{73}$$

while that for blue is given by the same expression, differing only in having subscripts B and the number 7.0×10^9 rather than 4.65×10^9.

The minimum received powers to give a final accuracy of 1 ppm in a 1 Hz bandwidth with this instrument are estimated to be about 1×10^{-13} W for red light and 6.6×10^{-15} W for blue. Graphs of required laser power versus distance are given in Fig. 31 for both colors and for both day and night measurements. With clearer conditions, such as in the mountains of Colorado, scattering losses of 0.2 dB/km for red light and 0.4 dB/km for blue may be more realistic, and the curves of Fig. 32 would result. We see that ranges of 10 km or more should be achievable in daytime using low-power lasers, while measurements over several tens of kilometers are possible at night.

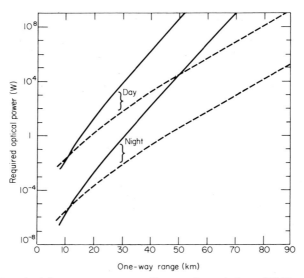

FIG. 31. Required laser power versus distance for red (---, 632.99 nm) and blue (——, 368.36 nm) light during day and night to achieve an accuracy of 1 ppm in corrected distance, assuming fully cw operation of the ESSA instrument and scattering losses of 0.5 dB/km for red and 1.0 dB/km for blue.

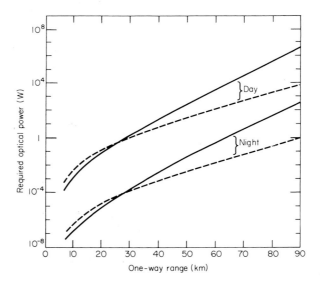

FIG. 32. Same as Fig. 31, except that scattering losses of 0.2 dB/km for red and 0.4 dB/km for blue are assumed.

8. *The Use of Pulsed Lasers*

It can be desirable for several reasons to pulse the modulator. If the modulator duty factor is D and the microwave power is increased to $1/D$ relative to that used in continuous operation, the required laser power is unchanged. A pulsed-modulator system can be significantly improved for a given average laser power, however, if the lasers are pulsed as well. If the modulator is operated at a 10% duty factor, for example, the lasers can be pulsed at a duty factor between 5 and 10%, depending on the path length and pulse duration (the modulator must be turned on for both transmitting and receiving the optical pulse). For the same average laser power, this gives a tenfold increase in effective optical power because all of the light is utilized rather than only 10% of it. Moreover, if the optical pulse length is short enough so that the transmitted and received pulses do not overlap in the instrument, the problem of backscatter by optical elements of the system can be much reduced.

9. *Transponder Systems*

At some increase in complexity, an operating range several times as large can be achieved for a given laser power by using a transponder rather than a retroreflector (Wood and Thompson, 1966). The light is then transmitted in only one direction over the path, the modulation is detected at the far end, and the signal is used to modulate light from a laser at that end that shines back to the starting point. The range achievable depends on the method of signal detection, of course, but if a light modulator and photomultiplier identical to those of the transmitter are used as described in the following section, the only changes in the preceding analysis will be that the geometrical attenuation is proportional to L^2 rather than to L^4, and the scattering attenuation factor contains L rather than $2L$ in the exponent. Hence, the power required from each laser will be considerably less and, more importantly, will increase much less rapidly with distance.

F. DESIGN OF A THREE-WAVELENGTH INSTRUMENT

To make the measurements of very high accuracy over the long paths required for such applications as determining patterns of large-scale strain accumulation and release in the earth's crust, three-wavelength systems having active elements at both ends of the path are required. Red and blue light modulated at 3 GHz and the unmodulated 3 GHz wave could be used as the three signals. We must measure the round-trip transit time for one signal, the difference in one-way transit time for the two optical signals, and the

difference between the one-way transit time of one optical signal and the microwave signal. For a path 50 km long in dry air at a pressure of 1013.25 mbar
and a temperature of 15° C, for example, the one-way phase delay relative to propagation in vacuum of 3 GHz modulation on a 633 nm carrier is
5.1×10^4 degrees. If the partial pressure of water vapor is 10 mbar but the
total pressure is the same, the atmospheric phase delay is reduced by 77 deg.
The change in phase delay caused by this same amount of water vapor for the
3 GHz microwave signal propagating directly is 8.1×10^3 deg. It was pointed
out in Section IV,C that an uncertainty of 9 mbar in the partial pressure of
water vapor gives rise to an uncertainty of 1 ppm in the corrected distance.
Hence, if we wish to measure the 50 km to an accuracy of 5 parts in 10^8, for
example, we must determine the average water vapor pressure to within
0.45 mbar, which requires measuring the microwave-optical phase difference
to an accuracy of

$$(0.45)(8.2 \times 10^3)/(10) = 370°$$

The microwave-optical measurement, then, does not need to be very accurate;
for this case we would only have to resolve the ambiguity in whole-wavelength
number for the two signals.

We could choose as the round-trip signal the microwave one, using a
circuit of standard design (Thomson and Vetter, 1958; Gilmer and Waters,
1967) to measure the round-trip transit time. Wood and Thompson (1968)
have described measurements of microwave-optical dispersion made with
such an instrument having only one optical wavelength. We choose here to
assume that the round-trip signal is the one least affected in phase by atmospheric density variations, that carried by the red light. A suitable system of
this type is shown in Fig. 33. Its basic principles are straightforward; in
tracing through the signals we need only remember that when two sinusoidal
signals are added and detected (the sum is squared and low-pass filtered),
the output is at the difference frequency, and its phase is the phase difference
of the original signals. We shall denote a signal of frequency ω and phase
angle φ by (ω, φ); hence the detection process applied to the sum of the
signals (ω_0, φ_0) and (ω_1, φ_1) gives the output $(\omega_0 - \omega_1, \varphi_0 - \varphi_1)$ if $\omega_0 > \omega_1$
and $(\omega_1 - \omega_0, \varphi_1 - \varphi_0)$ if $\omega_0 < \omega_1$. We fix the sign of the phase difference
by always writing the frequency difference to be positive. It can easily be
shown from the analysis of Section IV,B that this holds for the detection
of a modulation signal on an optical carrier by using a modulator and photomultiplier as well as for the simple detection of two microwave signals by
a diode.

The operation of phase-locked loops has been described in detail by
Gardner (1966).

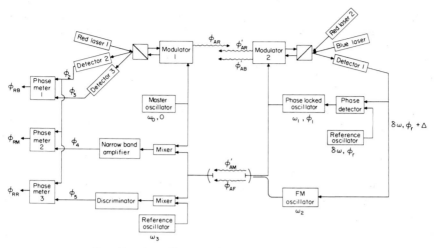

FIG. 33. Block diagram of three-wavelength system.

The master oscillator output is $(\omega_0, 0)$ and we assume that modulator 1 imposes this signal without phase shift on light passing through it. The light from red laser 1 is modulated and transmitted from left to right. Just before reaching modulator 2, the signal is $(\omega_0, -\varphi_{AR})$, where φ_{AR} denotes the phase shift of the signal on the red light caused by propagation over the atmospheric path. In modulator 2 the light is remodulated with a signal (ω_1, φ_1) $(\delta\omega, -\varphi_{AR} - \varphi_1)$. The difference frequency $\delta\omega = \omega_0 - \omega_1$ is normally chosen to be about 100 kHz, and we are assuming that ω_1 is less than ω_0. The loop causes the phase of this signal to match that of the reference oscillator, φ_r, to within some error Δ, so that

$$-\varphi_{AR} - \varphi_1 = \varphi_r + \Delta \qquad (74)$$

Note that the detector output carries no phase information about the path. The output of the phase-locked oscillator does carry this information; its phase is

$$\varphi_1 = -\varphi_{AR} - \varphi_r - \Delta \qquad (75)$$

Light from red laser 2 receives the modulation signal (ω_1, φ_1) in modulator 2 and is transmitted to the master terminal. Just before reaching modulator 1 this signal is $(\omega_1, \varphi_1 - \varphi'_{AR})$, where the path phase shift φ'_{AR} is different from φ_{AR} because the modulation frequency is ω_1 rather than ω_0. The light passes through modulator 1, where it is remodulated, to detector 2, from which the output signal is $(\delta\omega, \varphi_2)$. The phase φ_2 is given by

$$\varphi_2 = \varphi_{AR} + \varphi'_{AR} + \varphi_r + \Delta \qquad (76)$$

Light from the blue laser is also transmitted from the remote to the master terminal. This signal is also (ω_1, φ_1) upon leaving modulator 2, but its path phase shift is written φ'_{AB}. The output from detector 3 is $(\delta\omega, \varphi_3)$, where the phase is given by

$$\varphi_3 = \varphi_{AR} + \varphi'_{AB} + \varphi_r + \Delta \tag{77}$$

The outputs from detectors 2 and 3 are at the same frequency, and the output of phase meter 1, $\varphi_{RB} = \varphi_2 - \varphi_3$, gives the desired optical dispersion:

$$\varphi_{RB} = \varphi'_{AR} - \varphi'_{AB} \tag{78}$$

A sample of the microwave signal (ω_1, φ_1) is transmitted directly from the remote terminal to the master one. Its path phase shift is written φ'_{AM}. This signal is mixed with a sample of the signal $(\omega_0, 0)$ and detected, and the output is passed through a narrowband amplifier to eliminate a second signal having a different frequency but transmitted between the same pair of antennas. The amplifier output is $(\delta\omega, \varphi_4)$ where φ_4 is given by

$$\varphi_4 = \varphi_{AR} + \varphi'_{AM} + \varphi_r + \Delta \tag{79}$$

Phase meter 2 gives the microwave-optical dispersion, $\varphi_{RM} = \varphi_2 - \varphi_4$:

$$\varphi_{RM} = \varphi'_{AR} - \varphi'_{AM} \tag{80}$$

Because the phase-locked loop of the remote unit can have an error Δ, it is necessary to send a sample of the signal $(\delta\omega, \varphi_r + \Delta)$ back to the master unit to measure the round-trip phase shift for red light accurately. It is convenient to transmit this signal as frequency modulation on the output of a separate oscillator operating at a center frequency ω_3 that is at least 30 MHz different from ω_0, but not so much different that the same antennas cannot be used. The signal arrives with a path phase shift φ_{AF} that is small compared to the other atmospheric phase shifts because $\delta\omega$ is low. The signal is mixed with the output of a reference oscillator operating at frequency ω_3, detected, and demodulated by a discriminator having center frequency $\Delta\omega = \omega_3 - \omega_2$. The discriminator output is the signal $(\delta\omega, \varphi_5)$, where φ_5 is given by

$$\varphi_5 = \varphi_r + \Delta - \varphi_{AF} \tag{81}$$

Phase meter 3 then gives the round-trip phase shift for red light. Its output is $\varphi_{RR} = \varphi_2 - \varphi_5$,

$$\varphi_{RR} = \varphi_{AR} + \varphi'_{AR} + \varphi_{AF} \tag{82}$$

The offset φ_{AF} does not cause difficulty. For a 50-km path and a frequency $\delta\omega$ of 100 kHz, the total shift is 6×10^3 degrees, but the changes in the shift caused by changes in atmospheric conditions are small. A change in water vapor pressure of 10 mbar, giving a change of 45×10^{-6} in radio refractive index, changes φ_{AF} by only 0.27 degrees. The fact that φ_{RR} contains $\varphi_{AR} + \varphi'_{AR}$ rather than $2\varphi'_{AR}$ is easily corrected. In summary, once ambiguity is resolved the outputs of the three phase meters give the round-trip phase shift for red light, the optical dispersion, and the microwave-optical dispersion directly.

V. Velocity Measurement

A. INTRODUCTION TO OPTICAL DOPPLER METHODS

If one mirror of a Michelson interferometer is moved along the optical axis at velocity V, the irradiance at any point on the output plane varies at the frequency $v = 2V/\lambda$. For a wavelength of 633 nm, a frequency of 1000 fringes/sec corresponds to a mirror velocity of 0.3 mm/sec. It is equivalent, of course, to say that the light reflected by the moving mirror has suffered a Doppler shift in frequency of $2V/\lambda$. Because the fractional Doppler shift is very small, coherent detection is required. The same measurement of velocity could be made if the mirror were replaced with an optically rough surface or even with a flowing fluid containing scattering particles, although a receiver of very small area or very small angular field of view would be required. Just this technique is, in fact, commonly used in monostatic microwave Doppler radar systems for measuring wind velocity in storms and for measuring ionospheric electron and ion densities and temperatures. The mean velocity component of the scattering elements along the beam direction is given by the mean Doppler shift of the received signal, while the spectral width of the signal provides a measure of the range of scattering element velocities. The development of lasers makes possible the extension of these techniques to the optical spectral region, giving much greater spatial resolution; a volume as small as 1×10^{-6} cm^3 can be examined at a distance of a meter or more with a focused beam. In addition, improved precision may be possible in the velocity measurement because the absolute Doppler shift for a given velocity is much larger at optical than at microwave frequencies. The high sensitivity and noncontacting character of the method, along with the fact that only one vector component of the motion is measured, have proved attractive for a variety of applications. Velocity profiles and turbulence in fluid flow can be determined using focused bistatic systems, as in measurements of jets, wind tunnel flow, hydraulic flow, and atmospheric wind, while focused monostatic instruments are useful for localized measurements of surface vibration. We here give a simple analysis to summarize the principles and capabilities of such systems, considering specifically the measurement of fluid flow using aerosol scattering and later commenting on the very similar problem of vibration measurement using rough surfaces.

B. SCATTERING BY A SINGLE PARTICLE

Scattering by particles much smaller than a wavelength in size is adequately described by Rayleigh theory. Each particle acts as an electric dipole radiator and the angular distribution of the scattered light is independent of particle size and shape. The amount of light scattered by a single particle is very small; the scattering efficiency $Q_s = \sigma/\pi a^2$ is only about 3×10^{-12} for the molecules in normal air at a wavelength of 633 nm, where σ is the total scattering cross section and a is the particle radius. In scattering by spheres that are not small compared with the wavelength (Goody, 1964), the scattering is strongly forward-directed, may show several maxima, and varies less strongly with wavelength than in the Rayleigh case. The most important change for our purposes, however, is that the scattering efficiency is much larger, approaching a numerical value of 2 for large nonabsorbing particles. In practice, therefore, molecular scattering will be negligible if there is even one aerosol particle in the scattering volume; in fact, it is necessary to seed gas flows with small particles to ensure reliable operation if enough aerosols are not naturally present.

The Doppler shift given by a single scattering center may be found by considering the typical system geometry shown in Fig. 34. Light from the laser, at frequency ν_0 and wave vector $\mathbf{k}_0$, is incident on the scattering element at 0, which is moving at velocity $\mathbf{V}$ in a medium of phase refractive index n. The scattered light with frequency ν_s and wave vector $\mathbf{k}_s$ is collected at the square-law detector. Part of the original laser beam is split off by beamsplitter B_1, reflected by mirror M, and superimposed on the scattered light by beamsplitter B_2 after traversing an approximately equal path length. If

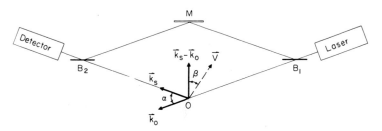

FIG. 34. Geometry of optical system for doppler shift measurement. The scattering center is at 0 and moves at velocity **V**. The reference beam is superimposed on the scattered light by beamsplitters B_1 and B_2 and mirror M.

the wavefronts are suitably matched at the detector, the output current will have a component at the difference frequency $\Delta v = v_s - v_0$. It can be shown by simple geometry that this Doppler shift Δv is given to first order (neglecting relativistic effects) by

$$\begin{aligned} \Delta v &= (1/2\pi)(\mathbf{k}_s - \mathbf{k}_0) \cdot \mathbf{V} \\ &= (2nV/\lambda_0) \sin{(\alpha/2)} \cos{\beta} \end{aligned} \tag{83}$$

where α is the scattering angle as normally defined and β is the angle between $\mathbf{V}$ and $(\mathbf{k}_s - \mathbf{k}_0)$. We note that only the magnitude of the component of $\mathbf{V}$ in the direction $(\mathbf{k}_s - \mathbf{k}_0)$ is measured; to determine the sign of this component it is necessary to use heterodyne rather than homodyne detection, offsetting the frequency of the reference beam so that the difference frequency will not pass through zero over the range of velocities measured. This is normally done with an acoustic diffraction modulator.

We also note that if the scattering particles are large, there will be a trade-off between Doppler shift, which increases with scattering angle, and the strength of the scattered signal, which decreases. [For a 1 μm water droplet the scattering cross section at 633 nm varies approximately as $\exp{(-\alpha/16°)}$.] Practical systems normally operate with small scattering angles, in the range 5° to 15°, especially if high velocities are to be measured. At an angle of 10° and a wavelength of 633 nm, the Doppler shift is 2.75 kHz/(cm/sec).

The other components of the vector velocity can be determined as well if two other detectors not lying in the plane defined by the laser, the scattering center, and the first detector are added. It is most convenient to do this by placing the three detectors symmetrically on a cone of angle α around the direction of the laser beam. The velocities obtained will not, however, be the orthogonal components unless a scattering angle of 70.5° is used so that the laser and the three detectors are located at the four vertices of a tetrahedron and the scattering volume is at the center. If only two, rather than three, of the vertices rest on the ground, the components directly measured have the normal horizontal and vertical orientation.

C. COHERENT DETECTION OF DIFFUSE LIGHT

We first find the signal-to-noise ratio given by a single small scattering particle, assuming that the signal and reference wavefronts are spatially coherent and accurately aligned. Only the results important for the present problem will be given; the fundamentals of optical heterodyne detection as well as practical details can be found elsewhere (Ross, 1966; Kerr, 1967). The root-mean-squared (rms) signal current at the frequency Δv is given by $i_S = (2I_S I_{LO})^{1/2}$, where I_S and I_{LO} are the direct currents that would be produced by the signal and reference (*LO*) waves alone. The rms noise current, assuming as usual that shot noise due to I_{LO} is the dominant noise, is given by $i_N = (2eI_{LO}B)^{1/2}$, where e is the electronic charge and B is the system bandwidth. The additional noise due to background light, such as scattered sunlight, is negligible for coherent detection in the visible spectral region. We can write the SNR, $\psi = (i_S/i_N)^2$, in terms of the intercepted optical signal power P_S by noting that for a detector of quantum efficiency η the current is given by $i_S = \eta e P_S/hv$, where hv is the energy of a single photon. Thus we find

$$\psi = \eta P_S/hvB \qquad (84)$$

If the laser power is P_0, we may write the *LO* and signal powers as

$$P_{LO} = C_r^2 P_0$$
$$P_S = QC_t^2 P_0 \qquad (85)$$

where C_r and C_t are the beamsplitter power reflectance and transmittance, respectively. The factor Q is the power scattering efficiency of the entire system including the scattering particle. It can be written

$$Q = (D/dR)^2 \sigma(\theta, \varphi) \qquad (86)$$

where d is the diameter of the laser beam (assumed to have uniform irradiance) at the scatterer, D is the collecting aperture diameter of the receiving optics, R is the distance from the scattering volume to the receiver, and $\sigma(\theta, \varphi)$ is the differential scattering cross section of the particle. The angles θ and φ are conventionally defined as indicated in Fig. 35. The quantity Q will obviously be small, and hence the maximum SNR will be achieved with $C_t \simeq 1$, when almost all of the laser power reaches the scattering volume and the *LO* beam is only intense enough to dominate the noise. For this case we have finally

$$\psi = (\eta P_0/hvB)(D/dR)^2 \sigma(\theta, \varphi) \qquad (87)$$

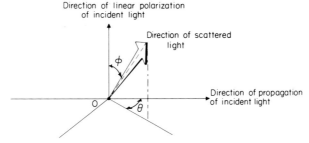

FIG. 35. Definition of the angles conventionally used in describing light scattering by a particle at O.

If the scattering volume contains a number of particles moving in different directions at different velocities, the resultant signal will, on the average, be larger than for one particle, but mutual interference effects will cause the heterodyne current to vary rapidly around the most probable value. For neutral particles having a mean separation of many particle diameters, and hence an adequately random spatial distribution, the signals for the individual scatterers add up as vectors in a two-dimensional random walk. The signal amplitude at the detector due to one particle is $(QP_0)^{1/2}$, and if there are on the average N particles in the scattering volume the resultant signal amplitude will be Rayleigh distributed with mean square value NQP_0. The heterodyne current is also Rayleigh distributed, its probability density given by

$$p(i_S) = (2i_S/I^2) \exp\left[-(i_S/I)^2\right], \qquad i_S \geq 0 \tag{88}$$

where $I^2 = \langle i_S{}^2 \rangle$ is the mean square value of the current, given by

$$I = (2I_{LO}\,I_S)^{1/2} \tag{89}$$

and I_S is given by

$$I_S = (\eta e/h\nu)NQP_0 \tag{90}$$

The mean value of the current is $\langle i_S \rangle = (\sqrt{\pi}/2)I$ and the variance is given by $\sigma^2 = \langle i_S{}^2 \rangle - \langle i_S \rangle^2 = (1 - \pi/4)I^2$, about 25% of the mean square value. The broad peaking of the Rayleigh probability density indicates that the heterodyne current will often differ substantially from the mean value. Although the average heterodyne current and hence the average SNR increase with the number of particles in the scattering volume, the constant ratio of variance to mean square indicates that the relative fluctuations in signal do not decrease with increasingly large N. If the scattering particles are in sufficiently rapid motion that the particle arrangement changes significantly during the measurement averaging time of the instrument, however, the resulting signal is unlikely to be far from the mean value.

The scattered signal from each particle appears at the Doppler-shifted frequency corresponding to its velocity component in the direction $(\mathbf{k}_s - \mathbf{k}_0)$. This velocity is due to both the Brownian motion of the particle and the gross motion of the medium. If the diameter of the scattering volume is small compared with the scale of turbulence of the medium and the sample averaging time is short compared with the characteristic time of the turbulence, the contribution of gross motion is the same for all particles and Brownian motion will be the principal source of the observed spectral width. The power spectrum of the heterodyne signal has the same form as the probability density function describing the number of scatterers at each velocity, which is Gaussian (one-dimensional Maxwellian) and centered around the frequency corresponding to the instantaneous velocity of bulk motion:

$$S(v) = S(v_m) \exp \left\{ -[(v - v_m)/[2 \sin (\alpha/2)/\lambda](2kT/m)^{1/2}]^2 \right\} \qquad (91)$$

Here $S(v)$ is the power spectral density at frequency v, v_m is the Doppler-shifted frequency due to the mean velocity, k is Boltzmann's constant, T is the absolute temperature of the surrounding gas, and m is the mass of the scattering particle. For aerosols this spreading is quite small. For a water droplet of 1 μm radius at a temperature of 300°K the rms value of one component of its velocity $(kT/m)^{1/2}$ is only 0.1 cm/sec, and the full width at half power of the Doppler spectrum for a scattering angle of 10° and a wavelength of 633 nm is only 650 Hz. This will normally be unobservable when large scattering volumes or long averaging times are used, for turbulence will dominate the width.

D. THE EFFECT OF FOCUSING

We now consider the effect of focusing the illumination and the receiver onto a common volume, maintaining a fixed number density ρ of scattering particles and changing the scattering volume. We assume that the instrument is bistatic and symmetrical, with transmitting and receiving optics of equal diameter, similarly focused, and equidistant from the scattering volume. For N particles in the scattering volume, the SNR is found by merely multiplying the right-hand side of Eq. (87) by N. We approximate the actual scattering volume by a sphere of diameter d, and hence $N = \pi d^3 \rho/6$. The solid angle of the receiver field of view is $\Omega_r = \pi d^2/4R^2$ and the area of the receiver is $A_r = \pi D^2/4$. We substitute these quantities into the expression for ψ and use the well-known antenna theorem $A_r \Omega_r = \lambda^2$, finding

$$\psi = (\eta P_0/hvB)(8/3\pi)(\rho\lambda^2\sigma(\theta, \varphi)/d) \qquad (92)$$

The point of most interest is that the SNR is maximized for a minimum value of d. This means that for a given working distance the largest practical optics should be used, and both transmitter and receiver should be focused to the minimum possible spot size. With diffraction-limited optics, d will be approximately equal to $2\lambda(R/D)$, although (R/D) will normally have to be of order of 10 to 100 to achieve a reasonable working distance. The conclusion that d should be minimized may be surprising, for we found earlier that the scattered signal is proportional to $\sqrt{N}$, but a qualitative explanation is easily given. The scattered signal power is proportional to the product of power density at the scattering volume (which is proportional to $1/d^2$), to the number of scatterers in the volume (d^3), and to the effective area of the receiver $(1/d^2$, by the antenna theorem); hence the received power and SNR are proportional to $1/d$.

Massey (1965) has analyzed the very similar problem of scattering from a rough surface, finding that the receiving aperture should be just large enough to resolve the spot focused by the illuminator on the surface. A larger receiving aperture gives neither improvement nor degradation. If the receiver is smaller than this, its field of view is larger than that necessary to collect light from the entire spot, and hence its effective aperture is smaller than optimum. Increasing the receiver aperture up to the point where the spot is just resolved therefore increases the signal, although increasing it further has no effect because one merely collects light from a decreasing fraction of the spot into an increasing solid angle and these two effects just cancel each other. If the transmitter and receiver have the same diameter and are at the same distance from the focused spot, the spot is automatically at the receiver's resolution limit and the scattered wave entering the receiver is spatially coherent. If in addition the surface roughness elements are small enough to scatter isotropically, one can find the heterodyne signal without a detailed scattering calculation by merely calculating the fraction of the incident light reaching the receiver, considering the reflectivity of the surface and the solid angle subtended by the receiver at the surface.

For measurements in which much of the path passes through the flowing medium, it is necessary to consider attenuation by the medium and also the wavefront distortion caused by variations in refractive index. To achieve the SNR and hence the sensitivity predicted here, the signal and reference wavefronts must be matched at the detector. For a given number density of scattering particles and a given working distance, Eq. (92) predicts that ψ will increase linearly with D. However, the improvement continues only until the aperture is approximately as large as the transverse phase coherence length. This limitation is not a significant problem for paths a few meters long through normal outdoor air (Fried, 1967), but can be for propagation through more highly turbulent media.

E. Numerical Examples and Experimental Results

The maximum range at which velocity measurements can be made is found by substituting $2\lambda/(R/D)$ for d in Eq. (92) and solving for R:

$$R = (\eta P_0/h\nu B\psi)(8/6\pi)\rho\lambda D\sigma(\theta, \varphi) \qquad (93)$$

For given characteristics of the flow and of the scattering particles the appropriate bandwidth B and minimum useful SNR ψ depend on the type of receiver used. In variable flow the mean Doppler shift may sweep over a range of many megahertz, while the Doppler bandwidth caused by Brownian motion of aerosol particles is normally only a few kilohertz. In turbulent flow the mean velocity will vary at a frequency determined by the characteristic time of the turbulence; the maximum rate of change of the mean Doppler shift depends on this frequency as well as on the strength of the turbulence.

The simplest way to measure velocity is to use a spectrum analyzer. The mean velocity can be estimated from the center of the displayed spectrum, while the observed spectral width will be caused by both Brownian motion and turbulence. Spectrum analyzers normally operate by scanning relatively slowly across the bandwidth of interest, however, and they are not suitable for tracking rapid changes in velocity. A second type of receiver more satisfactory for such measurement consits of a limiter and FM discriminator having an instantaneous bandwidth as large as the full frequency range over which the mean Doppler shift can vary. Such a receiver gives poor results, though, if the input SNR (calculated using the full bandwidth) drops below about 10 dB. The most satisfactory type of receiver if there are, on the average, many particles in the scattering volume is a tracking receiver in which a variable-frequency oscillator is phase-locked to the mean signal as shown in Fig. 36.

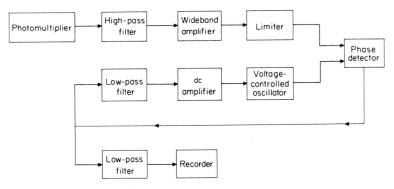

FIG. 36. Block diagram of tracking receiver for use in optical Doppler measurement of fluid flow.

The error signal in the loop determines the frequency of the variable oscillator and therefore can be used as a measure of the mean Doppler shift. For such a receiver the loop gain and instantaneous bandwidth need be only large enough to permit the phase-locked oscillator to follow the changes in mean frequency reliably, and the appropriate bandwidth B for Eq. (93) is given by the Doppler bandwidth or the maximum frequency at which the mean velocity changes, whichever is greater. It can be shown (Gardner, 1966) that a SNR in the loop of 6 dB is required for phase-lock to be achieved, and therefore the value of ψ appropriate in the range equation is 4. If the Doppler bandwidth is dominant it is possible to increase the precision of the final velocity measurement by low-pass filtering the loop output. The bandwidth that must be used in calculating the maximum range achievable is still the bandwidth of the loop, however, and not the final output bandwidth.

In finding the maximum range we assume the values $\eta = 0.2$, $P_0 = 1$ W, $\lambda = 488$ nm, $D = 15$ cm, $\psi = 4$ and then Eq. (93) becomes

$$R = (3.8 \times 10^{13})\rho\sigma(\theta, \varphi)/B \qquad (94)$$

where R is in centimeters. We immediately see that the method will be practical for laboratory measurements. For a highly turbulent flow $(B = 10$ kHz) seeded with a number density $\rho = 10^2$ cm^{-3} of 1 μm water droplets, for example, for which the differential cross section at $10°$ is about 5×10^{-8} cm^2, we find $R = 190$ meters. This indicates that excellent SNRs can be achieved with working distances of a few meters and flows that are seeded with quite low densities of reasonably large particles.

An analysis in which typical values for natural aerosol and molecular number densities were used (Owens, 1969) has shown that the optical Doppler method should be feasible as well for the measurement of wind velocity and turbulence in the open atmosphere. For small particles and low-velocity flow, so that the scattering is reasonably isotropic and the Doppler bandwidth is dominant over that caused by turbulence, we can go a step beyond Eq. (94) and give a simpler approximate formula. We replace $\sigma(\theta, \varphi)$ by an average differential cross section defined by $\langle\sigma(\theta, \varphi)\rangle = \sigma/4\pi$, where σ is given by $\sigma = Q_s\pi a^2$, Q_s is the scattering efficiency, and a is the particle radius, and set B equal to the full width at half-maximum of the Doppler spectrum for a $10°$ scattering angle. We then have

$$R = (1.14 \times 10^{16})\rho Q_s a^{7/2} \qquad (95)$$

For the same system parameters used above, and assuming that the natural aerosols are largely nonabsorbing, we find that the maximum range for wind measurements in clear air can be as large as 30 meters. In measurement through uniform haze, dust, or fog, the transmission loss along the propagation paths must also be considered. It can be shown easily from the definition of Q_s that the attenuation L in decibels per kilometer given by nonabsorbing particles is

$$L = (1.36 \times 10^6)\rho Q_s a^2 \qquad (96)$$

A medium haze $(\rho = 10^5$ cm^{-3}; $a = 0.1$ μm; $L = 6.8$ dB/km) actually gives very little improvement over clear air; the very small particles approximately double the amount of light scattered but also double the Doppler bandwidth.

Dust ($\rho = 10^4$ cm^{-3}; $a = 0.35$ μm; $L = 33.5$ dB/km) increases the range to about 100 meters, while fog [$\rho = 10^2$ cm^{-3}; $a = 3$ μm; $\sigma(10°) = 1.1 \times 10^{-7}$ cm^2; $L = 24.5$ dB/km] increases it to about 400 meters. The best results and the most reliable operation will be obtained, of course, by seeding the region to be studied with artificial aerosols. By using smoke candles to generate a small plume for which $\rho = 10^7$ cm^{-3} and $a = 0.1$ μm, a range of 2.4 km should be made possible. In practice the maximum range will be limited to values significantly less than this by turbulent wavefront degradation, absorption by the smoke particles, and other losses, but measurements should nevertheless be possible at ranges of a few hundred meters.

Further analysis of measurement error has been given by Davis (1968), while operating instruments have been built by several groups for the measurement of fluid flow and of surface vibration. Foreman *et al.* (1966) have described measurements with a 50 mW, 633 nm laser of mean velocities as high as 300 meters/sec at the center of a wind tunnel, using smoke candles, and also of the velocity profile in laminar water flow through a circular pipe. They have also measured the velocity of the exhaust from a solid-fuel rocket at a distsnce of 8 ft (Watson, 1967). Huffaker (1970) has described a three-axis instrument using a 1 W, 488 nm argon laser which has been used to measure mean velocity profiles and turbulence in a small subsonic jet and also in wind tunnel flow at Mach numbers in excess of 2.0. He has also measured atmospheric wind velocity at a range of 35 meters using a 20 W, 10.6 μm carbon dioxide laser and backscattering from natural contaminants. The maximum useful range predicted is about 500 meters. Fridman *et al.* (1970) have given further information about the same three-axis instrument, including basic theory, the choice of optimum particle concentration, and electronic design. Finally, Massey and Carter (1968; further details are given in Massey, 1966) have described an instrument for surface vibration analysis.

VI. Conclusion

The development of the gas laser has considerably broadened the range of practical applications for optical methods in metrology and geodesy. As an alignment tool the laser beam is convenient for both the precision alignment of large structures, such as aircraft assembly jigs and radio astronomy antennas, and for directional indication and automatic control in tunneling and grading. For the measurement of length, direct fringe-counting instruments are now available for use in realistic industrial environments. The overall accuracy is normally limited to about 1 part in 10^6 by uncertainty in refractive index, but better measurements are possible with good environmental control. In fact, the reproducibility given by the methane stabilization method may permit the helium–neon laser line at 633 nm to be defined as the fundamental standard of length. For longer geodetic paths, modulated-light methods are coming into wider use both as relatively inexpensive surveyor's tools and for long-distance measurements of very high accuracy. Velocity fields in fluid flow as well as surface vibration patterns can be measured with optical Doppler methods. Finally, three-dimensional measurements can be made by holographic interferometry for surface tolerancing optically rough objects and for testing lenses and mirrors for which no master surface exists. The convenience of laser methods will undoubtedly continue to lengthen the list of specific applications.

REFERENCES

Anderson, L. K., and McMurty, B. J. (1966). *App. Opt.* **5**, 1573.

Angus-Leppan, P. V., ed. (1968). *Prof. Conf. Refraction Effects in Geodesy and Conf. Electronic Distance Measurement, Univ. of New South Wales, Kensington, N.S.W., Australia.*

Baird, K. M., and Hanes, G. R. (1967). *In* "Applied Optics and Optical Engineering" (R. Kingslake, ed.), Vol. 4, pp. 309–361. Academic Press, New York.

Barger, R. L., and Hall, J. L. (1969). *Phys. Rev. Lett.* **22**, 4.

Bean, B. R., and Dutton, E. J. (1966). "Radio Meteorology." *Nat. Bur. Stand. (U.S.), Monogr.* **92**.

Bender, P. L. (1967). *Proc. IEEE* **55**, 1039.

Bergstrand, E. (1950). *Ark. Fys.* **2**, 119.

Betz, H. D. (1969). *Appl. Opt.* **8**, 1007.

Birnbaum, G. (1967). *Proc. IEEE* **55**, 1015.

Boyne, H. S., Hall, J. L., Barger, R. L., Bender, P. L., Ward, J., Levine, J., and Faller, J. E. (1970). *In* "Laser Applications in the Geosciences" (J. Gauger and F. F. Hall, Jr., eds.), pp. 215–225. Western Periodicals Co., North Hollywood, California.

Brillouin, L. (1960). "Wave Propagation and Group Velocity." Academic Press, New York.

Buck, A. L. (1967). *Proc. IEEE* **55**, 448.

Candler, C. (1951). "Modern Interferometers." Hilger & Watts, London.

Cook, H. D., and Marzetta, L. A. (1961). *J. Res. Nat. Bur. Stand., Sect. C* **65**, 129.

Curcio, J. A., Drummeter, L. F., and Knestrick, G. L. (1964). *Appl. Opt.* **3**, 1401.

Davis, D. T. (1968). *ISA Trans.* **7**, 43.

Dukes, J. N., and Gordon, G. B. (1970). *Hewlett-Packard Journal* **21**, 2.

Earnshaw, K. B., and Owens, J. C. (1967). *IEEE J. Quantum Electron.* **3**, 544.

Elterman, L. (1968). "UV, Visible, and IR Attenuation for Altitudes to 50 km." Environ. Res. Paper No. 285, AFCRL-68-0153. Air Force Cambridge Res. Labs., Bedford, Massachusetts.

Engelhard, E., and Vieweg, R. (1961). *Z. Angew. Phys.* **13**, 580.

Foreman, J. W., Jr., George, E. W., Jetton, J. L., Lewis, R. D., Thornton, J. R., and Watson, H. J. (1966). *IEEE J. Quantum Electron.* **2**, 260.

Foster, J. D. (1965). "Fringe Counting Laser Interferometers for Industrial Length Measurement." Rept. SCL-DC-65-92. Sandia Corp., Livermore, California.

Fridman, J. D., Kinnard, K. F., and Meister, K. (1970). *Proc. Electro-Opt. Syst. Design Conf., New York, 1969*, p. 128.

Fried, D. L. (1967). *Proc. IEEE* **55**, 57.

Gardner, F. M. (1966). "Phaselock Techniques." Wiley, New York.

Gilmer, R. O., and Waters, D. M. (1967). "A Solid-State System for Measurement of Integrated Refractive Index." ESSA Tech. Rept. IER 40-ITSA 40. U.S. Govt. Printing Office, Washington, D.C.

Goody, R. M. (1964). "Atmospheric Radiation." Oxford Univ. Press (Clarendon), London and New York.

Hall, J. L. (1968). *IEEE J. Quantum Electron.* **4**, 638.

Hernandez, E. N. (1970). Private communication.

Herriott, D. R. (1967). *Progr. Opt.* **6**, 171.

Herrmannsfeldt, W. B., Lee, M. J., Spranza, J. J., and Trigger, K. R. (1968). *Appl. Opt.* **7**, 995.

Huffaker, R. M. (1970). *Appl. Opt.* **9**, 1026.

International Association of Geodesy (1967). "Electromagnetic Distance Measurement." Hilger & Watts, London.

Kaminow, I. P., and Sharpless, W. M. (1967). *Appl. Opt.* **6**, 351.

Kaminow, I. P., and Turner, E. H. (1966). *Appl. Opt.* **5**, 1612.

Kerr, J. R. (1967). *Proc IEEE* **55**, 1686.

Lawrence, R. S., and Strohbehn, J. W. (1970). *Proc. IEEE* **58**, 1523.

Long, R. K. (1963). "Absorption of Laser Radiation in the Atmosphere." Antenna Lab. Rept. No. 1579-3. Dept. of Electrical Engineering, Ohio State Univ., Columbus, Ohio. (Clearinghouse No. AD 410571.)

Massey, G. A. (1965). *Appl. Opt.* **4**, 781.

Massey, G. A. (1966). Study of Vibration Measurement by Laser Methods. Unpubl. Tech. Rep. Sylvania Electronic Systems, Mountain View, California.

Massey, G. A., and Carter, R. R. (1968). *Shock and Vibration Bulletin* No. 37, Pt. 2, pp. 1–6. US. Naval Res. Lab., Washington, D.C.

Mielenz, K. D., Stephens, R. B., Gillilland, K. E., and Nefflen, K. F. (1966). *J. Opt. Soc. Amer.* **56**, 156.

Mollet, P., ed. (1960). "Optics in Metrology." Macmillan (Pergamon), New York.

Ochs, G. R., and Lawrence, R. S. (1969). "Measurements of Laser Beam Spread and Curvature over Near-Horizontal Atmospheric Paths." ESSA Tech. Rept. ERL 106-WPL 6. U.S. Govt. Printing Office, Washington, D.C.

Owens, J. C. (1967). *Appl. Opt.* **6**, 51.

Owens, J. C. (1968). *Bulletin Geodesique* **89**, 277.

Owens, J. C. (1969). *Proc IEEE* **57**, 530.

Peck, E. R. (1962). *J. Opt. Soc. Amer.* **52**, 253.

Peck, E. R., and Obetz, S. W. (1953). *J. Opt. Soc. Amer.* **43**, 505.

Rinner, K., and Benz, F., eds. (1966). "Handbuch der Vermessungskunde," Vol. VI. Metzlersche, Stuttgart.

Ross, M. (1966). "Laser Receivers." Wiley, New York.

Rowley, W. R. C. (1966). *IEEE Trans. Instrum. Meas.* **15**, 146.

Shurcliff, W. A., and Ballard, S. S. (1964). "Polarized Light." Van Nostrand, Princeton, New Jersey.

Smith, H. M. (1969). "Principles of Holography." Wiley, New York.

Steel, W. H. (1967). "Interferometry." Cambridge Univ. Press, London and New York.

Strohbehn, J. W. (1968). *Proc. IEEE* **56**, 1301.

Thayer, G. D. (1967). "Atmospheric Effects on Multiple-Frequency Range Measurements." ESSA Tech. Rept. IER 56-ITSA 53. U.S. Govt. Printing Office, Washington, D.C.

Thompson, M. C., Jr., and Janes, H. B. (1967). *Bulletin of the Seismological Society of America* **57**, 641.

Thompson, M. C., Jr., and Vetter, M. J. (1958). *Rev. Sci. Instrum.* **29**, 148.

Valley, S. L., ed. (1965). "Handbook of Geophysics and Space Environments," Ch. 3. McGraw-Hill, New York.

van Heel, A. C. S. (1965). *Progr. Opt.* **1**, 289.

Walsh, P. J., and Krause, I. (1966). *Proc. 8th Annu. Electron Laser Beam Symp., Ann Arbor, Mich.* p. 139.

Watson, H. J. (1967). Private communication.

Wood, E. A. (1964). "Crystals and Light." Van Nostrand, Princeton, New Jersey.

Wood, L. E., and Thompson, M. C., Jr. (1966). *Nature (London)* **211**, 173.

Wood, L. E., and Thompson, M. C., Jr. (1968). *Appl. Opt.* **7**, 1955.

THE LASER GYRO

Frederick Aronowitz

Systems and Research Center, Honeywell Inc.
Minneapolis, Minnesota

I. Introduction

One of the more promising applications of the laser is as a gyroscope (Heer, 1961; Rosenthal, 1962; Macek and Davis, 1963; McCartney, 1966; Killpatrick, 1967). The laser gyro is an integrating rate gyroscope in the unconventional sense, since it contains no spinning mass. The essential feature of the laser gyro is a ring-type cavity in which the laser radiation traverses a closed path. The laser cavity supports two independent, oppositely directed traveling waves that can oscillate at different frequencies. The frequencies of oscillation of the traveling waves are dependent on the rotation of the cavity with respect to inertial space. A measurement of the frequency difference between the two waves gives a direct measurement of the rotation of the laser cavity.

From a systems point of view, the laser gyro can be considered as just another black box. Power is applied and information is taken out and fed into a computer. This survey article provides further insight into the basic operation of the laser gyro.

Discussion of the laser gyro can be divided into three parts: (1) the basic concept involved in its operation (Section II), (2) the active laser medium, and (3) the cavity. This article deals mainly with the laser medium.

The cavity is discussed briefly in Section VII, following a description of the active laser medium. However, little emphasis is placed on the cavity since the problems involved in its construction are similar (although more severe) to those in the design and build of most lasers. The emphasis on the laser material and operation of the laser gyro bring to the surface potential problem areas that must be considered in the design and construction of the laser gyro.

The successful operation of the laser gyro, and its eventual acceptance as a device will be determined mainly by how well and how economically it can be designed and constructed.

II. Principle of Operation

A. PASSIVE SAGNAC INTERFEROMETER

The principle of operation of the laser gyro is best described by first considering a rotating ring interferometer, as first successfully demonstrated by Sagnac (1913). Since the effect is first order in v/c, classical theory will give the correct answer to first order (Ditchborn, 1959a). Strictly speaking, the special theory of relativity is not applicable, since the light must be considered on a rotating frame. The only rigorously correct theory is the general theory of relativity (Langerin, 1921; Landau and Lifshitz, 1951). However, for conceptual simplicity, the rotating interferometer will be considered, using classical theory.

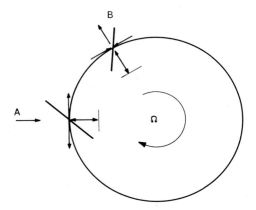

Fig. 1. Circular rotating (Sagnac interferometer).

Figure 1 shows an ideal circular interferometer of radius R. Light enters at point A and is split by the beamsplitter. In this ideal interferometer, the light is constrained to travel along the circumference of the circle. After traveling along the complete path, the light recombines at the original beamsplitter. When the interferometer is stationary, the transit time for the light to make a complete path is the same for both beams and is given by

$$t = 2\pi R/c \qquad (1)$$

where c is the velocity of light.

If the interferometer is rotated at a constant speed Ω, the closed path transit time is modified from that given by Eq. (1). In fact, the closed path transit time becomes different for light traveling with and against the direction of rotation. This occurs because of the fact that during the closed path transit time of the light, the beamsplitter, originally located at point A, moves to point B. Thus, with respect to inertial space, light traveling against and with the direction of rotation must traverse a smaller and greater distance, respectively, than when there is no rotation. Note that the speed of the light is considered to remain invariant. Then the closed path transit time for the light is given by the equations

$$2\pi R \pm X_\pm = ct_\pm$$
$$X_\pm = R\Omega t_\pm$$

or

$$t_\pm = 2\pi R/c \mp R\Omega \qquad (2)$$

The upper sign in Eq. (2) refers to the light traveling in the direction of rotation and X refers to the inertial space distance between points A and B. Note that Eq. (2) can be interpreted in terms of the speed of light being different for the two directions and the path length being the same.

The closed-path transit time difference for the light traveling in opposite directions is given by

$$\Delta t = t_+ - t_-$$

and from Eq. (2), we find, to first order

$$\Delta t = 4\pi\Omega R^2/c^2 \qquad (3)$$

This difference in closed-path transit time for light traveling in opposite directions gives rise to an optical path difference of $c\,\Delta t$, or from Eq. (3),

$$\Delta L = 4\pi\Omega R^2/c \qquad (4)$$

This is the basic equation for the rotating interferometer. It shows that the optical path difference is proportional to the area enclosed by the light and the rotation speed. Equation (4) does not take into account effects due to the presence of optically refracting materials in the path of the light beams. This latter case is treated in detail in a review article on the Sagnac effect (Post, 1967).

According to the general theory of relativity, a clock traveling on a rotating frame loses synchronization with one located on a stationary frame (Landau and Lifshitz, 1951). This loss of synchronization gives rise to a different closed-path transit time for light traveling in opposite directions on a rotating frame, or

$$\Delta t = \oint 2\Omega R^2 [1 - (\Omega R/c)^2]^{-1}\, d\varphi \qquad (5)$$

where the integral is taken over a closed contour. Neglecting second-order terms, Eq. (5) becomes

$$\Delta t = (2\Omega/c^2) \oint r^2\, d\varphi$$

or

$$\Delta t = 4A\Omega/c^2$$

where A is the area enclosed by the light. Thus Eq. (4) can be generalized for an arbitrary cavity configuration as

$$\Delta L = 4A\Omega/c \tag{6}$$

From the development of Eq. (5), the optical path difference given by Eq. (6) is independent of the location of the axis of rotation. It should also be noted that a measurement of the optical path difference enables an observer located on the rotating frame to measure the so called "absolute" rotation of his frame.

In the Michelson–Gale experiment, (Michelson and Gale, 1925) the rotation of the Earth was measured by use of a cavity rigidly attached to the surface of the Earth. The cavity configuration was rectangular with sides 2000×1100 ft. The measured path difference amounted to ~ 1300 Å or $\sim \frac{1}{4}$ fringe. The fringe shift was determined by comparison with a fringe pattern obtained with a much smaller area. In the experiment, only the component of rotation normal to the plane of the cavity was measured. For resonator cavities more suited to the laboratory, much higher rotation speeds are needed to give measurable fringe shifts.

B. ACTIVE RING LASER INTERFEROMETER

As discussed in Section II,A, the use of a ring resonator in the passive mode allowed the determination of the rotation (with respect to inertial space) of the resonator. The observer is located on the rotating frame. A light source, external to the cavity, is used and the quantity measured is the phase difference arising from the unequal path lengths for light traveling in opposite directions around the rotating cavity.

The difficulty in using the Sagnac interferometer as a practical device arises from lack of sensitivity, since the path difference for light traveling in the two directions is much less than a wavelength. The use of a laser as the external light source does not help. However, if the system is made into an active interferometer, the situation changes markedly. The improvement in sensitivity arises from the fact that the laser frequency is dependent on the cavity length.

Figure 2 is a schematic of a linear laser with two mirrors separated by a distance l and a ring laser with total perimeter L. In both cases the frequency of oscillation condition for the lowest order transverse mode is that the optical cavity length encloses an integral number of wavelengths. For the linear laser, the cavity modes consist of two oppositely directed traveling waves which compose a standing wave. The amplitudes and frequencies of the traveling waves are constrained to be equal. In the ring laser each cavity

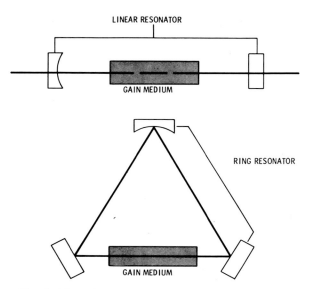

FIG. 2. Linear laser and ring laser cavity configuration.

mode also consists of two oppositely directed traveling waves. In this case the oppositely directed waves are independent, in the sense that they can oscillate with different amplitudes and frequencies. In fact, whether or not the ring laser could sustain stable oscillations in both directions was not answered until it was actually achieved (Macek and Davis, 1963).

If m represents the mode number (typically on the order of 10^5–10^6), the oscillation condition can be expressed as

$$m\lambda_\pm = L_\pm$$

or

$$v_\pm = mc/L_\pm \tag{7}$$

where $v_\pm$ represents the frequency of the wave which sees the cavity as being of length $L_\pm$, respectively. Thus small changes in the path length result in a small frequency change given by

$$\Delta v/v = \Delta L/L \tag{8}$$

Due to the high frequency in the optical region (10^{14} Hz), small length changes can result in large measurable frequency differences. Letting ΔL, as given by Eq. (6), represent the differential cavity length for the oppositely directed waves, the beat frequency can be found from Eq. (8) as

$$\Delta v = 4A\Omega/L\lambda \tag{9}$$

For a rotation of 10 deg/hr and for a ring laser with an equilateral triangular cavity of 13.2 cm per side operating at a wavelength of 0.633 μm, Eq. (9) gives a beat frequency of 5.9 Hz. Using heterodyne techniques, this beat frequency is readily measurable, although it amounts to only 10^{-14} of the value of the optical frequency.

From Eq. (7) it can be seen that thermal and mechanical instabilities can cause frequency variations far greater than the rotational beat frequency. Hence for the operation of the ring laser as a rotation sensor (laser gyro) it is necessary for both beams to physically occupy the same cavity.

C. READOUT IN THE LASER GYRO

In the laser gyro, rotation information is obtained by monotoring the oppositely directed waves. In the ideal case of a uniformly rotating laser, the frequencies of the waves are slightly different; the difference being given by Eq. (9). Thus a direct measurement of the beat frequency gives a number proportional to the rotation rate. Figure 3 shows a method of combining the oppositely directed beams to obtain readout. A small percentage (typically less than 0.1 %) of the energy of both beams is transmitted through one of the dielectric coated mirrors. The beams are made approximately colinear by a

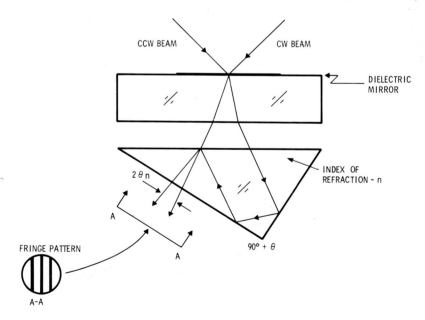

FIG. 3. Readout technique in the laser gyro.

90 degree corner prism to form a fringe pattern. The prism can be directly mounted to the mirror to minimize vibrations. Typically, a semitransparent coated mirror is used to match intensities.

The fringes are a measure of the instantaneous phase difference between the oppositely directed beams. For the case when the intensities are matched and the beams are nearly colinear (angular divergence of ε), the fringe pattern is given by

$$I = I_0[1 + \cos(2\pi\varepsilon x/\lambda + \Delta\omega t + \varphi)] \tag{10}$$

where $\Delta\omega$ is the angular beat frequency and φ is some arbitrary angle. Thus when the laser is not rotating, $\Delta\omega = 0$, and the fringe pattern is stationary. When the laser is rotated, the fringe pattern moves at the beat frequency rate. The fringe spacing is given by λ/ε. For a parallel substrate ε is given by

$$\varepsilon = 2n\theta$$

where n is the index of refraction of the prism and θ is the deviation of the prism angle from 90 degrees.

For a prism angle deviation of 15 arc sec and for the 0.633 μm He–Ne transition, the fringe spacing is 3 mm. Thus by the use of a detector whose dimensions are much smaller than the fringe spacing, a measurement of the rotation rate can be made by simply recording the rate at which intensity maximum moves past the detector. From Eq. (10) it can be seen that the sense of rotation determines the direction in which the fringe pattern moves. Thus by using two detectors spaced 90 degrees (a quarter fringe) apart and a logic circuit, both positive and negative counts can be accumulated to give rotation sense.

It should be noted that with this type of readout, the laser gyro is inherently an integrating rate gyro with a digital output. This can be seen from Eq. (9), where a time integration gives

$$N = (4A/\lambda L)\theta \tag{11}$$

where

$$N = \int_0^t \Delta v\, dt, \qquad \theta = \int_0^t \Omega\, dt \tag{12}$$

Thus with up–down counting the net number of accumulated counts depends only on the net angle through which the ideal gyro is turned. They are independent of rotation fluctuations.

Since 1 deg/hr corresponds to 1 arcsec/sec, the scale factor, given by Eq. (11) for a 13.2 cm (on a side) equilateral triangular configuration laser gyro oscillating on the 0.633 μm He–Ne transition, is 1 count corresponding to 1.7 arc sec. Thus by turning the gyro through one revolution, 0.76×10^6

counts are obtained. If the gyro, in the ideal case, was sitting in inertial space and turned through a complete revolution, first in one direction and then in the other, no net accumulation of counts would occur. If the experiment was repeated at the North Pole and the plane of the gyro was parallel to the Earth's surface, there would then be a net count accumulation. The counts would depend on the angle turned through by the Earth during the counting time. For example, if the total experiment took 10 seconds, then approximately 90 counts would have accumulated. If the experiment was repeated along the equator, no net accumulation of counts would occur. In this manner, the laser gyro has application as northfinder.

Figure 4 shows rotation data for a laser gyro located on a centrifuge (Killpatrick, 1967). The scale factor for this gyro was 10^3 counts/deg. The solid points were taken with the gyro located at the center of the centrifuge and the open points were obtained with the gyro located along the arm.

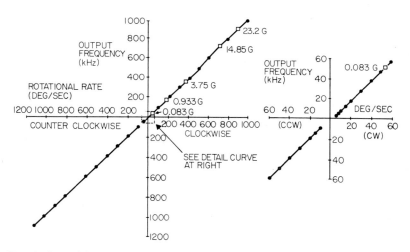

FIG. 4. Output frequency vs. rotation rate for the laser gyro. ●, Zero centrifugal g's; □, centrifugal g's as noted, scale factor $= 10^3$ counts/deg.

III. Error Sources in the Laser Gyro

A. SUMMARY OF ERROR TERMS

In the ideal stationary laser gyro, there are two oppositely directed traveling waves oscillating in a perfectly symmetric cavity. The optical paths are identical for both beams and both beams oscillate at the same frequency and with the same amplitude. When the laser gyro is rotated, the directional degeneracy on the optical path for each beam is removed and the frequencies of oscillation become different. The beat frequency as given by Eq. (9) is linear with respect to the rotation rate. Equation (9) can be written in terms of the instantaneous phase difference (ψ) between the oppositely directed wave as

$$\dot{\psi} = \Omega \tag{13}$$

The scale factor is incorporated into the units of Ω in Eq. (13).

The ideal laser gyro equation given by Eq. (13) is represented in Fig. 5a. Note that the axis can represent either counts versus angle, or beat frequency versus rotation rate. The slope in Fig. 5(a) is determined by the scale factor. Any effect which causes the input–output characteristics to deviate from the given straight line is considered to be an error source.

There are three types of errors which are critical in the design of the laser gyro. They are, as represented in Fig. 5, null-shift, lock-in, and mode pulling.

A null-shift error arises when the cavity is anisotropic with respect to radiation traveling in the two directions. This results in the optical paths being different for radiation traveling in both directions and hence the two

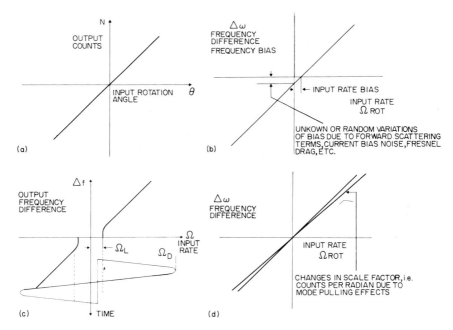

FIG. 5. Error sources in the laser gyro. (a) Ideal laser integrating gyro performance; (b) null-shift effects; (c) lock-in effects; (d) mode pulling effects.

waves oscillate at different frequencies. Unless the gyro is properly designed, null-shift errors can be orders of magnitude greater than the input rate.

Lock-in is a well-known phenomenon which is common to all coupled oscillator systems (Vander Pol, 1934; Kharkevich, 1959; Adler, 1946). The laser gyro can be considered as a coupled oscillator system in the sense that both waves can oscillate at their respective resonance frequency. There is mutual coupling between the waves such that at low input rates both waves lock to a common frequency (Macek *et al.*, 1963). In this region the system is not responsive to input rotations. The absence of points around zero rotation in Fig. 4 is a result of lock-in.

A third type of error that arises in the laser gyro is due to mode pulling effects (Lamb, 1964). In the derivation of Eq. (13) for the ideal beat frequency, an ideal empty cavity was assumed. In actuality the cavity contains a material which is the source of the laser radiation. Thus dispersion effects, both anomalous and normal, must be considered. Changes in the dispersive effects of the medium can result in a lack of stability and reproducibility of the scale factor, which can be critical for navigation and attitude reference applications.

Scale factor linearity (variation of scale factor as a function of rotation rate) is not considered to be among the most critical problem areas in the laser gyro. In the derivation of Eq. (13) cubic terms in rotation rate have been neglected and are negligible. Unlike conventional gyroscopes, better performance is expected from the laser gyro at high rotation rates. The inherent bandwidth capability of the laser medium far exceeds the bandwidth requirement capability in the accompanying electronic circuitry. Figure 4 shows linear performance results for rates exceeding 4×10^6 deg/hr.

Another potential problem area for gyroscopes in general is due to the effects of acceleration. Unlike rotating mass-type gyroscopes, there are no known acceleration effects on the laser gyro. Experiments with the laser gyro on a centrifuge have been performed with no unexpected results. Figure 4 shows limited results out to 23 g's.

B. Null-Shift Errors

Null shifts are nonreciprocal contributions to the index of refraction for the oppositely directed beams due to causes other than rotations. This causes a shift in the beat frequency versus rotation rate ideal curve. With a null shift it is then possible to get a beat frequency in the absence of any input rotation, as shown in Fig. 5(b). Equation (13) for the beat frequency then becomes

$$\dot{\psi} = \Omega + \Omega_N \tag{14}$$

where Ω_N is the effective rotation due to the null shift.

A well-known phenomenon which causes an anisotropy in the index of refraction is the Fresnel–Fizeau effect (Ditchburn, 1959b). It was found that the velocity of light v traveling through a moving medium of index of refraction n is

$$v = c/n \pm V(1 - 1/n^2) \tag{15}$$

where the plus and minus signs correspond to the case of the light traveling in and against the direction of the flow V.

At this point it should be noted that in the derivation of the beat frequency given by Eq. (9) for the case of a rotating ring laser, it was assumed that the cavity was empty. If the rotating cavity contains a co-moving medium, the equation for the beat frequency must be modified (Post, 1967). Every ring laser will contain, at the least, the laser material. In addition, optical elements such as windows and prism reflectors are sometimes contained in the cavity.

To modify the laser gyro beat frequency equation for the case of a co-moving material in the cavity, it is only necessary to replace the cavity path length L in Eqs. (7)–(9) by the optical path length, or

$$L \to \oint n\, ds \tag{16}$$

where the integral is over the closed cavity path. The differential transit time and differential path given by Eqs. (5) and (6), respectively, remain unchanged.

The null-shift beat frequency contribution for a medium moving with velocity V in the laser path can be written as

$$\Delta v_n = (2/\lambda)\left[\oint (n^2 - 1)V \cdot ds \Big/ \oint n\, ds\right] \tag{17}$$

For the case of a ring laser having a medium (of index n) flowing with velocity V along a distance d of the laser cavity, Eq. (17) reduces to

$$\Delta v_n = 2(n^2 - 1)V\, d/\lambda L \tag{18}$$

where L is the total optical cavity length given by Eq. (16).

Figure 6 shows the results of an experiment where moving solid, liquid, and gaseous media were separately inserted into a laser cavity (Macek *et al.*, 1964). Hence the ring laser has applicability to other areas, such as mass flow, density, flow profiles (Fenster and Kahn, 1968), and refractive index measurements.

Null shifts due to flowing media in the cavity path of the laser gyro are usually much too large for inertial grade instruments. For example, a 1 cm/sec flow of air ($n - 1 = 3 \times 10^{-4}$) along 1 cm of path in a ring laser with an enclosed area of 20 cm^2, gives rise to an effective rotation of 3 deg/hr.

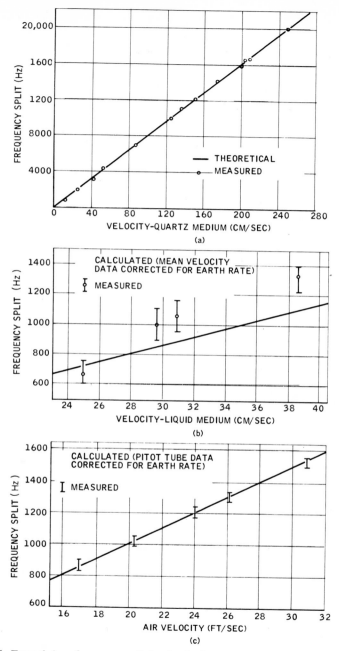

FIG. 6. Fresnel drag frequency splitting in the laser gyro; (a) solid medium (quartz), (b) liquid medium (CCl₄), (c) gaseous medium (dry air). From Macek *et al.* (1964).

A less obvious source of a Fresnel drag type null shift is the flow of the components of the gas in a dc excited discharge tube (Dessus *et al.*, 1966; Podorski and Aronowitz, 1968). In the He–Ne ring laser, with a single dc discharge tube, null shifts on the order of many hundreds of degrees per hour have been observed (Podgorski and Aronowitz, 1968). This is illustrated in Fig. 7.

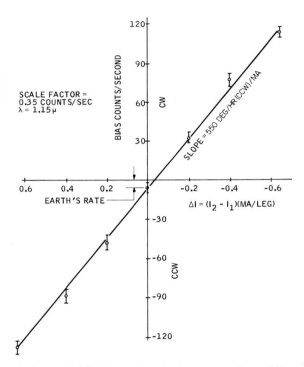

FIG. 7. Langmuir flow null shift due to dc excitation current. From Killpatrick (1967).

Contributions to the null shift arise from the electron flow, positive ion flow, and net neutral atom flows (cataphoresis and Langmuir flow). Calculations, which have been experimentally confirmed (Podgorski and Aronowitz, 1968), have shown that the dominant source of the discharge current null shift arises from a Langmuir flow of the neutral neon atoms that are excited to the two levels between which the stimulated emission occurs.

In cataphoresis the positive ions flow towards the cathode where they neutralize and build up a pressure. The pressure buildup causes a back flow of neutral atoms towards the anode. The null shift has been determined not to have the proper sign to be caused by cataphoresis. The Langmuir flow effect is of the proper sign. In the Langmuir (1923) flow effect, the discharge tube walls are found to have a negative charge. This allows a transfer of momentum from the positive ions (which are traveling toward the cathode) to the walls. This upsets the momentum flow balance between the electrons and the positive ions. The electrons then transfer some of their momentum to the gas particles as a whole. This causes a buildup of neutral gas atoms at the anode. This buildup in pressure causes a back diffusion of neutral gas particles towards the cathode. The back diffusion radial profile is parabolic while the flow due to the electron momentum transfer is uniform. Hence the resultant flow profile of the neutral atoms is towards the anode along the walls and towards the cathode along the center of the tube. The laser radiation is along the tube center.

Strictly speaking, the dc excitation null shift does not arise from the anisotropic index of refraction due to a moving medium, as given by Eq. (5). The null shift occurs due to anisotropic anomalous dispersion effects due to the atomic transition. A further discussion of the effect is deferred until after a discussion of the anomalous dispersion effects (Lamb, 1964; Aronowitz, 1965) of the gas.

Another source of null shift is nonreciprocal saturation effects in the active gain medium (Lee and Atwood, 1966). This causes a nonreciprocal contribution to the anomalous dispersion of the active laser medium. This effect can arise from any element in the cavity which can cause a nonreciprocal loss for the waves traveling in the two directions (Lee and Atwood, 1966). Nonreciprocal losses can occur due to anisotropic scattering effects. They can also occur from magnetooptic interations. For example, when two oppositely directed, linearly polarized beams impinge upon a Faraday cell and a half-wave plate in series, the loss is different for the two directions.

Magnetic fields have also been known to produce null shifts (Burrell et al., 1968; Hutchings et al., 1969). Figure 8 shows a plot of the null shift in a 1.15 μm He–Ne ring laser as a function of the strength of a transverse magnetic field (Aronowitz, 1968).

The magnetic field null-shift mechanism is not completely understood. In the single-mode case, the ring laser, in the presence of a magnetic field, is described by a set of eight coupled first-order nonlinear differential equations (Heer and Graft, 1965). No published results are available on the analysis of the equations.

It is known that a single-mode He–Ne linear laser with plane mirrors can oscillate with circularly polarized standing waves (Tomlinson and Fork, 1967). In the presence of a magnetic field, the degeneracy in both frequency and amplitude between the left and right circularly polarized fields is removed. A beat frequency results which is proportional to the strength of the magnetic field. Fields on the order of 10 gauss produce beats on the order of the null shifts which are observed in the laser gyro. Hence it is not unreasonable to expect Zeeman splitting effects to arise in the laser gyro.

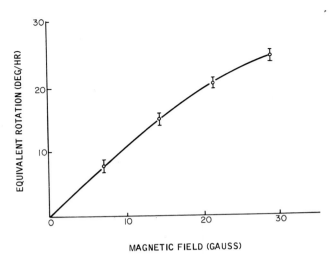

MAGNETIC FIELD (GAUSS)

FIG. 8. Magnetic field induced null shift in the He–Ne 1. 15 μm ring laser. From Aronowitz (1968).

C. LOCK-IN (FREQUENCY SYNCHRONIZATION)

As described in Fig. 5(c), when the rotation rate in the laser gyro is reduced below some critical value (called the lock-in threshold) the frequency difference between the oppositely directed traveling waves synchronizes to a common value (Macek et al., 1963). Thus, for rotation rates below the lock-in threshold, the laser gyro is not responsive to rotations.

Lock-in arises due to mutual coupling between the oppositely directed traveling waves (Basov et al., 1965; Bershtein, 1966; Aronowitz and Collins, 1966; de Lang, 1966; Zhelnov et al., 1966; Klimontovich et al., 1967a; Raterink et al., 1967; Wang, 1967; Tang and Statz, 1967; Whitney, 1969a; Aronowitz, 1969). The dominant source of the coupling is the mutual scattering of energy from each of the beams into the direction of the other. The effect is similar to lock-in coupling effects which have been long understood in conventional electronic oscillators (Vander Pol, 1934; Kharkevich, 1959; Adler, 1946). It is known that the frequency of a tank circuit can be perturbed by the injection of a small external voltage which is at a frequency close to that of the free running oscillator. As the frequency difference between the two signals is decreased or as the amplitude of the external signal is increased, the perturbing effect becomes greater. At some critical combination of the signal strength and frequency difference, the frequency of the free-running oscillator will lock to that of the external voltage.

For the analytically simple case of scattering of only one of the traveling waves into the direction of the other, the lock-in phenomenon can be represented with the aid of the vector-phase space diagram shown in Fig. 9 (Aronowitz, 1969). Let E_1 and E_2 represent the amplitudes of the two beams and let ψ be the instantaneous phase difference between the two. The vector diagram is represented on a set of axes rotating with the phase of field E_1.

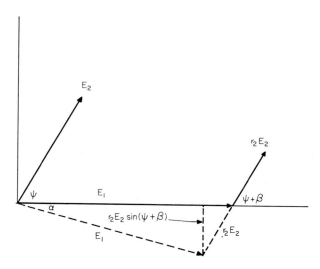

FIG. 9. Vector phase space diagram for frequency pulling due to backscattering.

Then $r_2 E_2$ represents the additional phase shift per pass picked up by beam E_1 due to scattering from beam E_2. The phase β is a constant phase angle arising from the scattering phenomena. Due to this additional phase shift per pass, the frequency of the radiation generated by stimulated emission will be decreased such that the net phase shift per pass $\Delta\varphi$, is still equal to an intégral multiple of 2π. The shift in phase is represented by α in Fig. 9 and is given by

$$\alpha = \Delta\varphi/\text{pass} = -\Delta\omega_1 \quad (\text{time/pass}) \tag{19}$$

The time for the radiation to make one pass is just the inverse of the longitudinal mode spacing, or (L/c). From Fig. 9 for $r_2 \ll 1$,

$$\alpha = r_2(E_2/E_1) \sin(\psi + \beta) \tag{20}$$

Combining Eqs. (19) and (20), the perturbation of the frequency of beam E_1 due to coupling by backscattering from beam E_2 is given by

$$\Delta\omega_1 = -r_2(E_2/E_1)(c/L) \sin(\psi + \beta) \tag{21}$$

For the case of the ring laser being rotated at a rate (Ω) much greater than the lock-in threshold (Ω_L), the effect of the backscattering coupling is small and ψ is obtained from the integration of Eq. (13) as

$$\psi = \Omega t \tag{22}$$

Thus as shown in Fig. 9, E_2 rotates around E_1 at the beat frequency and from Eq. (21), beam E_1 is frequency modulated at the beat frequency. The depth of modulation is proportional to the ratio of the backscattered amplitude over the oscillating amplitude and inversely proportional to the length of the cavity.

Modifying Eq. (13) to take into account the backscattering perturbation as given by Eq. (21), we find

$$\dot{\psi} = \Omega - \Omega_L \sin (\psi + \beta) \tag{23}$$

where

$$\Omega_L = r_2 (E_2/E_1)(c/L) \tag{24}$$

Equation (23) is an expression for the beat frequency of a rotating ring laser, modified to take into account coupling due to backscattering. If mutual backscattering were taken into account, the analysis would be similar (Aronowitz and Collins, 1966) and Eq. (23) would still hold. However, the expression for Ω_L and β would be more complicated. Any null shifts in the system can be considered to be included in the Ω term in Eq. (23).

Equation (23) is a standard differential equation which can be solved in a straightforward manner. The equation has two types of solutions, depending on whether the input rate is greater or less than the lock-in threshold.

First consider the case of input rates greater than the lock-in threshold. The solution of Eq. (23) is then

$$\tan \tfrac{1}{2}(\psi + \beta - \pi/2) = [(K + 1)/(K - 1)]^{1/2} \tan [\tfrac{1}{2}\Omega_L(K^2 - 1)^{1/2}t] \tag{25}$$

where

$$K = \Omega/\Omega_L > 1$$

Initial conditions were shown such that $\psi = \pi/2 - \beta$ at $t = 0$.

For large input rates, or $K \gg 1$, Eq. (25) reduces to

$$\psi = \Omega t + \pi/2 - \beta$$

which is the expected result for the beat frequency in the absence of backscattering coupling.

As previously noted, in the presence of backscattering coupling, the beat frequency is no longer constant, even with a constant input rate. However, the solution of Eq. (23), as given by Eq. (25), is periodic. The period of time over which ψ changes by 2π can be obtained from Eq. (25) as

$$T = 2\pi[\Omega_L(K^2 - 1)^{1/2}]^{-1} \qquad (26)$$

Using this time to define a frequency, we find

$$\Omega_b = [\Omega^2 - \Omega_L^2]^{1/2} \qquad (27)$$

This equation shows that the effective frequency difference between the oppositely directed traveling waves, defined in terms of the periodicity of the instantaneous phase difference, is reduced from the no-backscattering value due to the mutual coupling between the beams.

For values of $\Omega < \Omega_L$, the beams are frequency locked, or a constant phase difference exists between the oppositely directed beams. This results from a direct integration of Eq. (23). For the locked case, Eq. (23) predicts that the phase difference $\psi + \beta$ changes from $3\pi/2$ to zero to $\pi/2$ as Ω changes from Ω_L to zero to $-\Omega_L$, respectively.

For the case of rotations slightly above threshold, Eq. (25) becomes, for $K = 1 + \delta, \delta \ll 1$,

$$\tan \tfrac{1}{2}(\psi + \beta - \pi/2) = (2/\delta)^{1/2} \tan \Omega_L(\delta/2)^{1/2}t \qquad (28)$$

Except for times when the tangent function is approximately zero, the phase difference is $\psi + \beta = 3\pi/2$, which is the threshold value. Thus, slightly above lock-in threshold the phase remains essentially constant over a period and has a rapid jump of 2π.

The backscattering coupling effects can be illustrated with respect to Fig. 10, which shows a plot of the beat frequency as a function of rotation rate. For no backscattering, the beat frequency is just equal to the rotation rate, as represented by the 45 degree line. In the presence of backscattering, the beat frequency is given by Eq. (27) and is represented by the parabola. Note that the beat frequency is just an average value, taken over a period. As shown by Eq. (23), the instantaneous frequency varies between $\Omega \pm \Omega_L$ at all values of $\Omega > \Omega_L$. This is shown in Fig. 10 by the asymptotes $\Omega \pm \Omega_L$. For value of $\Omega \gg \Omega_L$, the beat frequency is almost uniformly varying between $\Omega \pm \Omega_L$. For values of Ω slightly above Ω_L, the system spends very little time at frequencies other than around $\Omega-\Omega_L$. Representative distorted waveforms are also shown in Fig. 10.

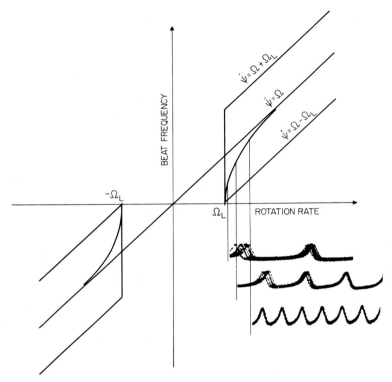

FIG. 10. Beat frequency as a function of input rate and distorted waveforms as a function of time. For rotations closer to the lock-in threshold, the waveforms become more distorted. At all rotation rates, the beat frequency ranges between $\Omega \pm \Omega_L$.

D. Scale Factor and Mode Pulling

The equation for the beat frequency in the absence of mode coupling and null shifts is given by Eq. (9) as

$$\Delta v = 4A\Omega/(\lambda L) \tag{29}$$

In Eq. (29), the A is the geometric area enclosed by the beams and L, as modified by Eq. (16), is the optical cavity length. In all applications it is necessary to know the scale factor, i.e., the relationship between the input rotation and the beat frequency. In certain applications it is necessary to have a preset scale factor, although in most cases it is enough to have any constant scale factor.

For the 0.633 μm He–Ne ring laser with an equilateral triangular resonator with 13.2 cm on a side, the scale factor is

$$\Delta\nu \quad (\text{Hz}) = 0.59 \, \Omega \quad (\text{deg/hr}) \tag{30a}$$

or

$$N \quad (\text{counts}) = 0.59 \, \theta \quad (\text{arc sec}) \tag{30b}$$

To consider the scale factor accuracy needed for a given gyro, consider an arbitrary counting time of 100 sec. Then from Eq. (30b) the number of counts is given by

$$N = 59 \, \Omega \quad (\text{deg/hr}) \tag{31}$$

For a system accuracy of 0.1 deg/hr, the count uncertainty is 6 counts. For this same count uncertainty, the scale factor must be known with increasing accuracy for higher rotation rates, or

$$\Delta s/s = \Delta\Omega/\Omega \tag{32}$$

Thus for a rotation rate of 10^4 deg/hr, the scale factor must be known and kept constant to one part in 10^5.

The difficulty in maintaining scale factor accuracy does not lie in the geometric dimensions, but rather in the index of refraction. Anomalous dispersion due to the atomic transitions causes a gain-dependent correction to the scale factor (Aronowitz, 1969). In the 1.15 μm He–Ne laser the correction is typically on the order of 10^{-2}–10^{-3}. For the high-gain 3.39 μm transition the correction causes changes on the order of the cavity length (Liu *et al.* 1969). The anomalous dispersion correction, more commonly called mode pulling, is a strong function of the operating characteristics of the laser. For a more detailed analysis, a study of the atomic transitions is necessary.

IV. Lock-In Compensation

A. REDUCTION OF BACKSCATTERING

As discussed in Section III on lock-in theory in the ring laser, the lock-in phenomenon is always to be expected, since it is not possible to completely remove all sources of coupling between the two beams.

From Eq. (24), an estimate of the lock-in threshold is given by $rc/(2\pi L)$, where L is the cavity length, c is the speed of light, and r is the fractional amplitude scattering coefficient. In current laser gyro designs, the dominant source of the backscattering is the multilayer dielectric mirror coatings. An estimate of the lock-in threshold can be made with the following assumptions.

It is assumed that a percentage r_s^2 of the light from one of the beams, when it strikes a mirror, is uniformly scattered into 4π radians. Only the part of the light which is scattered into the solid angle of the oppositely directed beam is effective in the coupling. Thus

$$(r/r_s)^2 = d\Omega/4\pi \tag{33}$$

Considering the solid angle being determined by the diffraction limit of the beam, Eq. (33) becomes

$$(r/r_s)^2 = \theta^2/16 = \lambda^2/(16d^2) \tag{34}$$

where d is the diameter of the laser beam. For the 0.633 μm He–Ne laser with a beam diameter of 0.05 cm and for mirror scattering of 0.01 % ($r_s = 10^{-2}$), Eq. (34) gives $r = 3 \times 10^{-6}$. For a total cavity length of 40 cm, the lock-in threshold is found from Eq. (24) to be approximately 300 Hz, or 500 deg/hr. This is a typical experimental value of the lock-in threshold of this type of laser gyro. The value used for the mirror scattering is within an order of magnitude of the state of the art, so much improvement is not expected from better mirrors.

An estimate of the way the lock-in threshold depends on the system parameters can be made by combining Eq. (24), (29), and (34) to give

$$\Omega_L = c\lambda^2 r_s/(32\pi Ad) \tag{35}$$

There is a weak parameter dependence in the beam diameter, but for a qualitative analysis, this can be neglected. In Eq. (35) it can be seen that lock-in threshold decreases with decreasing wavelength and increasing size of the ring laser.

With the above analysis of the backscattering coupling, lock-in thresholds will not be reduced to a sufficient degree with a more optimum design and better optical components. Some other technique must be used to overcome the dead zone.

Techniques have been proposed in which the coupling is reduced by spatially separating the two beams. However, any technique in which the two beams oscillate in separate cavities loses the major advantage of the laser gyro. Other techniques have been proposed in which the coupling is reduced by the oppositely directed beams being orthogonally polarized (de Lang, 1966; Smith and Watkins, 1962). This has not yet been accomplished. However, even if the ring laser were to operate with orthogonally polarized modes, it would be extremely difficult to get both modes to oscillate at the same cavity frequency. In passing through any optical element, residual and stress-induced birefringence will cause a null shift (Doyle and White, 1965). In addition, phase shift differences will occur on reflection (Rybakov *et al.*,

1968). Also, a three-mirror cavity will not be able to be used since the s-polarization radiation (electric field is perpendicular to the plane of incidence) picks up a phase shift of π at each reflection. Hence the set of longitudinal modes of s polarization are spaced $c/2L$ apart from the set of p-polarization (electric field in the plane of incidence) modes (Bagaev et al., 1966).

In the normal operation of the laser gyro, the laser is designed such that only one longitudinal mode (one pair of oppositely directed traveling waves) is above threshold at all times. This is to minimize mode interactions (Bershtein and Zaitser, 1966) which can give rise to spurious low-frequency oscillations and noise, and completely mask the rotation signal. In an alternate approach, to minimize the coupling between the oppositely directed beams, the ring laser has been operated with many longitudinal modes and phase-locked with an intercavity loss modulation technique (Buholz and Chodorow, 1967). When the laser was phase-locked in such a manner, the two beams traveled in pulses which were of length roughly 1/15 of the cavity length. Thus the two beams were coincident only when the pulses overlapped, and according to the proposed technique, better isolation between them could be achieved.

Preliminary experiments (Buholz and Chodorow, 1967) were performed with a 0.63 μm He–Ne laser with a cavity of length 411 cm (longitudinal mode spacing of 73 MHz). The results indicated that an improvement of approximately half an order of magnitude in lock-in threshold reduction was achieved. The improvement occurred for 14 modes being phase-locked, as opposed to operation with two modes self-locked. Lock-in threshold was reduced from $\sim$120 deg/hr to $\sim$30 deg/hr. However, from Eq. (35) for the lock-in threshold and for the size laser used, a value of twice Earth's rate could be obtained with a power backscattering of only 0.4%. With lower values of backscattering, lower lock-in thresholds should be obtainable with this size laser. Hence it is not obvious that any lock-in reduction can be obtained using the phase-locked system as opposed to the normal single-mode laser. This is in spite of the fact that the pulse crossed at points along the cavity length at which there was neither the active medium, the modulator, nor the mirrors. A possible explanation for the coupling may be that the scattering must be considered in terms of the multimode traveling waves, rather than the pulses.

B. STATIONARY NULL-SHIFT BIAS

In spite of the laser gyro having a dead zone with lock-in thresholds on the order of hundreds of degrees per hour, it is still possible to obtain measurements of rotation rates of less than 1 deg/hr. The technique used is to bias the laser gyro with an artificial input rotation such that zero rotation rate corresponds to a point well outside of the locked region. Hence at all times the system operates with a differential path and a frequency difference with respect to the oppositely directed beams.

The bias can be introduced by any technique which introduces an anisotropy in the index of refraction with respect to the oppositely directed beams. Techniques to introduce a bias are, as discussed in Section II,B on Null-Shift Errors In The Laser Gyro, flowing media, both passive (spinning wheels, flowing gases and liquids, etc.) (Macek et al., 1964; Bershtein and Zaitser, 1966) and active (Langmuir flow and cataphoresis) (Dessus et al., 1966; Podgorski and Aronowitz, 1968; Batifol and Pecile, 1966), magnetooptic nonreciprocal elements (Faraday cells) (Lee and Atwood, 1966; Hutchings et al., 1967, 1969; Macek, 1963), and additional physical rotation (Thomson and King, 1966).

The laser gyro has been applied as a northfinder (Catherin and Dessus, 1967) and a bias of ∼5 kHz has been obtained using the Langmuir flow effect in a dc discharge of 5 mA. The bias is large enough to move the beat frequency far enough away from the locked zone to ensure continual operation of the northfinder. However, for use as a gyroscope, the device would be sensitive to rotations in only one direction and would be unsatisfactory. For rotations in both directions rotations of 1–2 deg/sec would bring the laser into the highly nonlinear and even the locked region.

A bias of up to ∼35 kHz has been obtained in a 1.15 μm He–Ne laser (cavity length 220 cm) by flowing the active gas (discharge length 30 cm) at speeds up to ∼40 meters/sec. The bias is sufficiently high to operate the laser (at zero rotation rate) away from the locked region for certain applications. However the bias is not nearly high enough for most gyro applications and suffers from the serious handicap of being highly unstable. The magnitude of the bias is strongly dependent upon the flow characteristics of the gas in the tube and upon the characteristics of the discharge, i.e., the discharge current, gas mixture and gas pressure.

Experiments have been performed in which the laser was biased by a uniform mechanical rotation (Thompson and King, 1966). The rotation was stabilized to produce a constant 3.2 kHz beat frequency, corresponding to at least five times the lock-in rate.

The technique, which is probably used most often to provide a constant dc bias, is the introduction of an electrooptic nonreciprocal phase element into the cavity. As described with respect to Fig. 11, the element consists of a Faraday cell surrounded by two quarter-wave plates whose fast axes are orthogonal to one another. The wave plates are aligned such that the laser light, which is plane polarized, is incident upon the wave plates at an angle of π/4 with respect to the axis.

The heart of the nonreciprocal phase cell is the Faraday element. The

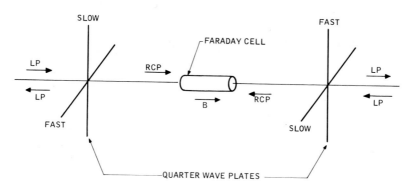

FIG. 11. Faraday cell nonreciprocal phase element. The linearly polarized light lies in the plane 45° with respect to the fast and slow quarter wave plate axis. For a positive material, the light traveling to the right sees an additional phase shift over that traveling to the left.

Faraday element is a magnetically active material (assumed positive) such that when circularly polarized light whose vector rotates in the same direction as the windings which produce the magnetic field traverse the materials an increase in optical path occurs over that which would occur if the polarization were of the opposite sense, or if the current were reversed. The additional phase is the same for light going in either direction, irrespective of the direction of the magnetic field. The results can be summarized as shown in Table I.

TABLE I

Polarization	Direction of light travel with respect to magnetic field	Additional phase
RCP	Parallel	Yes (φ)
LCP	Antiparallel	Yes (φ)
RCP	Antiparallel	No (0)
LCP	Parallel	No (0)

As described with respect to Fig. 11, the beam coming from the left is changed from linearly polarized to right circularly polarized (RCP) by the first quarter-wave plate. After passing through the Faraday element the light is still RCP but with an additional phase φ. After passing through the second wave plate the light is changed back to linear polarized light with the plane of polarization in the original direction. The beam coming from the left strikes the second wave plate and changes from linear polarized to RCP light. Since this light is now traveling antiparallel to the magnetic field, no additional phase is picked up as the light passes through the Faraday element. The first quarter-wave plate changes the light back to linear polarized light in the original plane. Note that only nonreciprocal phases have been considered. Reciprocal phase changes cancel when the phase difference is considered.

The differential phase φ is proportional to the magnetic field and the length of the cell. The proportionality constant, known as the Verdet constant, is typically on the order of 0.1 min arc/gauss/cm. The phase difference is equivalent to a path difference and from Eq. (8), gives rise to a bias frequency difference of

$$\Delta v = (c/L)\varphi/2\pi \qquad (36)$$

Hence, with reasonable magnetic field strengths, a bias on the order of 10^5–10^6 deg/hr is easily obtainable.

With such a large bias, there is the advantage of both a large input range and of minimizing scale factor nonlinearity. For example, Eq. (27) for the beat frequency can be linearized in the limit of the bias, plus input rate being much greater than the lock-in threshold, as

$$\Omega_b = \Omega[1 - \tfrac{1}{2}(\Omega_L/\Omega)^2] \qquad (37)$$

Thus, for lock-in thresholds on the order of 10^2 deg/hr and bias rates on the order of 10^5 deg/hr, scale factor linearities are obtainable which are on the order of 10^{-6}.

There are certain difficulties, other than those associated with the placement of any element in the laser cavity, which are involved with the use of such a nonreciprocal phase element. The bias rate is an effective input rate rate which must be subtracted to get useful information on the actual input rate. To get information at input rates of 0.1 deg/hr with a fixed bias of 10^5 deg/hr, a stability of 10^{-6} is needed. This implies a high degree of magnetic field stability and also thermal stability, since the Verdet constant is temperature dependent. The stability problem is the current limitation on the use of Faraday cells as fixed bias elements.

C. ALTERNATING NULL-SHIFT BIAS

A technique to overcome the bias stability problem is to operate the bias in both the positive and negative rotation rate direction (Killpatrick, 1967; Klimontovich *et al.*, 1967a), as illustrated in Fig. 5(c). The idea behind the technique is to minimize the (switching) time that the laser spends in the locked region. Since the laser gyro is basically an integrating rate gyro, only the net rotation rate appears in the output. The oscillating bias technique reduces the requirements on the absolute stability of the magnitude of the bias.

When the oscillating bias is sinusoidal, Eq. (23) for the beat frequency in the presence of backscattering coupling becomes

$$\dot{\psi} = \Omega - \Omega_L \sin{(\psi + \beta)} + \Omega_D \sin{\omega_d t} \qquad (38)$$

where Ω_D is the magnitude of the bias and ω_d is the dither rate.

In the general case, Eq. (38) cannot be solved in closed form. Computer solutions can be obtained, but they and their interpretation are complex. Figure 12 shows the resulting modification (Killpatrick, 1966) on the input–output laser gyro characteristics due to oscillating dither. The beat frequency is nonzero in the locked region and passes through zero rotation rate uniformly. A computer solution of Eq. (38) showing the scale factor deviation is given in Fig. 13 for a lock-in threshold of 300 deg/hr and a bias amplitude of 200,000 deg/hr. Above the bias amplitude rate, the scale factor deviation is identical to the deviation obtained in the absence of bias, as given by Eq. (37). Below the bias amplitude, the scale factor deviation is a positive constant which decreases with decreasing ratio of the lock-in threshold to bias amplitude. The analysis shows that the bias amplitude should be greater than the lock-in

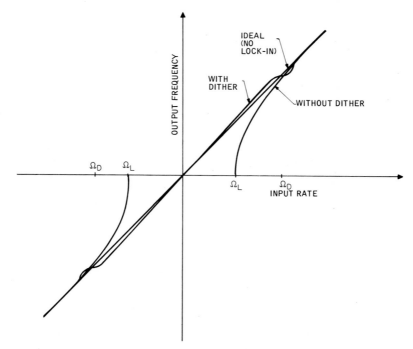

FIG. 12. Input–output laser gyro characteristics with dither, showing a smooth transition through the locked region. From Killpatrick (1966).

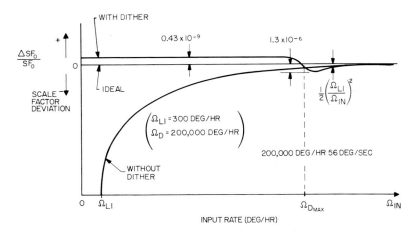

FIG. 13. Scale factor linearity with oscillating bias. The constant scale factor is the ideal case of no lock-in. Without dither the scale factor goes to zero, as given by Eq. (37). With dither, the scale factor is a constant (slightly greater than in the ideal case) for all rates below the maximum dither rate. Above the maximum dither rate, the scale factor is given by Eq. (37). From Killpatrick (1966).

threshold, and for minimum scale factor fluctuation, the ratio of the latter to the former should be as large as possible.

All the techniques discussed in the Section IV,B can be used to obtain an alternating bias. With respect to the choice of technique, one basic point should be kept in mind. The basic premise in the alternating bias technique is that the bias is perfectly symmetric. Any asymmetry will result in an effective net rotation per bias cycle and a dc drift term.

One bias technique avoids this problem. In mechanical bias, no long-term accumulated drift can occur since the motion is physically bounded. In addition, mechanical bias has another basic advantage. With the introduction of a large bias, high counting rate circuits and megahertz bandwidth electronics are needed. In mechanical bias, it is possible to design the readout system such that the motion of the fringe pattern due to the bias is compensated by the mechanical bias motion (Killpatrick, 1966). Hence bias counts are not detected and smaller bandwidth circuitry can be used.

The choice of the bias is one of the most important design questions in the laser gyro. Techniques are still highly proprietary, and new and better techniques are still being sought. It should be emphasized, however, that the lock-in problem is no longer as formidable as it was when originally investigated. Alternating bias techniques allow measurement of rotation rates of zero (to within an error, of course, which is currently less than 0.1 deg/hr). The problem has been shifted to the design of techniques which both minimize dc null shift errors and are economical enough to allow the laser gyro to compete on the market with more conventional gyroscopes.

A simple alternating mechanical bias for experimental purposes can be obtained by mounting the laser on a spring-mounted granite block and operating the entire system as a torsional pendulum. This was done (Carruthers, 1964) with a 0.633 μm He–Ne laser with an equilateral triangular cavity of one meter on a side (giving a scale factor of 3.7 counts/arc sec). Figure 14

ONE COUNT =0.27 ARC SEC I"=10⁻³ SECONDS

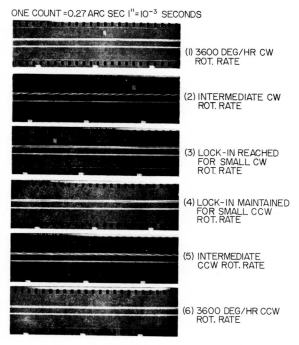

(1) 3600 DEG/HR CW
ROT. RATE

(2) INTERMEDIATE CW
ROT. RATE

(3) LOCK-IN REACHED
FOR SMALL CW
ROT. RATE

(4) LOCK-IN MAINTAINED
FOR SMALL CCW
ROT. RATE

(5) INTERMEDIATE
CCW ROT. RATE

(6) 3600 DEG/HR CCW
ROT. RATE

FIG. 14. Streak camera recording of fringe pattern motion for dithered laser gyro. The fringe motion is in the vertical direction. The slope of the fringes changes with changing the direction of rotation. Larger slopes signify larger rotation rates. From Carruthers (1964).

shows the motion of the fringe pattern at various rotation rates. The position of the visible fringes was recorded with a streak camera in such a manner that the film was moving in the horizontal direction while the horizontal fringes were moving in the vertical direction. This produced the twisted rope appearance shown, where the density of crossings, or slope, is proportional to the beat frequency. Successive fringes correspond to an angle of rotation of 0.27 seconds of arc. Figure 15 shows the output rotation of the laser as a

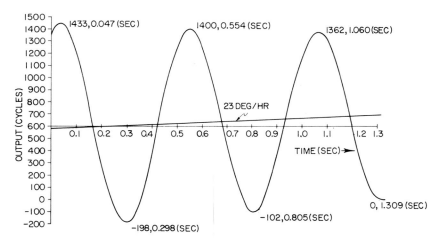

Fig. 15. Laser gyro rotation angle with dither. The data shown here was obtained from streak camera recordings, as shown in Fig. 14. The data points lie within the line thickness. The data shows the feasibility of measuring small inputs which are much less than the lock-in threshold.

function of time, as determined from the counting of fringes. The data covered a time span of ~1.1 sec and ~100 ft of film. The data points are within the thickness of the line. From the data, the maximum input was ~2000 deg/hr and even though the lock-in threshold was several hundred degrees per hour, a constant input rate of ~23 deg/hr was detected. This included the normal component of Earth's rate (10 deg/hr) plus a small null shift due to the fact that a single dc excited gain tube was used. The dither compensation scheme mentioned previously was not employed in obtaining this data. If it had been used, it would have removed the sinusoidal variation of the output phase angle shown in Fig. 15, leaving only the true buildup of phase angle due to the constant input rate that was present. Figure 16 shows the results of a 2-hour drift run (Killpatrick, 1966) where mechanical bias and compensation was used. The laser was operated on the He–Ne 1.15 μm transition and had a cavity length of 54 cm, giving a scale factor of 0.44 count/ arc sec. The results show, as expected, a continual buildup of counts due to the rotation of Earth. Actually, only the component of rotation normal to the surface at the experimental site was measured. This value of 11 deg/hr can be seen to correspond to the slope of the curve in Fig. 16, i.e., 4.7 counts/ sec divided by 0.44 count/arc sec gives 11 arc sec/sec. It should be noted that the lock-in threshold on this laser was ~2000 deg/hr. For this size laser and for the transition used, this value of lock-in threshold corresponds to that calculated from Eq. (35) for a mirror scattering of 0.05%.

The results shown in Fig. 16 are typical of those obtained with the laser

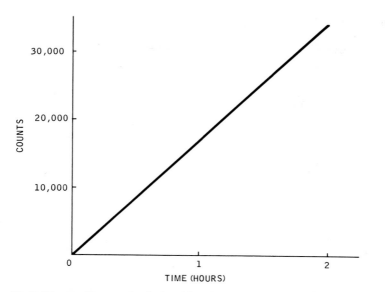

Fig. 16. Drift run with a mechanical ac bias. Automatic compensation was used such that no bias counts were detected. From Killpatrick (1966).

gyro. They show the potential of using the instrument for inertial grade applications in spite of the large lock-in thresholds.

The alternating bias technique allows the laser to remain unlocked over most of the dither cycle, and hence the gyro is responsive to any nonzero input rate. Cancellation of the bias dither electronically or automatically then allows the determination of the input. The errors which are inherent in the biasing technique are minimized with symmetry of the bias and increasing the percentage of time per dither cycle that the system is unlocked. Hence, an ideal ac bias scheme would use a perfectly symmetric square wave dither with as large a bias rate as possible and with as small a lock-in threshold as possible. In practice, compromises are made.

V. Dispersion Properties of the Active Medium

A. Distinction between Ring and Linear Lasers

In the investigation of the He–Ne laser, the model introduced by Lamb (1964) has met with much success in explaining experimental results. In Lamb's semiclassical self-consistent approach, an electromagnetic field is assumed to exist in the cavity. The electromagnetic field polarizes the moving atoms. A macroscopic polarization results, which is then used as a source term in Maxwell's equations to calculate a reaction field. The self-consistency gives rise to a set of equations which describes the amplitude and frequencies of the oscillating modes.

Lamb's linear laser theory has been generalized to account for the behavior of ring lasers by a number of authors (Aronowitz, 1965, 1969; Zhelnov et al., 1966; Klimontovich et al., 1967a; Raterink et al., 1967; Heer, 1964a; Gyorffy, 1966; Whitney, 1969b; Zeiger and Fradkin, 1966). In Lamb's treatment of a standing wave linear laser, the empty cavity normal mode eigenfunctions were chosen as a set of standing waves. In the ring laser, where the electromagnetic field is more realistically described by sets of oppositely directed traveling waves, it is then necessary to represent the empty cavity normal mode eigenfunctions by oppositely directed traveling waves. The treatment then follows that given by Lamb, with two exceptions.

The basic distinction between the ring laser theory and the linear laser theory is that in the ring laser the number of degrees of freedom of the system are doubled. This is due to the independence of the oppositely directed traveling waves. This leads to twice as many equations and added complexity in the analysis. In the simplest case of a single-mode (linearly polarized) ring laser, there are four equations describing the amplitudes and frequencies of each beam. In the limit of the amplitudes and frequencies being equal the four equations reduce to two equations that are identical to those given by Lamb for the description of a standing wave laser.

For the case of a ring laser in the presence of a magnetic field (Heer and Graft, 1965), eight equations are needed to describe the radiation of both polarizations. No analysis of the equations has been reported and very few experimental results (Burrell et al., 1968; Hutchings et al., 1969) have been published on the effects of magnetic fields on the dispersion properties of the active medium of the ring laser.

The second major distinction between the linear laser and the ring laser is the mode coupling problem. The self-consistent single-mode ring laser equations have been modified to account for the mutual backscattering coupling of energy from each of the beams into the direction of the other. As discussed in Section III,C, the backscattering coupling can, for the case of a rotating laser, modulate the frequency of each traveling wave at the beat frequency rate. At a critical backscattering magnitude, the two waves can be frequency synchronized. In addition, the backscattering has also been shown to modulate the amplitudes of the intensities of each wave at the beat frequency rate (Fenster and Kahn, 1966).

A second type of coupling between the oppositely directed beams can occur through the gain medium. For the case of homogeneous type transitions, the coupling is strong and when asymmetries occur between the two beams, mode competition occurs and only one traveling wave oscillates (Tang et al., 1964; Hercher et al., 1965; Rigrod and Bridges, 1965; Bass et al., 1968; Mocker, 1968). For the case of (predominantly) inhomogeneously broadened transitions, the coupling is ususally weak such that oscillation occurs in both directions (Macek and Davis, 1963). However, strong asymmetries can occur such that one of the traveling waves can be appreciably reduced in amplitude and even quenched (Lee and Atwood, 1966; Aronowitz and Collins, 1966; Hutchings et al., 1967). The assymmetry can be caused by a differential loss between the two directions (asymmetric scattering or a magnetooptic interaction) or a differential gain (frequency splitting due to anisotropic path length caused by rotation, Langmuir flow, Fresnel loss effects, Faraday effects, etc.). The mechanism for the competition is the gain medium. Oscillation of each mode results in gain saturation. The saturation extends over a large range of the atomic transition. Saturation due to the stronger mode can reduce the gain of the weaker below threshold such that it will not oscillate (Aronowitz, 1965).

Analysis has shown that for the single-mode low-gain He–Ne laser, the gain coupling is not of the type to cause locking effects (Aronowitz, 1965). For the single-mode case, combination tones, which could be generated by the nonlinear polarization (Lamb, 1964), do not exist at frequencies close to the oscillating frequencies. For the two-mode case, combination tones are generated such that the beat frequency at each mode is locked to a common value (Aronowitz, 1968).

B. RING LASER MODEL

The self-consistent treatment of the laser comprises two parts (Aronowitz, 1965, 1969). In the first part, Maxwell's equations (one dimensional with periodic boundary conditions) are expressed on a rotating frame (Heer, 1964b; Post and Yildiz; 1965; Yildiz and Tang, 1966; Khromykh, 1966). The wave equation is then obtained as

$$-\frac{1}{\varepsilon_0 \mu_0}\frac{\partial^2 E}{\partial z^2} + \frac{\omega}{Q}\frac{\partial E}{\partial t} + \frac{\partial^2 E}{\partial t^2} + \frac{a}{\varepsilon_0 \mu_0}\frac{\partial^2 E}{\partial z\,\partial t} = \frac{\omega^2 P}{\varepsilon_0} - \frac{\sigma_s}{\varepsilon_0}\frac{\partial E_s}{\partial t} \tag{39}$$

In the model it is assumed that the losses, averaged over the cavity length, can be expressed in terms of the passive Q of the cavity as

$$\sigma/\varepsilon_0 = \omega/Q$$

The cross term is proportional to the rotation (Ω) of the laser and is given by

$$a = 4A\Omega/(Lc^2) \tag{40}$$

where L is the cavity length and A is the area enclosed by the light. Only terms linear in a have been included, and since the macroscopic polarization is nearly monochromatic, the second time derivative of P has been replaced by $-\omega^2 P$. The last term on the right-hand side of Eq. (39) represents the effects of backscattering coupling, and E_s represents the backscattering field.

The solution of the wave equation is obtained by expanding the field into the set of empty-cavity normal mode eigenfunctions

$$E(z, t) = \sum_n [A_n(t)U_n(z) + \tilde{A}_n(t)V_n(z)] \tag{41}$$

with

$$U_n(z) = \sin K_n z \tag{42a}$$

$$V_n(z) = \cos K_n z \tag{42b}$$

$$K_n = 2\pi n/L \tag{42c}$$

The empty-cavity normal mode eigenfunctions satisfy the equation

$$\left[\frac{d^2}{dz^2} + \varepsilon_0 \mu_0 \Omega_n{}^2\right] \begin{pmatrix} U_n(z) \\ V_n(z) \end{pmatrix} = 0 \tag{43}$$

and by separation of variables, the set of coupled equations for the time-dependent coefficients of the empty-cavity normal-mode eigenfunctions are

$$\frac{d^2 A_n}{dt^2} + \frac{\omega}{Q_n}\frac{dA_n}{dt} + \Omega_n{}^2 A_n - ac^2 K_n \frac{d\tilde{A}_n}{dt} = \frac{\omega^2}{\varepsilon_0} P_n - \frac{\sigma_s}{\varepsilon_0}\frac{d}{dt} E_{sn} \tag{44a}$$

$$\frac{d^2 \tilde{A}_n}{dt^2} + \frac{\omega}{Q_n}\frac{d\tilde{A}_n}{dt} + \Omega_n{}^2 \tilde{A}_n + ac^2 K_n \frac{dA_n}{dt} = \frac{\omega^2}{\varepsilon_0} \tilde{P}_n - \frac{\sigma_s}{\varepsilon_0}\frac{d}{dt} \tilde{E}_{sn} \tag{44b}$$

where the P_n and E_{sn} are the respective Fourier components of the empty-cavity normal-mode eigenfunctions.

The A coefficients are expressed in terms of slowly varying time-dependent coefficients and are in the form such as to reduce to two oppositely directed traveling waves in an empty cavity, or

$$A_n(t) = E_{1n}(t) \cos \theta_{1n} + E_{2n}(t) \cos \theta_{2n} \tag{45a}$$

$$\tilde{A}_n(t) = E_{1n}(t) \sin \theta_{1n} - E_{2n}(t) \sin \theta_{2n} \tag{45b}$$

where

$$\theta_{in} = \omega_{in} t + \varphi_{in}(t) \qquad i = 1, 2. \tag{45c}$$

The Fourier components of the polarization are then written as an "in phase" and "in quadrature" term with respect to frequency "one," or

$$P_n(t) = S_{1n}(t) \sin \theta_{1n} + C_{1n}(t) \cos \theta_{1n} \tag{46a}$$

$$\tilde{P}_n(t) = \tilde{S}_{1n}(t) \sin \theta_{1n} + \tilde{C}_{1n}(t) \cos \theta_{1n} \tag{46b}$$

To represent the Fourier components of the scattering field, it is assumed that a fraction r_i of the fields E_i are scattered back into the direction of the other beam with an additional phase angle ε_i, or

$$E_2(\omega_2 t + \varphi_2) \longleftarrow \qquad \longrightarrow E_1(\omega_1 t + \varphi_1)$$

$$r_1 E_1(\omega_1 t + \varphi_1 + \varepsilon_1) \quad \longleftarrow \quad \longrightarrow r_2 E_2(\omega_2 t + \varphi_2 + \varepsilon_2)$$

Then the Fourier components of the backscattering fields can be written as

$$E_{sn} = r_{1n} E_{1n} \cos(\theta_{1n} + \varepsilon_{1n}) + r_{2n} E_{2n} \cos(\theta_{2n} + \varepsilon_{2n}) \tag{47a}$$

$$\tilde{E}_{sn} = -r_{1n} E_{1n} \sin(\theta_{1n} + \varepsilon_{1n}) + r_{2n} E_{2n} \sin(\theta_{2n} + \varepsilon_{2n}) \tag{47b}$$

Substituting Eqs. (45)–(47) into Eq. (44) and equating coefficients of $\sin \theta_{1n}$ and $\cos \theta_{1n}$ to zero, the four equations for the amplitudes and frequencies of the oppositely directed beams of each mode are obtained as

$$\dot{E}_{1n} + (\omega/2Q_n)E_{1n} = (\omega/4\varepsilon_0)(\tilde{C}_{1n} - S_{1n}) - (\sigma_s/2)r_{2n} E_{2n} \cos(\psi_n + \varepsilon_{2n}) \tag{48a}$$

$$\dot{E}_{2n} + (\omega/2Q_n)E_{2n} = (\omega/4\varepsilon_0)[(\tilde{S}_{1n} - C_{1n}) \sin \psi_n - (S_{1n} + \tilde{C}_{1n}) \cos \psi_n]$$
$$- (\sigma_s/2\varepsilon_0)r_{1n} E_{1n} \cos(\psi_n - \varepsilon_{1n}) \tag{48b}$$

$$(\Omega_{1n} - \dot{\theta}_{1n})E_{1n} = (\omega/4\varepsilon_0)(C_{1n} + \tilde{S}_{1n}) + (\sigma_s/2\varepsilon_0)r_{2n} E_{2n} \sin(\psi_n + \varepsilon_{2n}) \tag{48c}$$

$$(\Omega_{2n} - \dot{\theta}_{2n})E_{2n} = (\omega/4\varepsilon_0)[(C_{1n} - \tilde{S}_{1n}) \cos \psi_n - (S_{1n} + \tilde{C}_{1n}) \sin \psi_n] \tag{48d}$$
$$- (\sigma_s/2\varepsilon_0)r_{1n} E_{1n} \sin(\psi_n - \varepsilon_{1n})$$

where

$$\psi_n = \theta_{2n} - \theta_{1n} = (\omega_2 - \omega_1)t + (\varphi_2 - \varphi_1) \tag{48e}$$

is a slowly varying function of time.

In Eqs. (48c) and (48d) the empty-cavity frequencies Ω_n have been replaced by Ω_{in}, where

$$\Omega_{2n} = \Omega_n + \tfrac{1}{2}aK_n c^2 \tag{49a}$$

$$\Omega_{1n} = \Omega_n - \tfrac{1}{2}aK_n c^2 \tag{49b}$$

Equations (48) are the basic ring laser equations for the amplitudes and frequencies of each mode. The empty-cavity mode splitting is given by Eq. (49) and is seen to agree with Eq. (9). The dispersive effects of the active medium are expressed in terms of the Fourier component of the polarization.

The calculations of Fourier components of the polarization is the second part of the calculation. It is assumed that the electric field exists in the cavity and polarizes the atoms. The calculation uses quantum mechanics and density matrix concepts. A perturbation treatment is used in that the density matrix is expanded on powers of the interaction (Lamb, 1964). Hence the treatment is most valid for the case of low gain systems (Stenholm and Lamb, 1969) and even then, for the case of single-mode operation. Ring laser calculations have been made with the inclusion of terms up to the fifth power in the electric field (Klimontovich et al., 1967b). For a qualitative analysis of the dispersion effects, third-order theory is sufficient. Fifth-order terms are necessary for stability investigation (Klimontovich et al., 1967b).

C. Backscattering Contributions to the Self-Consistent Equations

In the analysis of the self-consistent equations, it can be seen that there are terms on the right-hand side of Eqs. (48) which are independent of the gain medium. These are the backscattering terms and they modify the properties of the empty passive cavity. It can be seen that by substituting Eqs. (48c) and (48d) into the derivative of Eq. (48e) and neglecting the polarization terms, we obtain the beat frequency equation

$$\dot{\psi} = \Omega + \sigma_s/2\varepsilon_0[r_2(E_2/E_1)\sin(\psi + \varepsilon_2) + r_1(E_1/E_2)\sin(\psi - \varepsilon_1)] \quad (50)$$

where Ω is the cavity splitting due to rotation. Equation (50) is identical to the lock-in Eq. (23), which was derived using only backscattering in one direction, with the association of the backscattering conductivity as

$$\sigma_s/2\varepsilon_0 = c/L$$

Thus the lock-in phenomenon has been formally obtained and shown to be (to first order) independent of the gain media. Of course the gain media is necessary for the laser in the first place and the backscattering results from laser energy which would otherwise be lost, being scattered back into the cavity. However, this becomes a matter of semantics. The important fact is that there are no gain terms, to first order, in the lock-in term in Eq. (50).

To higher order, the gain dependence comes in two ways. For low-gain systems, there is a strong gain dependence through the factor that expresses the ratio of the electric field intensity. This will be discussed more thoroughly in Section IV,B.

The second way in which gain dependence arises is through the polarization (Klimontovich et al., 1967a; Tang and Statz, 1967; Aronowitz, 1969). In the self-consistent treatment used in deriving Eq. (48), it was assumed that the backscattering fields exist and are treated as source terms in Maxwell's equations. However, they were not considered to aid in the polarization of the atoms. If they were, additional backscattering coupling terms would arise that are proportional to the gain. For low-gain systems such as the He–Ne 0.633 or 1.15 μm transitions ($g \sim 0.01$–0.1), these terms are one to two orders of magnitude smaller than the terms shown in Eq. (50). For high-gain systems such as the He–Ne 3.39 μm transition, these "higher order" gain terms are large enough such that the approximate backscattering model used in deriving Eqs. (48) breaks down. For a rough estimate of the lock-in threshold for the 3.39 μm laser, it would probably be sufficient to replace the backscattering coefficient r by $r \exp(g)$.

It should be noted that in some treatments of lock-in, the lowest order contribution, as shown in Eqs. (48) has been neglected (Klimontovich et al., 1967a; Tang and Statz, 1967). The first-order lock-in term then contains a gain (or loss) factor and predicts much lower lock-in thresholds than those that are experimentally obtained.

D. First-Order Theory—Threshold Operation and Mode Pulling

Using first-order perturbation theory (Lamb, 1964), the Fourier components of the polarization have been calculated (Aronowitz, 1965, 1969) with the following assumptions. The laser is low gain and the active medium is a gas. The transition is broadened due to the Doppler motion of the atoms and due to the finite lifetime of the states. Only collisions which abruptly change the phase of the emitting atoms are considered (Szoke and Javan, 1963, 1966). Soft collisions which affect the velocity distribution and phase shifts leading to asymmetry and energy shifts are not considered (Szoke and Javan, 1963, 1966; Fork and Pollack, 1965).

The self-consistent Eqs. (48) are found to be (neglecting the backscattering terms for brevity)

$$(2L/c)\dot{E}_j/E_j = \alpha_j \tag{51}$$

$$\omega_j + \dot{\phi}_j = \Omega_j + \sigma_j \qquad j = 1, 2 \tag{52}$$

where

$$\alpha_j = GZ_i(\xi_j)/Z_i(0) - \gamma_j \tag{53}$$

$$\sigma_j = [c/(2L)]GZ_r(\xi_j)/Z_i(0) \tag{54}$$

As in the case of the linear laser, the first-order theory gives the threshold conditions. Equation (51) shows that the threshold condition for each beam is independent of the other. From Eq. (53), α_j is the gain minus the loss for each beam. Z_i and Z_r are the imaginary and real parts, respectively, of the plasma dispersion function (Fried and Conte, 1961)

$$Z(\xi) = 2i \int_0^\infty \exp(-x^2 - 2\eta x + 2i\xi x)\, dx \tag{55}$$

where $\xi_i = (\omega_i - \omega_d)/Ku$ is a measure of the deviation of the oscillation frequency from the center frequency ω_d and $\eta = \gamma_{ab}/Ku$ is the relative value of the homogeneous broadening (natural plus collision width) to the Doppler broadening.

For the case of $\eta \ll 1$ an expansion of Eq. (55) gives

$$Z_i(\xi) = \sqrt{\pi} \exp(-\xi^2) - 2\eta[1 - 2\xi F(\xi)] + 0(\eta^2) \tag{56a}$$

$$Z_r(\xi) = -2F(\xi) + \sqrt{\pi}\, \xi \eta \exp(-\xi^2) + 0(\eta^2) \tag{56b}$$

with $F(\xi)$ given by

$$F(\xi) = \exp(-\xi^2) \int_0^\xi \exp x^2 \, dx \tag{56c}$$

$$\cong \xi(1 - 2\xi^2/3) \qquad \xi \ll 1. \tag{56d}$$

From Eqs. (52) and (54), it can be seen that the oscillation frequency is pulled from the empty-cavity frequency by the term σ, which is a measure of the anomalous dispersion of the active medium. The pulling is zero at the line center and increases with increasing detuning of the frequency from the center frequency. The pulling is always toward the line center.

What is of interest in the ring laser is not so much the pulling of both oscillations, but the difference in pulling. Thus an equation for the scale factor, analogous to Eq. (13), can be obtained from Eqs. (52) and (54) as

$$\dot{\psi} = \Omega \left\{ 1 + \left(\frac{c}{2L}\right)\left(\frac{G}{Ku}\right)\frac{Z_r'(\xi)}{Z_i(0)}\left[1 + \frac{1}{24}\left(\frac{\Omega}{Ku}\right)^2 \frac{Z_r'''(\xi)}{Z_r'(\xi)}\right]\right\} \tag{57}$$

In Eq. (57), the difference between the dispersion functions Z_r for each beam was obtained using a Taylor expansion (to cubic terms) about the average frequency $\xi = 1/2(\xi_1 + \xi_2)$. The frequency difference was written as $\xi_2 - \xi_1 = \Omega/Ku$. Thus it can be seen that the scale factor contains nonlinear terms. These terms are negligible, even for extremely high rotations. For rotation rates of 10^6 deg/hr, the scale factor correction is 10^{-9}. However, the first-order dispersion correction is not negligible.

The derivative of the dispersion curve, Z_r', is a bell-shaped curve opening upward and $Z_r' < 0$ over most of the operating range. Thus the scale factor is reduced from the empty cavity value. Near line center the reduction for the He–Ne 1.15 μm and 0.633 μm ring laser is 8×10^{-3} for a gain of 5 and 1%, respectively.

Figure 17 shows the scale factor as a function of tuning the length of a He–Ne 1.15 μm ring laser of cavity length 40 cm (Killpatrick, 1966). The data was taken by simultaneously mechanically dithering the gyro with a maximum input rate of 60 deg/sec and rotating uniformly at a rate of 40 deg/sec. The counts due to the dither were automatically compensated. The gain was approximately 1%, which when substituted into Eq. (57) gives a maximum scale factor change of 1.6×10^{-3}. This is in agreement with the data in Fig. 17.

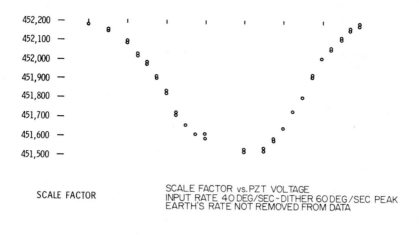

FIG. 17. Scale factor as a function of laser oscillation frequency in the He–Ne 1.15μm ring laser. A 1 : 1 mixture of ^{20}Ne : ^{22}Ne was used. The maximum output power lies at the minimum scale factor point. From Killpatrick (1966).

The analysis of the effect of the anomalous dispersion of the active medium on the scale factor shows the need for accurately controlling the cavity length. Standard-length control techniques (White, 1965) can be used to stabilize the laser frequency to the maximum of the power versus length tuning curve. This will ensure a constant scale factor with a value determined by the maximum differential mode-pulling correction. For systems with a need for an exact predetermined scale factor, this correction must be compensated for in the length design.

E. Second-Order Theory—Hole Burning

A second-order perturbation calculation (Lamb, 1964) gives the population inversion (averaged over the cavity length) as a function of the velocity distribution of the gas as (Aronowitz, 1965, 1969)

$$\Delta\rho(v) = \overline{N}W(v)[1 - 2I_1 \mathcal{L}(\xi_1 + v/u) - 2I_2 \mathcal{L}(\xi_2 - v/u)] \qquad (58)$$

The dimensionless intensity of each beam is

$$I_i = |\mu_{ab}|^2 E_i^2 / 2\hbar^2 \gamma_a \gamma_b \qquad (59)$$

where μ_{ab} is the electric dipole matrix element between the laser states and γ_a and γ_b are the decay rates of the two states. In Eq. (58) the Lorentzian function is defined as

$$\mathfrak{L}(x) = [1 + (x/\eta)^2]^{-1} \tag{60}$$

Equation (58) shows the saturated velocity distribution $\Delta\rho(v)$ to be equal to the unsaturated distribution $NW(v)$ with two Lorentzian holes (Bennett, 1962, 1964) "burnt" into the curve. The depth of each hole is determined by the strength of each beam and the width by the natural plus collision width. Except when the oscillation frequency is very close to line center, the holes are located on opposite sides of the velocity distribution. Hence both beams draw upon essentially different gain atoms.

To see this, consider the case of the oscillation frequency being less than the center frequency. Then for any atom to iteract with the radiation it must see the radiation as being resonance radiation in its own frame, and hence doppler shifted up in frequency. Thus each beam interacts with atoms moving toward the direction from which the beam is coming. The velocity spread is determined by the uncertainty principle.

F. THIRD-ORDER THEORY—GAIN SATURATION AND MODE PUSHING

A third-order perturbation calculation (Lamb, 1964) for the polarization brings in the effects of saturation on the dispersion properties of the active medium. The self-consistent equations for beam "one" are found to be (with the inclusion of the backscattering terms in ρ) (Aronowitz, 1965, 1969)

$$(2L/c)\dot{E}_1/E_1 = \alpha_1 - \beta_1 I_1 - \theta_{12} I_2 - 2\rho_2 \cos(\psi + \varepsilon_2) \tag{61a}$$

$$(2L/c)\dot{E}_2/E_2 = \alpha_2 - \beta_2 I_2 - \theta_{21} I_1 - 2\rho_1 \cos(\psi - \varepsilon_1) \tag{61b}$$

$$\omega_1 + \dot{\phi}_1 - \Omega_1 = \sigma_1 + \tau_{12} I_2 - (c/L)\rho_2 \sin(\psi + \varepsilon_2) \tag{62a}$$

$$\omega_2 + \dot{\phi}_2 - \Omega_2 = \sigma_2 + \tau_{21} I_1 - (c/L)\rho_1 \sin(\varepsilon_1 - \psi) \tag{62b}$$

where the new terms are given by

$$\beta_1 = GZ_i(\xi_1)/Z_i(0) \tag{63}$$

$$\theta_{12} = GZ_i(\xi_2)\,\mathfrak{L}(\xi)/Z_i(0) \tag{64}$$

$$\tau_{12} = [c/(2L)](\xi/\eta)GZ_i(\xi_1)\,\mathfrak{L}(\xi)/Z_i(0) \tag{65}$$

$$\rho_2 = r_2 E_2/E_1 \tag{66a}$$

$$\rho_1 = r_1 E_1/E_2 \tag{66b}$$

Analogous equations hold for the other constants and the other terms are as defined previously.

In the amplitude equations, the β_i terms show gain saturation for each beam on itself due to hole burning, and the θ_{ij} terms show gain saturation for each beam due to hole burning by the other beam. In the frequency equations, the τ_{ij} terms show a mode pushing correction to the oscillation frequency due to the hole burning correction in the dispersion curve. The correction results in a Lorentzian dispersion curve centered at each oscillation frequency with the opposite sign of the Gaussian dispersion curve which is due to the gain curve. Hence the nomenclature " mode pushing." Since the dispersion curves are odd functions a beam cannot mode push on itself.

The beat frequency equation obtained from Eqs. (62a and b) now becomes

$$(L/c)\dot{\psi} = \Omega' + \tau'_{21}I_1 - \tau'_{12}I_2 + \rho_2 \sin(\psi + \varepsilon_2) + \rho_1 \sin(\psi - \varepsilon_1) \qquad (67)$$

where Ω' and τ' signify a removal of the factor L/c, and Ω' contains the mode pulling terms, as discussed with respect to Eq. (57).

As previously discussed, the terms in ρ give rise to the frequency synchronization effect. The terms in τ give rise to a lock-in contribution, a null shift, and a scale factor correction. This can be seen most quickly if the system is considered to be locked. Then the term in τ_{ij} in Eq. (67) can be eliminated by solving the amplitude equations [given by Eq. (61)] for I_1 and I_2. The resulting terms in ρ_i contribute to the lock-in terms in ρ_i in Eq. (67). A seen from Eq. (53), the terms in α_i contain a loss term. If there is a loss difference for the two beams, the resulting term is equivalent to a null shift. The remainder of the terms give rise to a small-scale factor correction. The mode pushing correction is an order of magnitude smaller than the mode pulling correction.

With respect to the operation of the laser gyro, differential loss null shift is by far the most important part of the differential mode pushing term. For the simple case of the coefficients being symmetric with respect to the two beams, the null shift is

$$\Omega_N = (\gamma_2 - \gamma_1)\tau/(\beta - \theta) \qquad (68)$$

Substituting values of the coefficients from Eqs. (63)–(65) the null-shift bias is found to be

$$\Omega_N = (\gamma_2 - \gamma_1)[c/(2L)](\xi/\eta) \, \mathfrak{L}/(1 - \mathfrak{L}) \qquad (69a)$$

or

$$\Omega_N = (\gamma_2 - \gamma_1)[c/(2L)](\eta/\xi) \qquad (69b)$$

The null shift is found to be a dispersion-type curve, symmetrically located about the peak of the power versus oscillation frequency curve and is proportional to the differential loss. In the transition from Eq. (68) to Eqs.

(69a and b), one of the approximations made in deriving the self-consistent equations becomes of importance. The fact that the effects of "soft collisions" were neglected allows the maximum value of the Lorentzian factor to have the value unity. From measurements of the Lamb dip (McFarlane *et al.*, 1963) in power tuning experiments (Szoke and Javan, 1963, 1966) and from analysis (Gyorffy *et al.*, 1968), the effects of soft collisions cause the Lorentzian to have a wider width and to have pressure dependent amplitude reduction factors. This will eliminate the singularity in Eq. (69b).

Since Lamb dip experiments are sensitive to the factor $(1 + \Gamma \mathcal{L})$ (Γ is the pressure-dependent reduction factor) and the null shift is sensitive to $1 - \Gamma \mathcal{L}$ null shift experiments using the ring laser will be more sensitive to collision effects.

G. MODE COMPETITION AND TWO-ISOTOPE SYSTEM

Ring laser power tuning curves are different from those obtained with linear lasers in that competition between the two oppositely directed traveling waves can occur. For the active medium being composed of a single isotope, the two holes in the gain curve overlap as the oscillation frequency is tuned toward the center frequency. At the center frequency both beams are drawing upon the same gain atoms and any asymmetries in the system can cause extinction of one of the beams. Analysis (Aronowitz, 1965) of the third-order self-consistent amplitude equations shows that the two beams can coexist with a high degree of hole overlap.

Figure 18 shows power tuning curves (Aronowitz, 1971) for various gain excitations for a He–Ne (99.99% ^{20}Ne) ring laser of cavity length 43.1 cm (696 MHz mode spacing). At the center of the Lamb dip, over a range of ~9 MHz, strong mode competition occurs between the two beams. The data was taken with a ring laser with internal mirrors and nothing, other than an aperture, in the cavity. The total gas pressure was ~0.5 Torr. The width of the competition region was found to increase with increasing pressure and poorer quality mirrors. At maximum competition, extinction of the ccw beam did not occur. Figure 19 is a magnification of one of the center competition regions shown in Fig. 18. It was found that with the laser stationary (rotating at 11 deg/hr) the system was unlocked over a portion of the competition region. Similar results have been found by other workers (Hutchings *et al.*, 1967; Heer, 1964a; Lisitsyn and Troshin, 1967). The unlocking occurred as the laser, which was being tuned in the direction of decreasing frequency, was tuned just past the extremum point. As the tuning from the extremum point increased, the amplitude of the ac bias signal modulating the output power increased. The frequency started at a maximum and decreased until the

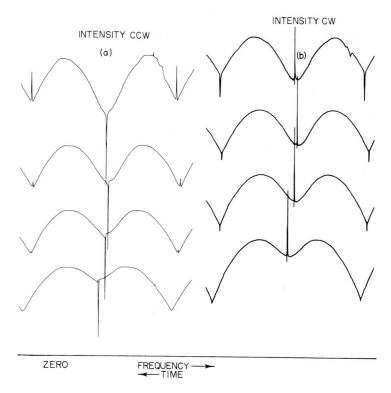

FIG. 18. Power tuning curves for various gain excitation for the He–Ne 0.633 μm ring laser. The ^{20}Ne isotope concentration was 99.99 %, the total gas pressure 0.5 Torr and mode spacing was 696 MHz. (a) The ccw beam; (b) shows the cw beam. At the center of the Lamb dip a strong mode competition strike occurred. Smaller mode competition was found for the case of two longitudinal modes being symmetrically spaced about the doppler center. Mode competition occurred between successive longitudinal modes such that only one mode oscillated (both traveling waves) at all times. Except for the competition spikes, Fig. 18 shows single mode data. The scale for each beam is only approximately the same. From Aronowitz (1971).

system locked, which occurred at the jump point. For each beam, the oscillations were out of phase by π.

The complete mechanism for the bias is not yet completely clear and more work is needed. There is some thought that the origin lies in the coupling of energy from one direction into the other by backscattering. However, according to the self-consistent amplitude and frequency equations given by Eqs. (61) and (62), backscattering coupling increases the lock-in threshold and

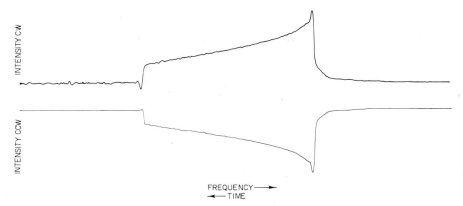

Fɪɢ. 19. Blow-up of center competition region from Fig. 18. From Aronowitz (1971).

reduces the possibility of bias beats. If, however, the backscattering were asymmetric for the twò directions and a differential loss existed, the equations predict a competition at line center. The competition would result in the differential mode pushing term acting as a bias, and if strong enough, could result in the unlocking of the system.

In another work, the polarization and the self-consistent equations have been calculated to the fifth order (Klimontovich et al., 1967). The fifth-order terms are shown to determine the stability of the system. It is shown that the possibility exists for coexistence of both waves, extinction of one of the waves, and a state in which energy is periodically pumped from one beam into the other.

A correlation of the differential loss and null shift bias has been experimentally observed (Hutchings et al., 1967). Figure 20 shows null-shift measurements and power tuning curves as a function of tuning the oscillation frequency of a He–Ne 0.633 μm ring laser of cavity length 75.4 cm (mode spacing of 398 MHz). In the power curves the mode competition was strong enough to extinguish one of the beams and was attributed to a differential loss of $10^{-6}(\Delta\gamma/\gamma = 3 \times 10^{-4})$. Using this value of differential loss, Eq. (69b) predicts a bias of a few kilohertz, which agrees with the data. In the experiment, the bias to unlock the laser was obtained from a Faraday cell. In Fig. 20 the dispersion-type bias is shown to reverse sign with a reversal of the competition. This was attibuted to a change in the sign of the differential loss, which changes the sign of the bias. When the Faraday bias was reversed, similar changes occurred.

The mode competition problem in the ring làser can be eliminated by reducing the gain medium coupling between the oppositely directed beams. This can be done quite simply by operating the laser with a mixture of

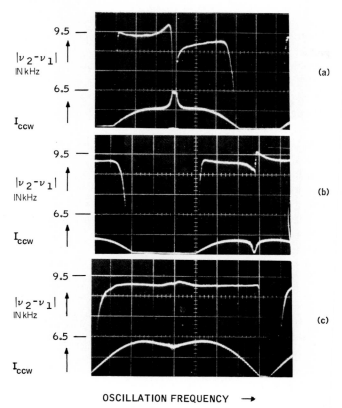

OSCILLATION FREQUENCY →

Fig. 20. Experimental displays of difference frequency and wave intensity for (a) the ccw dominent, (b) the ccw extinguished at the center of the gain curve, and (c) nearly identical traveling wave intensities. From Hutchings *et al.* (1967).

isotopes of the active medium (Aronowitz, 1965, 1969). For example, in the He–Ne ring laser, the center of the atomic transition of ^{22}Ne lies 875 MHz and 261 MHz higher than the center for ^{20}Ne for the 0.633 μm and 1.15 μm transitions, respectively.

Using the hole burning concept (Bennett, 1962) and with a mixture of two isotopes, saturation holes occur in the velocity distribution of each individual isotope. In the gain curves, since the centers of the gain due to each isotope are displaced, the holes can no longer completely overlap. This provides the needed stability for both beams to oscillate. The amount of additional isotope needed depends on the parameters of the system. For the He–Ne 1.15 μm transition a percent of the additional isotope is usually sufficient. For the He–Ne 0.633 μm transition, a somewhat larger amount is needed due to the larger isotope center transition separation.

In practice the He–Ne laser gyro is usually operated with a 1 : 1 mixture of the two isotopes. This gives a nearly symmetric gain curve with a peak midway between the centers of the two transitions. With the 1 : 1 isotope mixture, Lamb dips occur ± 130 and ± 437 MHz (1/2 the spacing between the centers of each isotope) about the peak gain frequency, for the He–Ne 1.15 μm and 0.633 μm transitions, respectively. Under the usual operating conditions, low gain for single longitudinal mode operation and high pressure for lifetime considerations, no Lamb dips are observed.

With the 1 : 1 isotope mixture, cavity length stabilization can be obtained at the peak gain frequency using standard-length control techniques (White, 1965). In addition to eliminating the competition problem, the 1 : 1 isotope mixture causes a reduction in the differential loss null shift, given by Eq. (68) at the operating point. This occurs since the presence of the second isotope causes a modification of all the coefficients in the amplitude and frequency self-consistent equations [given by Eqs. (61) and (62)] by simple superposition. For example, Eq. (65) is modified to become (Aronowitz, 1965, 1969)

$$\tau_{21} = \left[\frac{c}{2L} \frac{G}{Z_i(0)} \right] \left[f\left(\frac{\xi}{\eta}\right) \mathcal{L}(\xi) Z_i(\xi_1) + f'\left(\frac{\xi'}{\eta}\right) \mathcal{L}(\xi') Z_i(\xi_1') \right] \tag{70}$$

where primed frequencies are measured with respect to the second isotope center, and f and f' are the fractional amounts of each isotope component.

VI. Other Topics

A. Velocity Flow of the Active Medium

In Section III, Error Sources in the Laser Gyro, the concept of a null shift arising from a flow of the gas components was introduced. It was stated that the null-shift effect occurs due to a Fresnel drag effect for all atoms except the active atoms. Also the active atom null shift is by far the most dominant, and the effect is due to anomalous dispersion. With the determination of the effects of the active atoms by means of the self-consistent equations, the effects of a moving active atom can be seen quite simply.

The velocity distribution of the atoms, introduced in Eq. (58), for a Maxwellian distribution with a zero average velocity can be written as

$$W(v)\, dv = \exp\left(-w^2\right) dw / \sqrt{\pi} \tag{71}$$

where

$$w = v/u \tag{72}$$

For the case of the velocity distribution having some nonzero average v_0, Eq. (72) is modified by letting $w \to w - v_0/u$. This modifies the calculation of the polarization and all the self-consistent equations are modified by simply letting

$$\xi_1 \to \xi_1 - v_0/u \tag{73a}$$

$$\xi_2 \to \xi_2 + v_0/u \tag{73b}$$

For example, Eq. (58) for the hole burnt into the velocity distribution becomes

$$\Delta\rho(v) = \bar{N}W(v - v_0)[1 - 2I_1 \mathcal{L}(\xi_1 - v_0/u + v/u) - 2I_2 \mathcal{L}(\xi_2 + v_0/u - v/u)] \tag{74}$$

A better understanding of the effects of the velocity flow can be obtained by considering the modification in the gain distribution in frequency space. The gain curve is defined with respect to a "small" light signal which is amplified by the gain medium. Hence the gain curve is anisotropic with respect to direction, and two gain curves must be drawn, one for each beam. Figure 21 shows both beams, which have frequencies greater than the center frequency (only a single isotope is considered for simplicity), interacting with atoms on a rotating ring laser. The atoms are moving in the direction of the traveling waves such as to cause the atoms to see the radiation as being resonance radiation (downward Doppler shift). Since I_1 is moving in the direction of rotation, it has the lower of the cavity split frequencies. Locking effects are considered small and neglected.

Let v_0, which represents the net velocity flow, be (arbitrarily) in the direction of the rotation (Ω). Let b and c represent observers which measure the gain of the medium as seen by a test signal traveling in the direction of I_2 and I_1, respectively. Figure 21(b) represents the gain as measured by observer b. The dashed curve represents the unsaturated gain for the case of no net velocity flow. The heavy curve represents the gain when there is a velocity flow in the direction as indicated in Fig. 21(a). Since the atoms, on the average, are flowing away from the observer b, the center of the spontaneous emission is down shifted in frequency. Note that the v_- atoms (which mainly contribute to beam I_2) are moving toward the observer and hence spontaneously emit radiation at a frequency higher than those with zero velocity. Hence beam I_2 draws upon atoms on the high-frequency side of the gain curve and the saturation of these atoms is represented by the hole at frequency ω_2. Conversely, the v_+ atoms (which contribute to beam I_1) spontaneously emit on the low-frequency side (about doppler frequency ω, not the frequency of the maximum of the shifted gain curve) of the gain curve. The saturation of these atoms is represented by the image hole (saturation hole at other than an

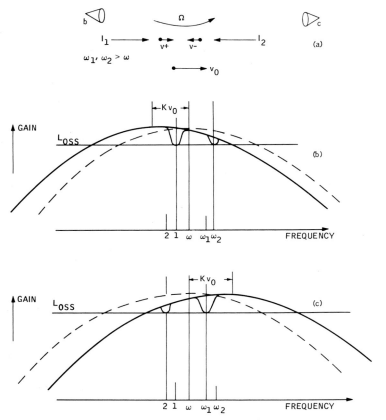

FIG. 21. Gain curves vs. frequency for (b) the beam traveling against the direction of rotation and (c) the beam traveling in the direction of rotation for the case of a net velocity flow of the active atoms. In (a) beams I_1 and I_2 are represented as interacting with atoms v_+ and v_-, respectively. Observers b and c measure the gain seen by beams I_2 and I_1, respectively.

oscillation frequency). It can also be seen that there is now a gain difference (different hole size) for the two oppositely directed traveling waves. The beam traveling in the direction of the velocity flow will have a greater gain.

Figure 21(c) represents the gain curve as seen by observer c. The physical interpretation of Fig. 21(c) is analogous to that used in Fig. 21(b) and the two curves are completely analogous. Note that the distances of the frequencies ω_1 and ω_2 from the shifted gain curves are in the proper direction to agree with the mathematical shifts, as given by Eqs. (73a and b).

Due to the dispersive properties of the active medium, the existence of a net velocity flow can cause a frequency splitting between the oppositely directed beams. As seen in Fig. 21, a velocity flow in the direction indicated shifts the gain maximum from the frequency which is equidistant from the two holes. This effectively changes the mode pushing for each beam, and it is seen that there will be a greater pushing of frequency ω_2 toward the gain maximum. This tends to reduce the rotational mode splitting. Hence, when the velocity flow is in the direction of the rotation, the frequency splitting contributions of the rotation and of the velocity flow tend to cancel. It should be noted that there will be a pushing effect which will be in the direction opposite to the pulling effect. However, in spite of the intensity difference, the pulling effect predominates.

To calculate the frequency splitting due to the velocity flow, the self-consistent frequency equations can be written from Eqs. (61) and (62) with the velocity flow frequency shifts given in Eq. (73). Making a Taylor expansion and dropping cubic terms, the beat frequency is found as (Podgorski and Aronowitz, 1968; Aronowitz, 1969)

$$\dot{\psi} = \Omega_R[1 - (A + A_1) - (B - B_1)I] - 2Kv[(A + A_1) + (B - B_1)I] \qquad (75)$$

where A = first-order mode pulling term, B = third order mode pushing term, I = average intensity of oppositely directed beams, A_1 = first-order term arising from third-order intensity difference, and B_1 = third-order term arising from third-order intensity difference.

B, A_1, and B_1 have been obtained by solving the intensity self-consistent steady-state equations. The factors for a two-isotope system can be found in Podgorski and Aronowitz (1968).

In Eq. (75), the effects of a velocity flow have the same frequency dependence as the mode pulling and pushing correction to the rotational frequency splitting term. This is expected since both effects are caused by the same physical phenomena—mode pulling and pushing corrections to the anomalous dispersion due to an anisotropy of the index of refraction.

Figure 22 shows the correction to the beat frequency Ω_R for the case of a velocity flow of 10 cm/sec and 1 cm/sec being either parallel or antiparallel to the direction of the rotation. The well-shaped curve is simply the superposition of the terms A, B, A_1, B_1. The dominant contribution is due to the differential mode pulling (term in A). The first-order intensity difference term (term in A_1) gives the dominant correction to the term in A giving the flat well-shaped curve seen in Fig. 22. It is noted that for the 1 cm/sec velocity flow, the mode pulling correction and velocity flow terms almost cancel. For the 1 cm/sec case in Fig. 22, the scale has been expanded by a factor of 5. In Fig. 22, the units along the y axis correspond to a digital output, i.e., a number such as 77,000 counts per 7.7 second interval corresponds to 11,000 Hz. The scale factor for this ring laser is 0.35 count/sec = 1 deg/hr. Hence the rotation of 109,400 counts/7.7 seconds corresponds to 11.3 deg/sec.

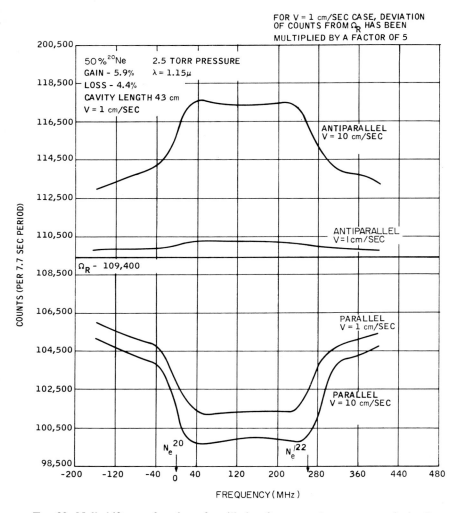

FIG. 22. Null shift as a function of oscillation frequency due to a net velocity flow both parallel and antiparallel to the direction of rotation, as given by Eq. (75).

Figure 23 shows experimental data illustrating the velocity flow null shift obtained in a He–Ne 1.15 μm ring laser with a 1 : 1 ^{20}Ne : ^{22}Ne isotope mix. The velocity flow was obtained by Langmuir flow caused by an unbalanced dc excitation current. The Langmuir flow causes an atom flow along the laser beam from the anode to the cathode. When the rotation was in this direction,

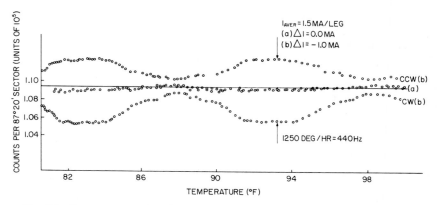

FIG. 23. Counts versus mode position for balanced current (a) and current unbalance (b) of 1.0 mA. The temperature scale is only an approximate indication of frequency. The data are for the tuning of two longitudinal modes across the doppler gain curve. Both curves (a) and (b) were positioned by overlapping the peaks of the output power which occurred at approximately 83° and 93° F. The horizontal line shows the expected value of the counts in the absence of mode pulling effects. From Podgorski and Aronowitz (1968).

the results were in agreement with Eq. (75). Reversing the current unbalance reversed the sign of the null shift, and doubling the current unbalance approximately doubled the null shift.

Depending on the application, the Langmuir velocity flow effect can be used to provide lock-in compensation. The big disadvantage is large errors occurring from insufficient bias magnitude. This is offset by the simplicity of the bias mechanization.

B. LOCK-IN THRESHOLD VARIATION WITH GAS PARAMETERS

In the operation of the laser gyro, performance is maximized with minimum lock-in threshold. It has been found experimentally (Aronowitz, 1969; Aronowitz and Collins, 1970) that the lock-in threshold can vary by as much as an order of magnitude, depending on the operating conditions of the laser. An analysis (Aronowitz, 1964; Aronowitz and Collins, 1970) of the self-consistent amplitude and frequency equations given by Eqs. (61) and (62) explains this lock-in threshold variation.

The equations can be simplified with the substitutions

$$\psi = \varphi + \pi + \tfrac{1}{2}(\varepsilon_1 - \varepsilon_2) \tag{76a}$$

$$\varepsilon = \tfrac{1}{2}(\varepsilon_1 + \varepsilon_2) \tag{76b}$$

Then the four equations describing the electric fields and frequencies of the oppositely directed waves can be simplified to three equations describing the intensities and frequency difference, or

$$(L/c)\dot{I}_1 = I_1[\alpha_1 - \beta_1 I_1 - \theta_{12} I_2 + 2\rho_2 \cos(\varphi + \varepsilon)] \tag{77a}$$

$$(L/c)\dot{I}_2 = I_2[\alpha_2 - \beta_2 I_2 - \theta_{21} I_1 + 2\rho_1 \cos(\varphi - \varepsilon)] \tag{77b}$$

$$(L/c)\dot{\varphi} = \Omega' + \tau'_{21} I_1 - \tau'_{12} I_2 - [\rho_2 \sin(\varphi + \varepsilon) + \rho_1 \sin(\varphi - \varepsilon)] \tag{78}$$

The prime signifies division by c/L.

For steady-state operation, Eqs. (77a and b) can be solved for the two intensities I_1 and I_2 and substituted into the mode pushing term in Eq. (78). The resulting lock-in equation is of the form

$$(L/c)\dot{\varphi} = \Omega' - \Omega_L \sin(\varphi + \delta) \tag{79}$$

where, for the case of equal saturation coefficients for each beam,

$$t = 2\tau'/(\beta - \theta) \tag{80a}$$

$$\Omega_L = [\Omega_{LO}^2 + \Omega_A{}^2]^{1/2} \tag{80b}$$

$$\Omega_{LO} = 2(r_1 r_2)^{1/2}(\cos \varepsilon + t \sin \varepsilon) \tag{80c}$$

$$\Omega_A = (\rho_2 - \rho_1)(1 + t^2)^{1/2} \tag{80d}$$

$$\delta = \tan^{-1}[(\rho_2 - \rho_1)/(\rho_2 + \rho_1)] \tan(\varepsilon - \chi) \tag{80e}$$

$$\chi = \tan^{-1} t \tag{80f}$$

$$\rho_2 = r_2(I_2/I_1)^{1/2}, \qquad \rho_1 = r_1(I_1/I_2)^{1/2} \tag{80g}$$

The lock-in threshold frequency is $(c/L)\Omega_L/(2\pi)$. In Eq. (79), equal losses have been assumed for both beams. Otherwise a differential loss null shift would occur, but it could be incorporated into the Ω' term.

As long as $\Omega' < \Omega_L$, steady-state solutions of the self-consistent equations exist and Eq. (79) gives the phase difference between the oppositely directed beams. For simplicity, consider the case when there is symmetry between the two directions with respect to the backscattering coefficients ($r_1 = r_2 = r$) and consider the case for $I_1 = I_2$. Then Eq. (79) gives the phase difference as

$$\varphi = \sin^{-1}(\Omega'/\Omega_{LO}) \tag{81}$$

Thus, as the rotation rate ranges from $-\Omega_{LO} \to +\Omega_{LO}$, φ ranges from $-\pi/2 \to +\pi/2$, passing through zero at $\Omega' = 0$. Note that if the π were omitted in the substitution given by Eq. (76a), the range of φ would be in the second and third quadrants. Hence phase jumps of π are possible if in the course of an experiment the sign of the Ω_L term changes.

As seen from Eqs. (77), the assumption of equal beam intensities as $\varphi(\Omega)$ varies is invalid. For ε in the first quadrant and for increasing rotation rate, cos $(\varepsilon + \varphi)$ decreases and cos $(\varepsilon - \varphi)$ increases and then decreases. This changes the net gain, and the intensities are expected to vary with increasing rotation rate. Figure 24 shows steady-state computer solutions of Eqs. (77a

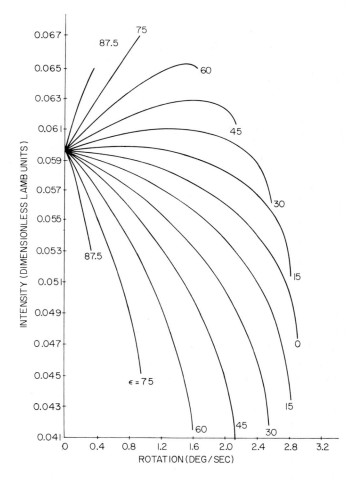

FIG. 24. Intensities of the two oppositely directed beams as a function of rotation rate (for rotations less than the lock-in threshold) for various backscattering angles ε. The beam traveling in the direction of rotation initially decreases with increasing values of rotation. The curves end abruptly at the lock-in threshold. The parameters were chosen for the Ne–Ne 0.633 μm ring laser.

and b) and (78) for the two intensities as a function of rotation rate, for various values of ε. For ε in the first quadrant, the beam which decreases in intensity is the one traveling in the direction of rotation. The curves end at the lock-in threshold. For brevity, the intensity-phase interaction for the case of rotation rates less than the lock-in threshold has been called "winking" (Aronowitz, 1969; Aronowitz and Collins, 1970).

Referring to Eqs. (80b)–(80d), it can be seen that the lock-in threshold depends on the scattering parameters through r and ε, and on the gas parameters through I and t. It can be seen that the lock-in threshold is not a fixed quantity, but rather a dynamical function of the rotation rate. For low rotation rates and for symmetric backscattering, the intensities are nearly equal and the lock-in threshold is essentially determined by the Ω_{LO} term, as given by Eq. (80c). As the rotation rate increases, the winking increases and the magnitude of the Ω_A term, given by Eq. (80d), increases. The Ω_A term is proportional to the intensity difference divided by the geometric mean. As the laser excitation increases, although the intensity difference increases, the relative winking decreases. Hence lock-in threshold is expected to increase as excitation threshold is approached (Hutchings *et al.*, 1969; Aronowitz, 1969; Aronowitz and Collins, 1970; Belenov *et al.*, 1966). Figure 25 shows computer solutions of the steady-state self-consistent equations for the intensities of the oppositely directed beams as a function of rotation rate. The lock-in threshold is also plotted as a function of the gain/loss ratio. The winking is seen to be an appreciable fraction of the zero rotation rate value. As discussed, the absolute winking increases with increasing excitation, although the relative winking decreases. This is reflected in the increasing lock-in threshold with decreasing excitation.

The oscillation frequency dependence on lock-in threshold is seen from Eqs. (80a–g) to arise from the t factor and is predominantly determined by the mode-pushing coefficient τ. Figure 26 shows computer solutions of the lock-in threshold Ω_{LO} and Ω_L as a function of frequency tuning, for various values of scattering phase angle ε. The Ω_{LO} curve is an odd function since τ is an odd function of frequency. For values of ε close to $\pi/2$, the asymmetry is most pronounced. A plot of the output power for zero rotation rate is also shown. For frequency detuning such that the oscillation is closer to threshold, the Ω_A term is seen to increase in its contribution to the lock-in threshold Ω_L. It should be noted that the slope of the Ω_{LO} curve would reverse at zero frequency for the 1.15 μm transition. This would occur due to the much smaller frequency separation between the transition centers of each isotope.

Figure 27 shows winking data for various excitation currents, taken with a He–Ne ring laser of cavity length 43 cm, operating on the 0.633 μm transition (Aronowitz, 1969; Aronowitz and Collins, 1970). The laser was filled

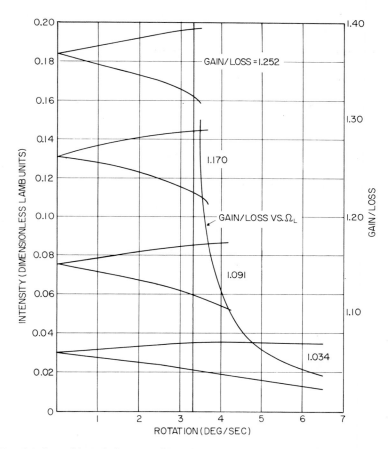

FIG. 25. Intensities of the oppositely directed beams as a function of rotation (for rotations less than the lock-in threshold) for various values of gain. The beam traveling in the direction of rotation decreases with increasing rotation. The curves end abruptly at the lock-in threshold. A plot of lock-in threshold as a function of gain/loss ratio is also shown. The vertical asymptotic corresponds to Ω_{LO}. The parameters chosen were for the He–Ne 0.633 μm ring laser, filled with a 1 : 1 ratio of ^{20}Ne : Ne^{22}.

with a 1 : 1 mixture of ^{20}Ne : ^{22}Ne. The winking was such that the beam traveling in the direction of rotation (for both directions) decreased. The results compare quite well with the computer solution shown in Fig. 25. At the lock-in threshold there was a sharp jump in both intensities toward the zero rotation value.

Figure 28 shows lock-in threshold data (Aronowitz, 1969; Aronowitz and

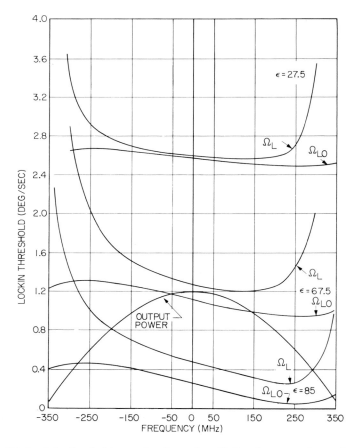

FIG. 26. Lock-in threshold as a function of oscillation frequency for various values of the backscattering angle ε. The corresponding output power curve is also plotted. Parameters are for the He–Ne 0.633 μm ring laser filled with a 1 : 1 ratio of ^{20}Ne : ^{22}Ne.

Collins, 1970), taken with a similar laser, as a function of oscillation frequency for two values of discharge current. The results are in agreement with Figs. 25 and 26, showing lock-in threshold to be asymmetric and increasing with operation closer to threshold. The data for Fig. 28 were obtained using the sharp jump in the winking at the lock-in threshold. Corroboration of the unlocking was made by direct observation of the rotation signal.

In both the analysis of the lock-in threshold and the experimental data shown, the time history was such as to cross from the locked to the unlocked region. The fact that the winking increased the lock-in threshold and that the

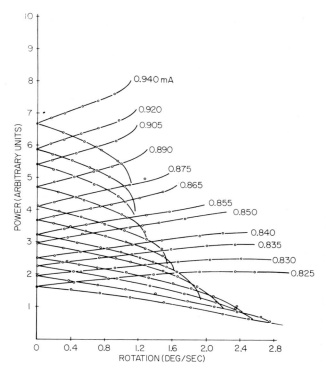

FIG. 27. Experimental data for the intensities of the oppositely directed beams as a function of rotation rate for various values of discharge current. The beam traveling in the direction of rotation decreased with increased rotation. The solid lines are smooth curves drawn through the data points and they end at the lock-in threshold. The data were for the He–Ne 0.633 μm ring laser filled with a 1 : 1 mixture of ^{20}Ne : ^{22}Ne. From Aronowitz and Collins (1970).

winking was found to cut back sharply as the system unlocked implies that lower lock-in thresholds would exist in going from the unlocked to the locked region (Hutchings *et al.*, 1969; Aronowitz, 1969; Belenov and Oraevski, 1968). This was indeed found to be the case. When the system unlocked with a sharp cutback in winking, the rotation signal was observed to be sinusoidal. At that point it was possible to reduce the rotation rate and the system remained unlocked. As the rotation rate continued to decrease, the waveform of the rotation sign was observed to have the characteristic lock-in-type distortion and further reduction of rotation causes the system to lock. This hysteresis was directly observed in a beat frequency measurement, as shown in Fig. 29 (Hutchings *et al.*, 1969).

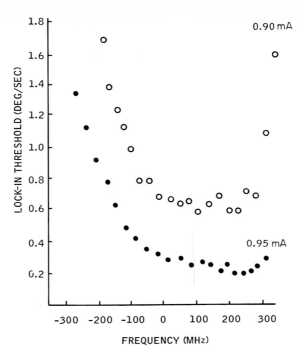

FIG. 28. Experimental values of lock-in threshold as a function of oscillation frequency for two values of discharge current. The data were for the He–Ne 0.633 μm ring laser filled with a 1 : 1 mixture of ^{20}Ne : ^{22}Ne. Zero frequency corresponds to the frequency at which the ouput power was a maximum. From Aronowitz and Collins (1970).

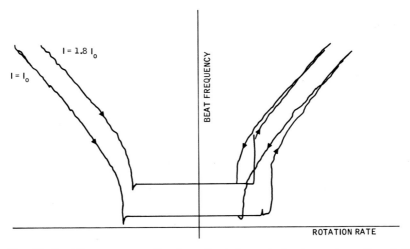

FIG. 29. Beat frequency as a function of rotation rate for two values of excitation current. The arrows indicate the direction of tuning, showing the lock-in hysteresis. The data were for the He–Ne 0.633 μm ring laser with a 1 : 1 mixture of ^{20}Ne : ^{22}Ne. From Hutchings et al. (1969).

VII. Laser Gyro Construction

A. LASER TRANSITION

The discussion on the construction of the laser gyro has been put off until the operation of the laser gyro has been completely discussed. With an understanding of the principles of operation and also some of the difficulties, it becomes easier to see the reason for current design techniques. However, it should be emphasized that the laser gyro has not yet evolved into the stage where it can be stated that there is a best way to construct it. Improvements, some minor and some radical, are still being made and will continue to be made in the coming years. However, some techniques in the construction are still basic, and will probably remain so.

The starting point in all laser gyros is the choice of the laser transition. At this date, in all known practical devices, the decision has been to use the gaseous He–Ne laser. The low-gain 0.633 μm and 1.15 μm transitions are preferred.

At first sight, solid state lasers appear attractive due to size considerations, ruggedness, and high power. Some solid-state ring lasers have been built using ruby (Tang et al., 1964) and neodymium (Bass et al., 1968). However, the spectral purity of the laser radiation cannot compare to that of the gas laser. In addition the neodymium laser has been shown (Bass et al., 1968) to be unstable with respect to radiation propagating in both directions. Another problem in using solid-state devices is the backscattering coupling arising from both the surface and the crystal itself.

The solid-state laser advantage of size and ruggedness is only an apparent advantage since gas lasers have been built with total cavity lengths of 10 cm and rugged enough to withstand many hundreds of g loading.

The reasons for the use of the He–Ne 0.633 μm and 1.15 μm laser is that to date, it has the best overall characteristics. First and foremost, the transitions have been, relatively speaking, very well investigated. The laser has high spectral purity, cw output, sufficient gain, good stability, high reliability, a long lifetime, a small stable Langmuir flow null shift, requires low input power, and can be made both rugged and compact.

A gas ion ring laser using argon has been constructed (Rigrod and Bridges, 1965) and the results have shown the unsuitability of the ion laser as a laser gyro. The difficulty arises from the high velocity flow of the active medium which causes instability problems between the oppositely directed traveling waves.

In the He–Ne ring laser, the 3.39 μm transition is not suitable for use as a laser gyro. The main difficulty arises due to the very high gain. This causes scale factor stability and magnetic field-induced null-shift problems (Burrell *et al.*, 1968). In addition, due to the high wavelength of the transition, detectors are not as convenient to use, the scale factor sensitivity is reduced, and the lock-in threshold is much higher.

In general, with increased detector sensitivity, scale factor sensitivity and reduced lock-in threshold, it is preferable to work with the He–Ne 0.633 μm transition as opposed to the 1.15 μm transition.

B. Mode Structure and Cavity Considerations

In terms of laser gyro performance and ease of operation, cw operation as opposed to pulsed or mode-locked operation (Buholz and Chodorow, 1967) is best. Single-mode operation is necessary. With operation of more than a single mode, low-frequency noise arising from mode coupling and combination tones can seriously restrict the operation of the ring laser as a rotation sensor. Operating the multimode laser as a mode-locked laser will tend to eliminate much of the noise (Buholz and Chodorow, 1967), although there is no advantage to be gained over the single-mode laser.

Restriction to only a single longitudinal mode can be accomplished by "near threshold" operation. Since the laser is usually stabilized to the frequency at which the gain curve is a maximum, the gain restriction is much less stringent than if "all frequency" operation were allowed. Even with an unstabilized laser, it is possible to operate a ring laser single mode with a larger excitation than a linear laser. Operating with the 0.633 μm transition mode, competition has been observed (Aronowitz, 1971) with the ring laser such that only a single longitudinal mode (both traveling wave components) oscillates.

The ring laser can be restricted to only a single transverse mode by means of an aperture. The analysis applicable to the linear laser can be applied almost directly to the ring laser (Collins, 1964). The basic distinction is that the ring laser is astigmatic with respect to the plane and normal to the plane of the laser. Hence all design calculations must be done twice and the aperture is ellipitical in shape. The mode structure of the ring laser cavity has been analyzed in detail (Collin's 1964), using techniques similar to those used for the linear laser.

In practice, the simplest configuration is the triangle. The triangle is simple in the sense that three optical components are fewer, and hence better, than four. In addition, the three-sided ring laser has the property of closure in the plane of the laser (Doyle, 1964). By this is meant that any alignment of the three mirrors results in a closed path in the laser plane. Unfortunately, this is not the case normal to the laser plane, and azimuth alignment is critical.

The laser radiation can be turned at corners by either mirrors or prisms (Lee and Atwood, 1966; Hutchings *et al.*, 1969). To minimize mode coupling by backscattering, the dielectric mirrors must be of the highest quality. In principle, internal reflecting prisms can be made with lower scattering characteristics. However, they are more expensive than mirrors and alignment is more difficult. In addition, prisms have the disadvantage of having residual and stress-induced birefringence, which in the presence of magnetic fields, can cause null shifts (Doyle, 1964).

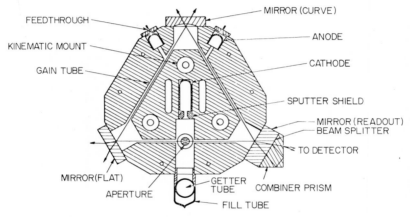

FIG. 30. Schematic drawing of a solid quartz block laser gyro. (The diagrams are published with the permission of Honeywell, Inc.)

To minimize both mode coupling effects due to backscattering and magnetic field null shifts due to natural and stress-induced birefringence, it is desirable to have as few optical elements in the cavity as possible. In principle and in practice, it is possible to operate the laser gyro with internal mirrors, and only an aperture in the cavity. Figure 30 shows a schematic of such a laser (Laser Gyro, 1966). For rigidity, the housing is constructed from a solid piece of fuzed quartz, into which holes have been drilled for the gain tubes and feedthroughs. The laser is prealigned in that the surfaces are polished and the dielectric mirror substrates are attached by optical contact. Two balance dc discharges are used to cancel null shifts due to Langmuir flow effects. Figure 31 shows a solid quartz block ring laser.

With this type of laser gyro, biasing can be done by mechanical dither.

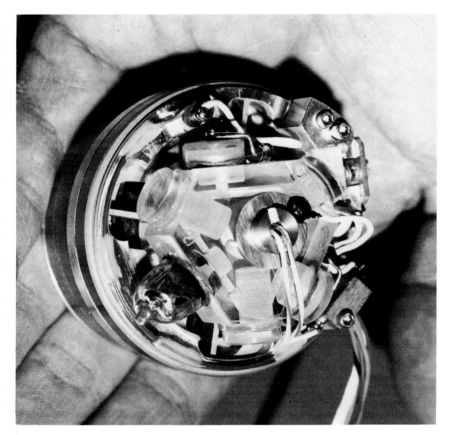

FIG. 31. Quartz block laser gyro. (The diagrams are published with the permission of Honeywell, Inc.)

For biasing of the Faraday cell type, it is necessary to employ windows to contain the discharge such that the cell can be introduced into the cavity. With windows and external mirrors there are sealing problems, and hence there are disadvantages with respect to contamination and lifetime. However, this is an engineering problem and is not basic to the laser gyro. It should be emphasized though, that in a system with external mirrors, it is absolutely necessary to work with a completely enclosed and preferably evacuated cavity. This is necessary to eliminate Fresnel drag-type null shifts and to reduce backscattering from contaminants in the air external to the gain tubes.

Using the solid-block concept it has been possible to construct a three-axis laser gyro in a single quartz block housing as shown in Fig. 32 (Laser Gyro, 1966).

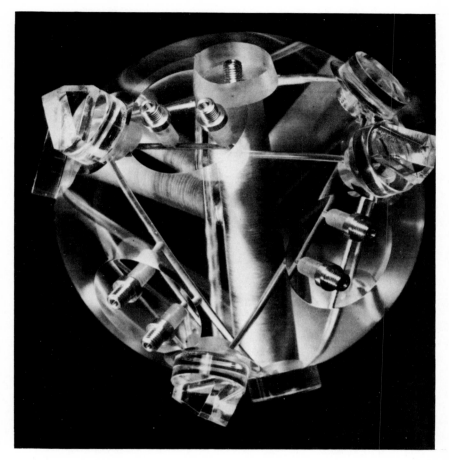

FIG. 32. Three axis quartz block laser gyro. (The diagrams are published with the permission of Honeywell, Inc.)

VIII. Applications of the Laser Gyro

The laser gyro is an unusually promising device, both in actual hardware and in concept, for many applications (Phelps, 1968). There are inherent features in this type of gyro which offer worthwhile benefits to a variety of guidance, control, and navigation problems.

The advantages of the laser gyro apply mainly to the strapped-down rather than gimbaled type of intertial system. In this type of system the gyros (and accelerometers, if required) are rigidly attached to the vehicle. There is no stable element in the conventional sense with gimbal or other isolation from vehicle angular motion.

The vehicle attitude is computed by a digital (special-purpose) computer by continuous updating of the transformation between the vehicle and reference coordinate system using the rate or incremental angle outputs from three orthogonal laser gyros. The computer, which is a relatively low cost and small size (20 cubic inches for some applications) unit, performs the functions of gimbals and is in effect an "electronic gimbal" system.

The advantages of strapped-down systems are several; size and weight, reliability, maintainability, environmental capability, and cost, when compared with gimbaled counterparts.

The disadvantages of strapped-down systems in the past arose mainly from the conventional gyros rather than the system concept. The conventional gyros when operated in a strapped-down mode have a definite angular rate and performance limitations due to the necessity for continuous rebalance by a magnetic torquer to counteract the intertial torques. In addition, drift trimming (i.e., correction for gyro null shift) prior to a mission is much more difficult with strapped-down systems since the input axis cannot be rotated as in the gimbaled system case.

The laser gyro can provide the characteristics needed for further development and exploitation of strapped-down systems, particularly for applications which demand high turning rates. The laser gyro can provide linear output at rates of 10^4 deg/sec since there are no inertial forces as in conventional gyros. The limitation is only that of providing the high-speed pulse circuitry to count the fringes. Further, the laser gyro is inherently stable on a run-to-run null-shift basis so that the need for drift trimming is much reduced, and reaction time (warm-up time, stabilization, and initialization time, etc.) is improved.

The laser gyro characteristics of interest to the system designer are drift, scale factor, size–weight, power, cost, environment capability, reaction time, and reliability.

Drift characteristics which are of importance include random, long-term and run-to-run stablity and g and g^2 effects. Scale factor characteristics include range (maximum input rate), plus and minus symmetry, nonlinearity, stability, and absolute accuracy.

The laser gyro does have drift rate errors similar in a broad sense to that of conventional gyros. The long-term run-to-run stability and the thermal effects are similar in character to conventional gyros. No attempt is made to compare numerical values with conventional units because of the diversity of available instruments and the specifics of the particular application limitations. Generally speaking, the values for laser gyros are lower for instruments of comparable cost and moderately severe environments.

The random drift of a laser gyro is, at present, generally higher than for its conventional gyro counterparts. The cause of this drift is well known and future improvements are expected. The random drift is nearly a pure white noise so that the net effect is, of course, much reduced for long application times. The numerical values are quite dependent on the specific test procedure and are best expressed as a drift angle versus time value of the form $\theta(t) = K(t)^{1/2}$.

There are no known (theoretically or experimentally) g and g^2 effects of practical importance in a properly designed laser gyro since there is no mass or momentum involved in the angular rate measurement. This, of course, greatly simplifies the design task, particularly for accurate missile or boost guidance applications.

The thermal and reaction time effects are of course related. The reaction time, per se, of a laser gyro is instantaneous since the lasing action begins at the instant of turn-on. Drift rate effects are caused by small changes in the cavity length (a fraction of a wavelength) which can occur with temperature, so that in principle the gyro could have a drift rate error at the instant of turn-on from a low-temperature condition. As a practical matter, however, the solid-block construction from a single low-temperature-coefficient material minimizes this effect. The temperature required to change the cavity length by one wavelength is of the order of 50°–100° F so that thermal control requirements are quite moderate. As a further refinement, one mirror is mounted on a piezoelectric element, and the path length is controlled precisely to remove even the small effects of temperature. The control signal can be derived from either the amplitude or frequency of the lasing action since these are affected by length change of the cavity. The action of the piezoelectric length control is instantaneous in practical terms.

Random, long-term, and run-to-run drift investigations have shown demonstrated results of less than 0.1 deg/hr. No g and g^2 effects have been observed.

The scale factor of the dithered laser gyro is shown in Fig. 13. The maximum nonlinearity occurs at input rates equal to the maximum dither rate and is typically less than one part in 10^4. The nonlinearity decreases with both increasing dither rate and decreasing lock-in threshold.

Of more importance to systems applications, since the angular motion for many applications is periodic, is the $\pm$ symmetry of the scale factor to prevent rectification of the angular motion. In the laser gyro, as compared with conventional gyros, the scale factor is absolutely symmetric. This property is inherently verified by the dither lock-in compensation, since symmetry must be present to prevent rectification.

There are a number of trade-offs involved in applying the laser gyro to a specific application. The laser gyro, while offering many advantages, is not necessarily the choice of all systems. Some of the inherent advantages of the laser gyro have been discussed above. The main disadvantages of the laser gyro which may be important in some applications are

(1) Relatively large size compared with conventional gyros (e.g., 4 in. diameter by 2 in. compared with 1.7 in. diameter × 3 in. conventional gyros).

(2) Very low drift rates have not been demonstrated. For very precise Earth-bound navigation applications, the required drift rates have not been achieved by the laser gyro, although advances in the technology are expected which may yield these results in the future. For high-accuracy boost guidance applications, the freedom from g to g^2 effects can reduce comparable overall system accuracies to that obtainable with state-of-the-art conventional gyros.

(3) Very long lifetimes have not been demonstrated. The 5000 hour operating lifetime, which is the current state-of-the-art is quite sufficient for many applications. However, some space applications do require much longer operating lifetimes. Additional R and D efforts are required to determine the extent to which lifetime can be extended.

An example of an application where the laser gyro is an obvious choice is a severe environment missile application. Some of the salient requirements which the laser gyro system can meet are

(a) Turning rates—several hundred deg/sec

(b) Vibration—hundreds of g's

(c) Size (3-axis gyro package)—7.5 in. diameter × 9 in.

(d) MTBF—11,000 hours

In this type of application there is sufficient vehicle angular motion to eliminate the need for dither to compensate for lock-in. Applications of this type (as well as more moderate environments) are ideal for the laser gyro. The required accuracy of the altitude reference can be met by the laser gyro for most guidance problems.

The laser gyro, at the present state of development, offers potential advantages for strapped-down system applications for a wide variety of guidance, navigation, and control problems. The benefits of the laser gyro to the system mechanization are primarily cost, reaction time, performance stability, and performance in high rate and acceleration environments.

ACKNOWLEDGMENTS

I wish to express my appreciation to J. Killpatrick, T. Podgorski, and B. Doyle for their aid and for valuable discussions on many aspects of the work described here.

REFERENCES

Adler, R. (1946). *Proc. IRE* **34**, 351.
Aronowitz, F. (1965). *Phys. Rev. A* **139**, A635.
Aronowitz, F. (1969). Ph. D. Thesis, New York Univ., New York.
Aronowitz, (1968). Unpublished observations.
Aronowitz, F. (1971). To be published.
Aronowitz, F., and Collins, R. J. (1966). *Appl. Phys. Lett.* **9**, 55.
Aronowitz, F., and Collins, R. J. (1970). *J. Appl. Phys.* **41**, 130.
Bagaev, S. N., Troitskii, Y. V., and Troshin, B. I. (1966). *Opt. Spectrosc.* (*USSR*) **21**, 420.
Basov, N. G., Belenov, E. M., and Letokhov, V. S. (1965). *Soviet Phys. Dokl.* **10**, 236.
Bass, M., Statz, H., and DeMars, G. A. (1968). *J. Appl. Phys.* **39**, 4015.
Batifol, E., and Pecile, D. (1966). *C. R. Acad. Sci., Ser. B* **263**, 446.
Belenov, E. M., and Oraevskii, A. N. (1968). *Soviet Phys. Dokl.* **13**, 411.
Belenov, E. M., Markin, E. P., Morozov, V. N., and Oraevskii, A. N. (1966). *Soviet Phys. JETP Lett.* **3**, 32.
Bennett, W. R., Jr. (1962). *Phys. Rev.* **126**, 580.
Bennett, W. R., Jr. (1964). *Quantum Electronics, Conf., Paris, 1963*, p. 441. Columbia Univ. Press, New York.
Bershtein, I. L. (1966). *Soviet Phys. Dokl.* **7**, 607.
Bershtein, I. L., and Zaitser, Y. I. (1966). *Soviet Phys. JETP* **22**, 663.
Buholz, N., and Chodorow, M. (1967). *IEEE J. Quantum Electron.* **3**, 454.
Burrell, G. J., Moss, T. S., and Hetherington, A. (1968). *Infrared Phys.* **8**, 199.
Carruthers, J. (1964). Unpublished observations.
Catherin, J. M. and Dessus, B. (1967). *IEEE J. Quantum Electron.* **3**, 449.
Collins, S. A., Jr. (1964). *Appl. Opt.* **3**, 1263.
de Lang, H. (1966). *Appl. Phys. Lett.* **9**, 205.
Dessus, B., Catherin, J. M., and Migne, J. (1966). *C. R. Acad. Sci., Ser. B* **262**, 1691.
Ditchburn, R. W. (1959a). "Light," p. 339. Wiley (Interscience), New York.
Ditchburn, R. W. (1959b). "Light," p. 333. Wiley (Interscience), New York.
Doyle, B. (1964). Unpublished observations.
Doyle, W. M., and White, M. B. (1965). *J. Opt. Soc. Amer.* **55**, 1221.
Fenster, P., and Kahn, W. K. (1966). *Electron Lett.* **2**, 380.
Fenster, P., and Kahn, W. K. (1968). *Appl. Opt.* **7**, 2383.
Fork, R. L., and Pollack, M. A. (1965). *Phys. Rev. A* **139**, 1408.
Fried, B. D., and Conte, S. D. (1961). "The Plasma Dispersion Function." Academic Press, New York.
Gyorffy, B. (1966). Ph. D. Thesis, Yale Univ., New Haven, Connecticut.
Gyorffy, B. L., Borenstein, M., and Lamb, W. E., Jr. (1968). *Phys. Rev.* **169**, 340.
Heer, C. V. (1961). *Bull Amer. Phys. Soc.* **6**, 58.
Heer, C. V. (1964a). *Symp. Unconventional Inertial Sensor, Polytech. Inst. Brooklyn.*
Heer, C. V. (1964b). *Phys. Rev. A* **134**, 799.
Heer, C. V., and Graft, R. D. (1965). *Phys. Rev. A* **140**, 1088.
Hercher, M., Young, M., and Smoyer, C. B. (1965). *J. Appl. Phys.* **36**, 3351.
Hutchings, T. J. Winocur, J., Durrett, R. H., Jacobs, E. D., and Zingery, W. L. (1967). *Phys. Rev.* **152**, 467.
Hutchings, T. J., Winocur, J., and Zingery, W. L. (1969). *5th Symp. Unconventional Inertial Sensors, Nav. Appl. Sci. Lab., Brooklyn, New York*, p. 199.
Kharkevich, A. A. (1959). *Electronic Design*, May 27.

Khromykh, A. M. (1966). *Soviet Phys. JETP* **23**, 185.
Killpatrick, J. (1967). *IEEE Spectrum* **4**, 44.
Killpatrick, J. (1966). Unpublished observations.
Klimontovich, Y. L., Kuryatov, V. N., and Landa, P. S. (1967a). *Soviet Phys. JETP* **24**, 1.
Klimontovich, Y. L., Landa, P. S., and Lariontsev, E. G. (1967b). *Soviet Phys. JETP* **25**, 1076.
Lamb, W. E., Jr. (1964). *Phys. Rev. A* **134**, 1429.
Landau, L., and Lifschitz, E. (1951). "Classical Theory of Fields," p. 281. Addison-Wesley, Reading, Massachusetts.
Langerin, M. P. (1921). *C. R. Acad. Sci.* **173**, 831.
Langmuir, I., (1923). *J. Franklin Inst.* **196**, 751.
Laser Gyro Comes in Quartz. (1966). *Electronics* **39**, 183.
Lee, P. H., and Atwood, J. G. (1966). *IEEE J. Quantum Electron.* **2**, 235.
Lisitsyn, V. N., and Troshin, B. I. (1967). *Opt. Spectrosc. (USSR)* **22**, 363.
Liu, C. S., Cherrington, B. E., and Verdeyen, J. T. (1969). *J. Appl. Phys.* **40**, 3556.
McCartney, E. J. (1966). *J. Inst. Navigation* **13**, 260.
Macek, W. M. (1963). Unpublished observations.
Macek, W. M., and Davis, D. T. M., Jr. (1963). *Appl. Phys. Lett.* **2**, 67.
Macek, W. M., Davis, D. T. M., Jr., Olthvis, R. W., Schneider, J. R., and White, G. R. (1963). "Optical Masers," p. 199. Polytech. Inst. of Brooklyn Press, Brooklyn, New York.
Macek, W. M., Schneider, J. R., and Salamon, R. M. (1964). *J. Appl. Phys.* **35**, 2556.
McFarlane, R. A., Bennett, W. R., Jr., and Lamb, W. E., Jr. (1963). *Appl Phys. Lett.* **2**, 169.
Michelson, A. H., and Gale, H. G. (1925). *Astrophys. J.* **61**, 140.
Mocker, H. (1968). *IEEE J. Quantum Electron.* **11**, 769.
Phelps, K. (1968). *Meeting of the American Astronautics Society, Denver.*
Podgorski, T. J., and Aronowitz, F. (1968). *IEEE J. Quantum Electron.* **4**, 11.
Post, E. J., and Yildiz, A. (1965). *Phys. Rev. Lett.* **15**, 177.
Post, E. J. (1967). *Rev. Mod. Phys.* **39**, 475.
Raterink, H. J., Stadt, H. V. D., Velzel, C. H. F., and Dijkstra, G. (1967). *Appl. Opt.* **5**, 813.
Rigrod, W. W., and Bridges, T. J. (1965). *IEEE J. Quantum Electron.* **1**, 298.
Rosenthal, A. (1962). *J. Opt. Soc. Amer.* **52**, 1143.
Rybakov, B. V., Skulachenko, S. S., Chumichev, R. F., and Yudin, I. I. (1968). *Opt. Spectrosc. (USSR)* **25**, 317.
Sagnac, G. (1913). *C. R. Acad. Sci.* **157**, 708.
Smith, R. C., and Watkins, L. S. (1962). *Proc. IEEE* **53**, 160.
Stenholm, S., and Lamb, W. E., Jr. (1969). *Phys. Rev.* **181**, 618.
Szoke, A., and Javan, A. (1963). *Phys. Rev. Lett.* **10**, 521.
Szoke, A., and Javan, A. (1966). *Phys. Rev.* **145**, 137.
Tang, C. H., and Statz, H. (1967). *J. Appl. Phys.* **38**, 323.
Tang, C. H., Statz, H., De Mars, G. A., and Wilson, D. T. (1964). *Phys. Rev. A* **136**, 1.
Thomson, A. F. H., and King, P. G. R. (1966). *Electron Lett.* **2**, 382.
Tomlinson, W. J., and Fork, R. L. (1967). *Phys. Rev.* **164**, 466.
Vander Pol, B. (1934). *Proc. IRE* **22**, 1051.
Wang, C. C. (1967). *Proc. Symp. Mod. Optics, Polytech. Inst. Brooklyn.*
White, A. D. (1965). *IEEE J. Quantum Electron.* **1**, 349.
Whitney, C. (1969a). *Phys. Rev.* **181**, 542.
Whitney, C. (1969b). *Phys. Rev.* **181**, 535.
Yildiz, A., and Tang, C. H. (1966). *Phys. Rev.* **146**, 947.
Zeiger, S. G., and Fradkin, E. E. (1966). *Opt. Spectrosc. (USSR)* **21**, 217.
Zhelnov, B. L., Kazantsev, A. P., and Smirnov, V. S. (1966). *Soviet Phys. JETP* **23**, 858.

MACHINING AND
WELDING APPLICATIONS

Lelland A. Weaver

Westinghouse Research Laboratories
Churchill Borough, Pittsburgh, Pennsylvania

I. Introduction

When the laser was first introduced in the early 1960s, it was anticipated that a new era of scientific and technological advancement had been born. Such expectations have since proved to be well-founded, but in the early days of laser development considerable disappointment was expressed when these advances did not occur immediately. As an example, the pulsed ruby laser was widely publicized as being capable of drilling into any known material; output energies were often described in terms of the number of razor blades which could be penetrated by the focused laser beam. But when lasers did not demonstrate high average power capability they were largely discounted as prospective industrial processing tools, except for specialized applications requiring small holes and welds using pulsed solid-state laser systems (Haun et al., 1968). Early gas lasers such as the He–Ne or Xe type operated at power levels of less than 1 mW, and therefore were categorically eliminated as possible materials processing instruments.

In the intervening years, scientific discovery and technological advances have completely invalidated this assessment of the laser's role in industrial processing. Pulsed solid-state lasers now operate at peak power levels in excess of 10^{13} W (Gobeli, 1969), and continuous power levels of up to 1100 W have been attained by solid-state lasers.[1] Entirely new families of gas lasers have been discovered with continuous power outputs of up to 60 kW (Gerry, 1970). But despite these advances and the development of reliable commercial laser equipment, many misconceptions based upon the early technology still persist. Continuous and pulsed lasers *can* compete economically with traditional material processing techniques, and are being employed at present in many manufacturing operations (Cohen and Epperson, 1968; Gagliano et al., 1969; Smith, 1969; Bod et al., 1969).

Of the hundreds of laser systems developed up to this time, only a handful are in actual use as laboratory or industrial tools. For industrial machining and welding a minimum continuous power level or peak focused power density is required for the laser to be useful at all. This limits the suitable devices to about five basic systems: optically pumped ruby, glass Nd^{3+}, and YAG: Nd^{3+}, and the high power ArII and CO_2 gas lasers. These systems are all commercially available, and are currently undergoing continual development and improvement. The theory and operation of these five lasers are described in Sections II and III, and several of the most recent developments in the high power continuous laser technology are presented. This includes a discussion of high power Kr arc lamps used to pump YAG, the high flow-transverse mirror CO_2 laser, and the large bore high power ArII laser discharge tubes. Semiconductor and liquid lasers are not considered in this review because of their present low average power capabilities. As these devices are further developed, however, they might be of interest for small machining and welding requirements.

The physical processes involved in laser machining and welding are basically thermal in origin. Thus most of the physical effects have been observed and utilized before the advent of the laser. But it is the unique qualities of

---

[1] See Holobeam, Inc., Paramus, N. J., advertisement in *Laser Focus* (1970) 6, 2.

this "heat" energy which distinguish laser techniques from the prior art; this includes extremely high pulsed power densities, very small focused spot sizes, and the fine degree to which the radiant beam can be controlled in power level, duration, and location. Fundamental physical interaction processes, reviewed in Section IV, are often utilized more effectively with laser energy, or can be applied to new sets of materials. Two of the more recently developed laser machining techniques are discussed as examples of this: the gas jet assisted CO_2 laser cutting of metals with minimum heat affected zone, and the thermal fracture of materials such as rock with CO_2 lasers. Specific examples of laser machining and welding have been summarized in detail elsewhere (Cohen and Epperson, 1968; Gagliano et al., 1969), and no attempt is made here to duplicate this. Section V therefore concentrates on some of the general material properties of interest in laser techniques, and outlines some of the physical models and unknowns encountered at very high laser power densities. It is apparent that such phenomena as light trapping, oxide formation, and plasma plume production greatly affect the nature of the laser beam interaction, and low power density behavior cannot simply be extrapolated to high power density interactions. Our knowledge of laser devices and laser beam interactions is extending rapidly, but much work remains to be done before lasers can be employed in materials processing to their full potential.

II. High Power Gas Laser Systems

Lasers that employ electrically excited gases as the active medium have operated at the highest efficiency and continuous output power of any lasers to date. This is primarily due to the fact that low pressure gas discharges can be built in very large sizes without degradation of the laser properties. The gas discharge remains optically homogeneous and virtually lossless at the lasing wavelength even when the optical path length is several meters long, and in many cases the laser gain remains high at elevated beam power densities. Consequently, gas discharge lasers of extremely long length have been constructed, the longest being a 9 kW unit having a total folded discharge length of 600 ft (Horrigan et al., 1968). Since the laser medium is gaseous, very little optical distortion occurs at high heat loads as in a solid, and excess heat may be removed by pumping the gas continuously through the discharge tube. This pumping is also effective in removing undesirable decompositional products which may be produced within the laser at high power levels. Thus it is the gaseous discharge lasers which possess the characteristics necessary for very high continuous output operation (i.e., output powers in excess of 1 kW cw).

There are basically three distinct families of gas lasers, divided according to the nature of the lasing species. The most familiar is the group of neutral gas lasers in which the laser transition occurs between excited states of a neutral gas. A large number of such lasing systems has been discovered (Bennett, 1965; Bridges and Chester, 1965), perhaps the most widely used being the familiar He–Ne gas laser. The red 632.8 nm transition in neon has proved to be especially convenient for general optical alignment purposes; such units may be purchased commercially for under $100. Literally hundreds of laser transitions from the ultraviolet to the infrared have been isolated, providing the greatest wavelength selection of any type of laser system. Typically, neutral gas lasers operate at power levels less than 100 mW, and are therefore of little use for heavy industrial processing.

Laser transitions between the vibrational–rotational levels of neutral molecular gases constitute yet another group. These lasers are characterized by high efficiency operation in the infrared portion of the spectrum, with continuous power outputs in excess of several watts. The carbon dioxide laser (Patel, 1964a,b) is the most prominent member of this group, having a power capability in the kilowatt range. Because of their high efficiency and continuous output power, molecular gas lasers have found wide application in the machining and welding of various materials.

A further class of gas lasers employs the excited states of ionized gases as the laser medium. These lasers require very high current density electric discharges to produce the ionized species, and typically operate at low efficiency. However, quite high continuous output powers are available in the visible and near ultraviolet. The positive ion of argon produces the highest known continuous power in the visible,[2] and ion lasers have yielded the shortest wavelength continuous laser radiation to date (Dowley, 1968).

For purposes of industrial processing, the carbon dioxide laser is of prime interest because of its high continuous power capability, and the argon ion laser because of its substantial continuous output in the visible part of the spectrum. Both of these devices are available as finished products from a variety of manufacturers, and many are presently in use in laboratories and factories. These two types of lasers will be described in greater detail in the following sections. Table I summarizes the operating characteristics to be described, and compares them with those of a He–Ne gas laser.

A. CARBON DIOXIDE LASER

The possibility of producing very high continuous power levels first became evident in 1964 with the development of the $CO_2:N_2:He$ laser (Patel, 1964a,b). Within a few years the output power of these lasers soared

[2] See *Laser Focus* (1969) **5**, 20.

TABLE I

PROPERTIES OF COMMON GAS LASER DEVICES

Type of laser	wavelength (microns)	Output power	cw Tube efficiency (%)	Linear power generation rate	Volume power generation rate
CO_2 : N_2 : He					
Conventional cw	10.6	10 kW	17	0.06 kW/meter	0.06–0.25 W/cm³
High Flow cw	10.6	1 kW	12	1 kW/meter	1–9 W/cm³
Q switched	10.6	100 kW	—	20 kW/meter	40 W/cm³
Pulsed	10.6	200 kW	—	80 kW/meter	18 W/cm³
ArII					
(all lines)	0.4880– 0.5145	120 W	0.1	60 W/meter	0.5 W/cm³
He–Ne					
(red only)	0.6328	<200 mW	0.1	35 mW/meter	0.04 mW/cm³

from a few milliwatts to hundreds of watts, and recently a carbon dioxide laser capable of 9 kW was reported (Horrigan et al., 1968). This is several orders of magnitude greater than other continuous sources of laser radiation, and is comparable to the power levels of present-day electron beam welders (Schumacher, 1968). Moreover, these lasers are more efficient than any other type; typical tube efficiencies range between 15 and 20%.

The laser transition occurs between the 00^01 and 10^00 vibrational levels of the carbon dioxide molecule, as indicated in the energy level diagram of Fig. 1. The energy difference between these levels corresponds to an output wavelength of 10.6 μ. Nitrogen molecules in the discharge are excited by electronic collisions to the $v = 1$ vibrational level shown in Fig. 1, and since dipole radiation to the ground level is quantum mechanically forbidden from this state, the $v = 1$ population becomes quite large. Because the 00^01 vibrational level in CO_2 lies only 18 cm^{-1} away, this $v = 1$ excitation in N_2 is very effectively transferred to the upper laser level in CO_2 through super-elastic collisions with ground state CO_2 molecules. Thus the 00^01 level in CO_2 is preferentially populated, creating an excess of molecules in the upper laser level as compared with the lower laser level. This is one of the necessary conditions for laser action to occur. After lasing at 10.6 μ, the CO_2 molecule decays to the 01^10 level, and subsequently radiates to the ground state. The helium in the discharge assists in collisional processes which maintain the population inversion, and improves heat conduction to the walls.

A schematic diagram of a 150 watt CO_2 : N_2 : He laser is shown in Fig. 2, and is typical of the type of laser which can be purchased commercially. The

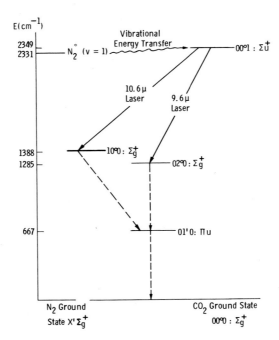

FIG. 1. Vibrational energy level diagram for the carbon dioxide and nitrogen molecules.

premixed gases, consisting of about 0.5 Torr of CO_2, 1.5 Torr of N_2, and 8.0 Torr of He, are conducted into the discharge section of the laser and pumped continuously through the tube. This prevents decompositional products in the gas mixture from accumulating and inhibiting laser action.

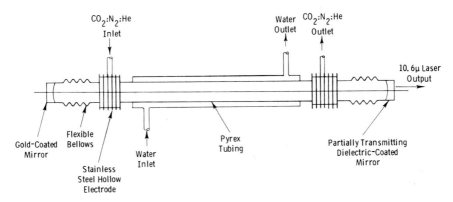

FIG. 2. Schematic diagram of a conventional electric discharge $CO_2 : N_2 : He$ laser.

The discharge tube is water-cooled, having a 2.5 cm diameter bore and a 2 meter length; a dc potential of ~ 10 kV is maintained between the electrodes, drawing ~ 100 mA through the discharge.

At each end of the discharge tube is an adjustable mirror attached through a flexible bellows to the tube. One mirror is almost totally reflecting at 10.6 μ, consisting of a gold deposit on Pyrex or stainless steel. The output mirror has a partially transmitting dielectric coating deposited on a germanium substrate. Thus some 20% of the laser energy within the discharge section is permitted to leak out through the germanium mirror, constituting the useful output beam of the device. Between 120 and 150 W of continuous output power at 10.6 μ is available from a laser of this size, with the tube efficiency being about 15%. Higher power devices are constructed by zigzagging many such discharge modules back and forth between optical folding assemblies which reverse the beam direction. Typically, an output power of ~ 60 W/meter of discharge length is available from such high power units. Nighan and Bennett (1969) have shown that this is a natural consequence of the division of electrical energy between ionization processes which sustain the discharge, and vibrational excitation which leads to laser power generation. Under typical discharge conditions $\sim 42\%$ of the energy transferred to a $CO_2:N_2$ laser mixture resides in vibrational modes favorable for lasing at 10.6 μ, corresponding to an energy storage of ~ 0.147 W/cm^3. Since the quantum efficiency of the laser transition is $\sim 41\%$, this analysis suggests that ~ 0.06 W/cm^3 of laser power is available from the electrically excited mixture. For a tube cross-sectional area of 10 cm^2, this corresponds to a linear power generation of 60 W/meter of discharge. Although a volume power generation as high as 0.25 W/cm^3 has been reported (Deutsch et al., 1969), 60 W/meter is typical of high power devices, and is relatively insensitive to tube diameter over a broad range. Thus conventional lasers in the kilowatt range are physically large, and the water, gas, and electrical support systems tend to be unwieldy.

Recent developments in molecular gas laser technology have shown, however, that high laser power levels can be obtained from physically compact devices. By employing separate injection of an rf heated $N_2:He$ mixture into an axial 200 meters/sec CO_2 flow, Cool and Shirley (1969) demonstrated that 10.6 μ gains as high as $\alpha = 0.0415$ cm^{-1} could be achieved. By comparison, the conventional electric discharge CO_2 laser gain is $\alpha \gtrsim 0.01$ cm^{-1}. Moreover the optical gain in this flowing gas laser was observed to be virtually constant over the tube cross section, implying that uniformly high gain independent of tube diameter had been achieved. For the first time it became apparent that CO_2 laser power levels could be increased by methods other than merely lengthening the discharge tube.

A kilowatt high flow CO_2 laser embodying these principles has recently

been described by Tiffany *et al.* (1969). The laser, depicted schematically in
Fig. 3, employs a mirror configuration whose optical axis is transverse to the
gas flow. Electrical energy is supplied to the laser mixture through internal
electrodes, and as the gas flows through the mirror cavity at ~30 meters/sec
the 10.6 μ laser beam is extracted through a partially transparent output
mirror. A gas-to-water heat exchanger then cools the laser gas to ambient
temperature, and a 6000 ft^3/min blower recirculates the gas around the loop
to be used again. The distance between the mirrors is 1 meter and the laser

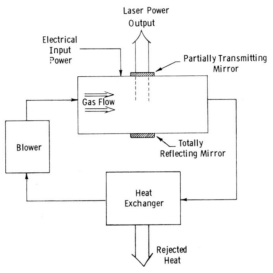

FIG. 3. Block diagram of a high flow, closed cycle electrically excited CO_2 laser.

beam diameter is ~4 cm; this corresponds to a volumetric power generation
rate ~0.9 W/cm^3, substantially greater than a conventional electric discharge
device. Thus the unit is physically compact, producing 1100 watts of laser
power from a 1 meter active medium length (1.1 kW/meter) at 10% overall
efficiency. Even higher volumetric yields have been achieved by Deutsch
et al. (1969), who report 9 W/cm^3 from a longitudinal flow device. They
obtained 140 W of laser power at 12% tube efficiency from a discharge cell
only 10 cm long. Hill (1971) recently obtained 20 kW of continuous output
power from a closed-loop electrically excited CO_2 laser system having active
medium dimensions of 5.6 × 76 × 100 cm^3, the highest average power reported from an electrically pumped laser.

The addition of purely thermal energy to the laser gas is also effective in
producing high output power levels from small volumes. Initial efforts
generated only very low power outputs (Fein *et al.*, 1969), but recently

Bronfin *et al.* (1969) reported 50 W from a volume 5 cm in length and 0.8 cm^2 in cross section corresponding to 12.5 W/cm^3. This was obtained by heating N_2 to 1300°K at 1 atm and expanding it through a supersonic nozzle. The CO_2 was mixed with the nonequilibrium N_2 flow to obtain a population inversion within the CO_2; 10.6 μ laser radiation was extracted by a mirror system transverse to the flow. Gerry(1970) has reported a continuous output of 60 kW from a combustion-fired gas dynamic laser with a thermal-to-optical conversion efficiency of $\sim 1\%$. Thus both thermal and electrical excitation schemes are capable of producing extremely high volumetric power yields in high flow devices, and can generate >1 kW from active medium lengths of ~ 1 meter.

Molecular gas lasers are unique among members of the gas laser family in that they can be Q switched to produce high peak power pulses of laser energy (Hocker *et al.*, 1966). This technique, common in solid-state pulsed lasers, cannot normally be applied to most gas lasers because of the very short spontaneous lifetimes of their upper laser levels as compared to the net population inversion pumping rate. Gases such as CO_2, however, possess vibrational lifetimes sufficiently long to permit the storage of laser inversions within the active medium during the pumping period. If properly aligned mirrors are suddenly exposed to provide optical feedback within the active medium, a very rapid lasing of the overpumped medium occurs. Commonly one of the CO_2 laser mirrors is allowed to rotate rapidly so that optical alignment of the two mirrors occurs periodically. Using rotating mirror Q switches with CO_2 lasers, scientists have produced 10.6 μ pulses of 100 kW peak power and 50 nsec pulsewidth at a repetition rate of 400 pulses per second.[3] An alternate approach is to pulse the gas discharge with extremely high voltages. Such techniques, using 500,000 V pulses, have produced laser outputs of 200 kW peak power in 5 J pulses at a 42 pps repetition rate (Hill, 1968). Recently Beaulieu (1970) announced pulsed laser operation in a Transversely Excited Atmospheric pressure (TEA) laser with peak power levels in excess of 20 MW. These high peak power laser pulses possessing high average power are very useful for certain cutting and machining applications, and greatly extend the capability of the conventional continuous output device.

B. Argon Ion Laser

The family of gaseous ion lasers is distinctive because of its variety of visible and ultraviolet laser transitions, and its ability to produce significant amounts of visible laser power on a continuous basis. The argon ion laser,

---

[3] See, for example, the Westinghouse 180 watt CO_2 laser with rotating Q-switch attachment.

discovered in 1964 (Bridges, 1964; Bennett *et al.*, 1964a,b; Gordon *et al.*, 1964), is the most prominent member of this group and in recent years output powers as high as 120 W have been obtained from laboratory devices (Herziger and Seelig, 1969; Banse *et al.*, 1969) Krypton and neon ion lasers operate at lower power levels, but extend farther into the ultraviolet range of the spectrum (Bennett, 1965).

Figure 4 illustrates a partial energy level diagram of the singly ionized argon atom, denoted as ArII. It is thought that these states are obtained in a gaseous discharge by a two-step process in which the neutral argon atom is first ionized by direct electron impact, and then the positive ion is excited to various energy levels by subsequent electronic collisions. Since these excited states are some 20 eV above the neutral argon 15.8 eV ionization potential, the lasing system is inherently energetic, requiring a large number of high

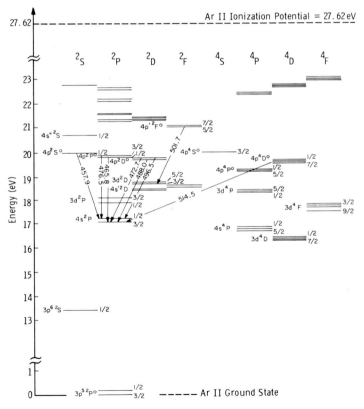

FIG. 4. Partial energy level diagram of the ArII ion showing the common blue–green laser transitions.

energy electrons to obtain substantial upper laser level population. Laser action commonly occurs on eight visible lines between 457.9 nm and 514.5 nm in the blue-green portion of the spectrum, terminating on the $4s^2P_{1/2}$, $4s^2P_{3/2}$, and $3d^2D_{3/2}$ states of the ArII ion. Ions in these levels subsequently decay to the ion ground state through ultraviolet emission (~ 70 nm). The strongest individual laser emission is obtained on the 514.5 nm and the 488.0 nm lines, although all eight blue-green laser lines can oscillate simultaneously with a single set of dielectric mirrors.

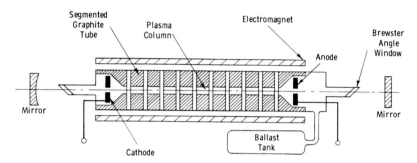

FIG. 5. Schematic diagram of a segmented bore argon ion laser.

Figure 5 illustrates a schematic representation of an argon ion laser. The discharge tube must be specially constructed to withstand the high current density dc discharge required for ArII excitation. Quartz tubing is often employed, but most commercial units now use a segmented graphite or BeO construction designed to resist high heat loadings and bore erosion. The discharge tube is water-cooled, and provision is made for gas circulation within the segmented tube to prevent accumulation of neutral argon near the anode due to electrophoretic effects (Chester, 1968a,b). A high current density discharge is maintained by a dc potential between the heavy duty anode and cathode. Since currents of about 5 A are required, an axial magnetic field is applied to the tube to stabilize the discharge and keep it away from the tube walls. Brewster angle quartz windows serve as a vacuum seal, and dielectric-coated mirrors, whose reflectivity is peaked near the operating wavelengths, are placed at either end of the tube. If operation at a single wavelength is desired, a dispersive prism can be situated within the optical cavity to discriminate against unwanted laser oscillations.

Recently Herziger and Seelig (1969) have reported high power ion laser performance in a discharge regime which differs from that normally employed. The discharge tube is a large bore (> 10 mm i.d.) quartz tube which requires no externally applied magnetic field. The optimum electron temperature was found to be 3.5 to 4 eV, and the tube operating current was ~ 300 A (265 A/cm^2). This device produced some 120 W of continuous output power with all visible ArII lines oscillating; this is the highest power level reported to date. In addition ~ 20 W were obtained in the visible KrII lines, and ~ 1.5 W in the ArIII (3638 Å, 3511Å) and KrIII (3507 Å) ultraviolet lines. Devices of this nature, in addition to others under development,[4] indicate that substantially higher continuous outputs in the visible might soon be available.

At present, commercial units are available with efficiencies of $\sim 0.1\%$ and a power output of ~ 12 W with all blue-green lines lasing simultaneously. Using a prism, single line operation at 514.5 nm can be obtained comprising about 50% of this total output. Visible wavelength lasers with high continuous output power are potentially attractive for industrial processing because of the much smaller spot size available in a focused beam at shorter wavelengths, and the excellent coupling of visible wavelengths into most metals. Although commercially available ArII lasers do not have sufficient continuous power capability for heavy machining and cutting applications, they can be applied to low energy industrial processes. As commercial units are constructed above the 100 W level in coming years they should be employed profitably as machining and welding tools.

III. High Power Solid-State Laser Systems

The solid-state optically pumped laser produces the highest energy and peak power output of any existing pulsed laser system. These unique features result in part from the very high density of laser ions available in solid materials. Concentrations of $\sim 10^{20}$ laser ions/cm^3 are typical for solid hosts, whereas gaseous lasers usually operate with fewer than $\sim 10^{18}$ laser particles/cm^3. Moreover, solid laser materials can be excited very rapidly with high energy flash lamps, and Q-switching techniques can be employed to extract the stored laser energy in a giant pulse of short duration. Energies of 5000 J have been obtained in a single pulse of laser radiation (Young, 1967) and peak power levels of 10^{13} W have been reported (Gobeli, 1969). Recently, ultrashort laser pulses of duration 2.5×10^{-13} sec have been produced in solid laser materials (Shapiro and Duguay, 1969). In addition to the pulsed and Q-switched modes, solid-state lasers can be operated continuously at power levels of ~ 1100 W.[5] These characteristics make solid-state optically pumped lasers particularly useful for industrial processing.

[4] See *Laser Focus* (1969) **5**, 20.
[5] See Holobeam, Inc., Paramus, N. J., advertisement in *Laser Focus* (1970) **6**, 2.

The active medium employed in these lasers is a solid crystalline or glass material doped with a lasing ion such as Cr^{3+} or Nd^{3+}. Since these materials are electrical insulators, direct electrical excitation of the laser species is not possible as in a gas discharge laser. Thus, the intense optical energy radiated from a lamp is used as the primary energy source, and the laser rod can be thought of as an optical transducer which absorbs the incoherent pump light and converts it into a directed beam of coherent laser light. The output beam can be focused to power densities many orders of magnitude greater than can the light from the pump source, and can propagate over great distances with beam divergence close to the theoretical minimum. Thus the laser light output is of much greater utility for industrial processing than the pump light which produces it.

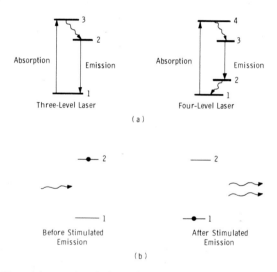

FIG. 6. (a) Absorption and emission of three and four level laser systems. (b) The stimulated emission process.

It is convenient to divide the class of optically pumped solid-state lasers into three and four level laser systems, as shown in Fig. 6(a). The absorption of pump light in a three level system excites ground state ions to level 3, which subsequently decays through rapid nonradiative processes to the upper laser level. Lasing occurs to the ground state, as illustrated in Fig. 6(b), provided that an excess of ions exists in the upper laser level. This requires that greater than 50 % of the ground state ions can be excited in order to create a population inversion with respect to the ground level. Thus, three level lasers possess inherently high pumping requirements, and usually operate on a pulsed basis. The well-known ruby laser is a three level system since laser action terminates on the ground state of the Cr^{3+} ion.

In the four level system the absorbed pump light excites the ground state ions to level 4, which then decays to the upper laser level 3. Laser action occurs to level 2 if a population inversion between these levels exists, and the ion is then deexcited to the ground state. The important difference is that only a small fraction of the ground state ions need be excited to create the population inversion between levels 3 and 2, as opposed to greater than 50% with the three level system. Consequently, pump requirements and lasing thresholds are greatly reduced in four level systems. The Nd^{3+} ion is the most important member of this group, since it lases at the highest peak and continuous power level of any optically pumped laser. Of the many solid-state laser materials discovered to date, only three have found general application for industrial processing. These are ruby (crystalline Al_2O_3 doped with Cr^{3+}), glass (barium crown or high silicate glass doped with Nd^{3+}), and YAG (crystalline $Y_3Al_5O_{12}$ doped with Nd^{3+}). Table II compares some

TABLE II

PROPERTIES OF COMMERCIALLY AVAILABLE SOLID-STATE LASER MATERIALS

Material (active ion)	Output wavelength (μ)	Mode of operation	Output	Thermal conductivity (W/cm°C)	Dimensional availability length × diam. (in.)	Cost ($/in.)
Ruby Cr^{3+}	0.6943	Pulsed	500 J	0.11	12 × 1	300–400
		Q switched	10^9 W			
Glass Nd^{3+}	1.06	Pulsed	5000 J	0.002	72 × 2	100
		Q switched Oscillator– amplifier	5×10^{10} 1.7×10^{13}			
YAG Nd^{3+}	1.06	Continuous Pulsed Q switched	1100 W 10 J 2×10^7 W	0.03	5 × 0.25	1000

of the physical properties and performance characteristics of these laser materials. It is seen that these materials can·generate extremely high output power in the red and near-infrared portion of the spectrum, and are available in reasonable physical sizes. The operation of these laser systems is described in the following sections.

A. Ruby Laser

Ruby was the first material in which laser action was demonstrated, and has continued to be an important source of high power laser emission. The material is crystalline sapphire (Al_2O_3) doped with $\sim 0.05\%$ Cr^{3+}, and can be grown in lengths up to 12 in. with good optical quality. It is an extremely hard and durable material with high thermal conductivity, permitting effective cooling of the laser rod. Laser characteristics are quite dependent upon the rod temperature, so that efficient cooling is necessary to insure consistent operation of the laser. Pumping thresholds are usually quite high, since the chromium ion constitutes a three level laser system.

The three level diagram in Fig. 6(a) is representative of the laser cycle in Cr^{3+}. Absorption of pump lamp energy in the green part of the spectrum excites ground state ions to a band of energy levels above the upper laser level. Nonradiative decay to the ^2E level in Cr^{3+} then occurs, and a population inversion with respect to the ground state is created at sufficiently high pumping rates. This excess population radiates through stimulated emission at 694.3 nm to the ground state. Since this is a three level laser system, pulse or Q-switched operation is customary, although continuous outputs have been obtained (Bridges, 1964; Bennett *et al.*, 1964a).

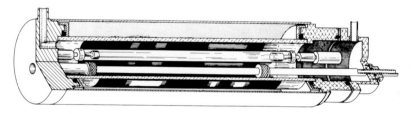

FIG. 7. Pulsed laser head showing laser rod and pump lamp within a cylindrical reflecting enclosure.

Figure 7 shows the geometric arrangement of the ruby laser rod and pumping lamp. Rod and lamp are placed parallel to one another within a reflecting cylinder which concentrates the lamp radiation onto the laser rod. A circularly cylindric reflecting enclosure is shown here, but often elliptical or double-elliptical cylinders are used (Nelson and Boyle, 1962; Evtuhov and Neeland, 1965). The flash lamp, filled with ~ 150 Torr of xenon gas, is quartz-jacketed and of rugged construction. Both rod and lamp are cooled by a continuous flow of deionized water. Electrical energy stored within external capacitor banks is discharged through the flash lamp, and light absorbed by the ruby rod creates the necessary population inversion. Usually the ends of the rod are polished and coated with highly reflecting dielectric layers, although external resonators are also employed. The red laser pulse is extracted through the partially transmitting coating at one end of the rod.

The intensity and duration of the flash lamp radiation determines the pulse length and energy of the output beam. Systems of this type normally produce pulses of up to 400 J and pulse widths between 0.1 and 10 msec. Pulse lengths greater than 1 msec are desirable for pulsed welding applications, and most commercial units have external lamp circuitry capable of extending pulse lengths into this range. For Q-switched operation a synchronized electrooptic shutter is placed within the resonators and such systems can produce peak output powers of over 10^9 W. Beam divergence is usually ~ 1 mrad, and operating efficiency is between 0.1 and 1 %.

B. Glass Laser

Glass rods doped with Nd^{3+} were developed as laser materials in 1961 (Ciftan *et al.*, 1961; Bowness *et al.*, 1962; Snitzer, 1961), and have yielded the highest peak power of any laser to date (Gobeli, 1969). Barium crown glass or high silicate glasses are commonly used, and glass laser rods over 72 in. in length have been fabricated with excellent optical quality. Moreover, glass laser materials are relatively inexpensive to produce. Several glass laser rods are shown in Fig. 8, with the ends polished flat or into a corner-cube reflector. The neodymium ion lases at 1.06 μ, and since it is a four level system the pumping requirements for pulsed operation are quite modest. The major disadvantage of glass laser materials is their low thermal conductivity, which largely prevents their use for high average power applications. Thus glass: Nd^{3+} lasers are usually operated at low repetition rates in the pulsed or Q-switched mode.

The four level diagram of Fig. 6(a) serves to describe absorption and emission in Nd^{3+}. Pump lamp energy in bands near 530 nm, 580 nm, and 750 nm is absorbed by the Nd^{3+} ion, and excites the ion to levels corresponding to level 4 in Fig. 6(a). These ions then decay through nonradiative processes to the $^4F_{3/2}$ upper laser level, and lase at 1.06 μ to the $^4I_{11/2}$ level. This terminal laser level lies some 2200 cm^{-1} above the ground state, so that lasing can occur with only a small portion of the ground state ions excited. Further nonradiative decay from the lower laser level to the ground state completes the lasing cycle. In pulsed operation, the glass: Nd^{3+} laser head arrangement is similar to that shown in Fig. 7 for ruby. Rod and lamp are situated parallel to one another within an optical coupling cavity, and electrical energy stored within capacitors is discharged through a high pressure xenon lamp. Dielectric coatings on the ends of the glass rod serve as mirrors.

Glass laser systems are capable of generating very high energy pulses in

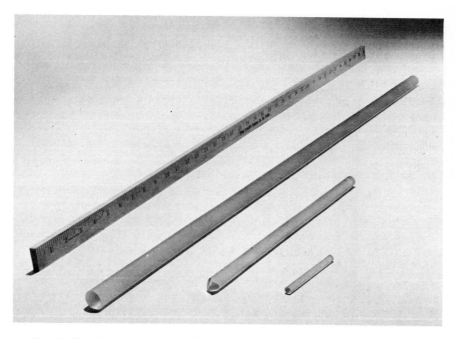

FIG. 8. Glass laser rods with optically polished ends, for use in high power pulsed laser devices.

short lengths of time (Young, 1969). The highest laser energy reported to date is 5000 J obtained from a 30 mm by 1 meter laser rod pumped by four xenon flashlamps (Young, 1967, 1969). The pulse duration of this device was ~ 3 msec, which corresponds to the length of the flashlamp irradiation. This high energy, long pulse mode of operation is very desirable for the pulsed welding of metals. Q switching is accomplished through a variety of methods (Collins and Kisliuk, 1962; McClung and Hellwarth, 1962; Soffer, 1964), producing peak pulsed power outputs as high as 5×10^{10} W. Recently an oscillator–amplifier combination of glass rods produced the highest peak power obtained to date (Gobeli, 1969), some 1.7×10^{13} W. Ultrashort pulses of 2.5×10^{-13} sec, corresponding to ~ 70 wavelengths of 1.06 μ light, have also been generated in glass lasers (Shapiro and Duguay, 1969). And the highest beam "brightness" of any known source was produced by a glass laser (Hagan, 1969) generating a radiance of 2×10^{17} W cm^{-2} sr^{-1}. Thus the glass laser exceeds all other sources in its ability to produce peak power levels and source radiance; this quality not only makes it useful for pulsed welding and machining, but for gas breakdown and thermonuclear reaction experiments as well.

C. YAG Laser

One of the best hosts developed for the Nd^{3+} laser ion in YAG, an acronym for yttrium aluminum garnet $(Y_3Al_5O_{12})$. This crystalline material doped with Nd^{3+} possesses many favorable physical characteristics which make it unique among solid-state laser materials. YAG has good thermal conductivity and can be grown with excellent optical quality; it is hard and durable. Unfortunately it cannot be fabricated in lengths greater than ~ 5 in., and is quite expensive. This restricts YAG to much lower energy operation than glass. Since it contains a four level laser ion its pumping threshold is low. Because of these qualities $YAG:Nd^{3+}$ is the only solid-state laser material that has generated significant amounts of continuous laser power, over 1100 W at 1.06 μ.

Absorption of pump light and emission of laser energy in $YAG:Nd^{3+}$ occurs in the same fashion as described for glass: Nd^{3+}. For continuous operation the radiant emission from a high power lamp is used to excite the laser ions in the YAG crystal. Figure 9 illustrates a unique cw laser arrangement employing a gold-coated spherical reflecting surface to couple the lamp radiation into the rod. For small laser rod lengths, spheres from 4 to 10 in. diameter provide excellent imaging of the lamp onto the rod when both are situated side by side near the center of the sphere. Thus up to 86% of the lamp emission is incident upon the laser rod for the geometry shown (Church and Liberman, 1967). Typically, the laser rod is between 3 and 5 mm in diameter and between 30 and 75 mm in length, with the lamp being approximately

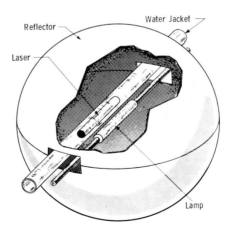

FIG. 9. Continuous $YAG:Nd^{3+}$ laser head showing laser rod and pump lamp within a spherical reflecting enclosure (Church and Liberman, 1967).

the same size. Dielectric coated mirrors outside the sphere provide optical feedback into the laser rod, and the laser energy at 1.06 μ is extracted through one of these mirrors.

Three different types of lamps have been used to pump YAG: the tungsten filament lamp, a K–Hg lamp, and high pressure Xe or Kr arcs. The broadband emission from tungsten corresponds to black body radiation at about 3200°K, but the Nd^{3+} ion in YAG has a narrow linewidth absorption band which consequently converts very little of this energy into laser light. In addition, the tungsten filament is quite fragile. This combination of spectral mismatch and fragility renders the tungsten filament YAG laser a low power, low efficiency laboratory device. A more suitable approach has been the use of arc discharge lamps that are mechanically rugged and dependable, and whose emission spectra can be controlled with appropriate additives and operating conditions. Liberman et al. (1969) demonstrated a K–Hg arc lamp whose line emission closely matches the absorption bands in YAG: Nd^{3+} at the operating arc core temperature of $\sim 4000°K$.

Since the potassium is corrosive and the temperature high, sapphire envelopes are necessary. These lamps have produced 10 W of laser output with an input of 420 W, yielding an overall efficiency of 2.4%. Although these lamps are efficient, they are presently expensive and cannot be operated at high power levels for long periods of time. Water-cooled Xe and Kr lamps provide better spectral matching than tungsten, and can be operated at high power levels. Several investigators (Liberman, 1969; Koechner, 1969a,b) have reported continuous output powers in excess of 100 W at 1.06 μ using Kr pumping. The highest power reported is 1100 W,[6] and commercial units are available (Koechner, 1969a,b) having 250 W at 2.1% efficiency. These systems use a double elliptical cylindrical cavity to couple the Kr lamp emission to the laser rod, as shown in Fig. 10. The two pump lamps lies along the common focus. Beam divergence at full power is $\sim$ 12 mrad, so that when the beam is focused with a 1 in. focal length lens power densities of $\sim 2 \times 10^5$ W/cm^2 can be obtained at 1.06 μ. These power densities can be used to cut metallic foil and vaporize most materials. The present power capability of these devices is no longer limited by the pumping lamps, but by the laser rod; thermal distortions in the rod cause excessive beam divergence and can fracture the rod.

With a rotating mirror Q switch (Smith and Galvin, 1967) and tungsten lamp pumping, peak pulses of 6 kW at 1200 pps have been obtained. Recently an acoustooptic modulator Q switch has been described (Chesler et al., 1969) which produces 1 kW peak pulses at a 5000 pps rate from a continuously

[6] See Holobeam, Inc., Paramus, N. J., advertisement in Laser Focus (1970) 6, 2.

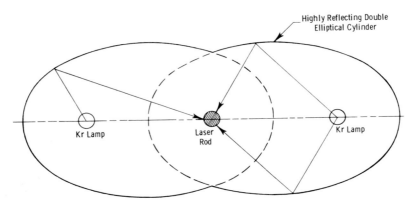

Fig. 10. Geometric arrangement of the laser rod and two pump lamps within a double elliptical cylinder reflecting enclosure.

pumped YAG laser. Both continuous and repetitively pulsed $YAG:Nd^{3+}$ lasers are attractive for industrial processing because of their compactness, versatility, and average power capability in the near infrared.

IV. Material Processing Mechanisms

Traditional methods of processing materials have depended primarily upon bringing various forms of mechanical, electrical, or chemical energy into contact with the workpiece. In recent years, however, the "directed energy source" concept has provided hope of performing these operations without intimate contact between energy source and workpiece. Such sources include high power lasers, electron beam, and ultrasonic devices capable of supplying power densities in excess of 10^6 W/cm^2 to surfaces remote from the source. This raises the attractive possibility of eliminating knives, drills, abrasive wheels, flames, chemicals, and electrodes from certain industrial operations, thereby reducing maintenance, replacement, and direct labor costs. Thus it is appropriate to inquire into the behavior of materials subjected to intense concentrations of essentially "thermal" energy in excess of $\sim 10^5$ W/cm^2. Only those effects of interest to machining and welding will be considered here, although many other useful thermally induced phenomena occur (i.e., optical absorption edge shift, refractive index changes, electrical conductivity changes).

Melting. If sufficient heat is applied to a solid, its temperature is increased to the melting point T_M of the material. With the addition of the heat of fusion W_F for the material, the solid is transformed into the liquid state.

Cutting and drilling are accomplished if the liquid is removed by gravity or convective flow, or by a jet or gas. An example of this type of cutting with a CO_2 laser is shown in Fig. 11, where a 3/4 in. thick sample of Lucite has been separated by a melt-cut at ~ 4 in./min. Welding is accomplished if the liquid formed at the juncture of two separate pieces is permitted to solidify (Platte and Smith, 1963).

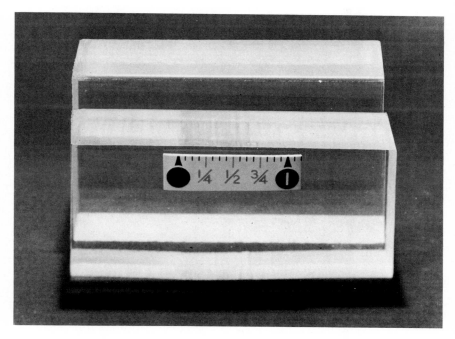

FIG. 11. Sample of lucite cut with a focused CO_2 laser beam (from Haun *et al.*, 1968).

Evaporation. The liquid created upon melting of a solid can be increased in temperature to its evaporation point T_E by the application of sufficient heat. At this temperature, addition of the heat of evaporation W_E transforms the liquid into a gas or vapor which can be blown way from the heating zone by a jet of inert gas.

Sputtering. During the process of evaporation hot vapors boiling from the liquid can impart kinetic energy to small volumes of liquid within the melt. Thus small globules of liquid can acquire sufficient energy to overcome surface tension forces at the vapor: liquid interface and be ejected from the heated zone. Material displaced in this manner is often considerable, and upon solidification can form a crater around the heated zone.

Evaporation of Entrapped Water. Many materials such as wood or rock contain either pockets of entrapped water, or water molecules chemically united to the molecular structure of the material. Intense heat can break these molecular bonds and evaporate the water and other compounds contained within the sample. These volatilized products exert great internal pressures upon the material, producing microfractures and ejecting particles of matter.

Heating of Entrapped Gases. Porous materials contain gaseous voids which upon heating can produce large internal pressures due to expansion of the heated gases. These forces can irreversibly weaken the sample by causing microfractures and by ejecting particulate matter. Figure 12 illustrates the

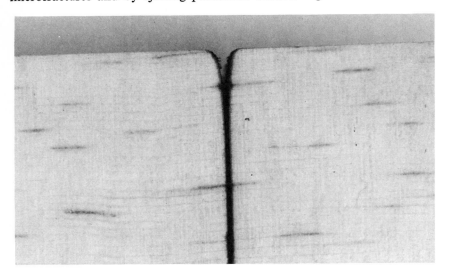

FIG. 12. Cross section of a wood sample cut with a focused CO_2 laser beam (from Haun *et al.*, 1968).

cross section of a 3/4 in. thick sample of wood cut at ~ 8 in./min with a focused CO_2 laser beam. The cutting action is a combination of entrapped water evaporation, gas heating, and chemical reaction induced by the laser heating.

Chemical Reactions. Intense heating can promote irreversible chemical reactions which result in the weakening or removal of material. Oxidation (i.e., burning) converts solids and liquids into volatile gases, which readily escape from the heated zone. Steel can be cut by the exothermic chemical reaction between the steel and an oxygen jet (Sullivan and Houldcroft, 1967; Adams, 1968), with the concentrated heat source merely initiating and sustaining the reaction. Often the products of chemical reactions are structurally weak or of increased volume, leading to material fracture from thermal or expansive stresses.

Phase Changes. Concentrated heat can alter the molecular arrangement of a material and so change the metallurgical phase (i.e., the change of α-quartz to β-quartz upon heating) (Browell and Hetherington, 1964). These products are often weaker or of increased volume, causing fracture from thermal or expansive stresses.

Thermal Stresses. If a material is heated unevenly, gradients in local temperature are produced which can lead to fracture. This follows from the tendency of most solid materials to expand upon heating. Large temperature gradients in a material therefore produce large expansion differentials. Thermally induced stresses within a material can cause it to fail through fracture (Moavenzadeh *et al.*, 1968).

Shock Wave Propagation. Particularly in the case of high peak power pulsed laser systems, it is suspected that beam energy propagates into the irradiated material by means of a traveling shock wave (Haun, 1968). This impulse of acoustical energy, if excessive, can cause structural weakening and microfractures contributing to material failure.

Since lasers can be considered to be sources of concentrated "heat" energy for the purposes of industrial machining and welding, many successful laser applications are obvious extensions of older "thermal" techniques. For example, melting, evaporation, and sputtering of metals with laser beams follow naturally from the prior art of machining and welding with torches and arcs. Most of the early laser applications were concerned with these fundamental interactions and many economically feasible operations have been isolated. These include (Cohen and Epperson, 1968; Gagliano *et al.*, 1969) microcircuit welding, plastic strip cutting, diamond die drilling, and resistor trimming. Figure 13 illustrates another such application—the repair of an electron tube by focusing a pulsed ruby laser through the glass envelope onto the faulty connection designated by the arrow. In this case a 0.030 in. diameter Kovar wire was welded to a 0.010 in. thick steel tab to repair the tube without breaking the vacuum seal. Recently several laser-age versions of well-established material processing techniques have been developed, and merit special attention due to their novelty and effectiveness.

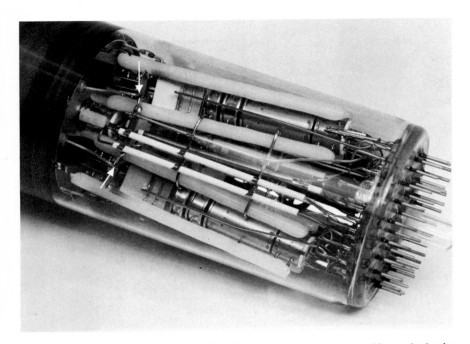

FIG. 13. Electron tube circuit welding through the glass envelope with a pulsed ruby laser. The white arrow designates the repaired connection.

A. GAS JET-ASSISTED LASER CUTTING

For many years the property of exothermic chemical reactions has been exploited in the oxyacetylene torch cutting of metals. The heat from the torch initiates melting and oxidation of the metal, but it is the large amount of heat released by this oxidation process which actually performs the cutting. The convective flow of the gas stream is effective in blowing the molten oxide away from the cutting area. A similar combination of laser heating in the presence of an oxygen jet was proposed by Sullivan and Houldcroft (1967) for the exothermic CO_2 laser cutting of metals. The experimental arrangement is shown in Fig. 14. The 10.6 μ output from a CO_2 laser is directed downward toward the workpiece by reflection from a plane mirror and passes through a focusing lens. This lens forms part of a small pressure chamber into which oxygen is fed. Both the focused laser beam and the oxygen jet emerge coaxially through a nozzle at the bottom of the pressure chamber. The workpiece is translated past this focal point to effect a cutting traversal.

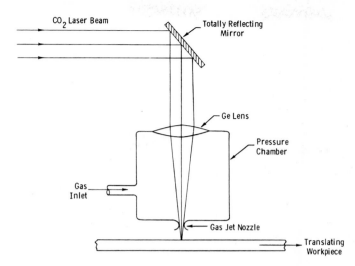

FIG. 14. Schematic diagram of the apparatus used to cut materials with a focused CO_2 laser beam and a coaxial gas jet.

Metals which possess a low thermal diffusivity can sustain sufficiently high temperatures to melt the oxide, providing this melting point is not too high. Adams (1968) demonstrated that mild steel, stainless steel, and titanium possess such properties by cutting them with an oxygen jet assisted CO_2 laser beam of 250 to 400 W. Cutting rates varied from 15 in./min for the stainless steel to >100 in./min in titanium. Other investigators[7] have since improved upon this performance, cutting commercially pure titanium 0.020 in. thick at 600 in./min with 135 W of laser power. A particularly attractive feature of these cuts is the very narrow kerf width: 0.015 in. for the 0.020 in. thick titanium. Typically, the heat-affected zone is very small, often less than 0.010 in. Thicknesses of 0.39 in. titanium have been cut at 100 in./min, as well as 0.010 in. zircaloy at 600 in./min. Holes have been burned through 1/8 in. thick boron filament and titanium-clad boron, materials which are otherwise difficult to drill (Bod et al., 1969). Metals such as copper and aluminium have thermal diffusivities about an order of magnitude higher than titanium, and therefore have not been cut using this method. However, thin sheets of copper 0.010 in. thick have been cut using Cl_2 as the reactive gas with the CO_2 laser beam (Adams, 1968).

A variation of this method employs an inert gas in the pressure chamber to purge the workpiece with a high velocity jet of nonreacting gas (Adams,

[7] See "CO_2 Applications," available from Coherent Radiation Laboratories, 932 East Meadow Drive, Palo Alto, California, 1969.

1968).[8] Gases such as N_2 and Ar have been employed to inhibit burning which might otherwise damage the workpiece. Polyester carpet, wood, paper, and plastics have been cut with an inert gas jet assisted CO_2 laser.[8] The inert gas jet also cools the cut edges and blows away accumulated debris. Both the reactive and inert gas jet methods have extended CO_2 laser cutting techniques into areas not previously considered feasible, and should yield improved results as higher laser power levels are employed.

B. LASER-INDUCED THERMAL FRACTURE

Many brittle materials will fracture when subjected to large temperature gradients—for example, a cold drinking glass plunged into hot water. Recently CO_2 laser beams have been employed to establish high localized gradients in brittle materials, and thereby induce mechanical failure. (Gagliano *et al.*, 1969; Bod *et al.*, 1969). The fracture separates the material along a line defined by the laser-heated zone, and no material is removed through melting, evaporation, or sputtering. Since the focused CO_2 laser beam is capable of exceptional heat localization and ease of movement, these fractures are induced in a controllable fashion. Materials which possess a high coefficient of thermal expansion, a low thermal diffusivity and low mechanical strength are good candidates for this process.

Rock samples have been subjected to the radiation of an unfocused 0–5 kW CO_2 laser beam (Williamson *et al.*, 1968), and were found to weaken through internal thermal fracture. It is thought that this weakening occurs due to microfractures induced by expansive heating of entrapped water and gaseous vapors. In addition, gross fractures are induced in the bulk samples due to excessive laser-induced thermal gradients. Rectangular bars of granite and marble were irradiated for periods ranging up to 32 sec, corresponding to total energy inputs between 1000 and 30,000 J. Structural weakening of the samples was observed after a few thousand J, roughly independent of the power level employed. Between 10 and 190 J/cm^3 of rock volume was required to produce thermal weakening to half strength using the CO_2 laser beam. This compares with 260–390 J/cm^3 required to fragment marble or granite with a jackhammer, and ~ 6600 J/cm^3 using flame jet piercing (Schumacher, 1968; Schumacher and Taylor, 1969). Similar results have been obtained with high power electron beams, where the specific energy requirement is 117–315 J/cm^3 for granite (Schumacher, 1968; Schumacher and Taylor, 1969). Thus preliminary CO_2 laser experiments with laboratory rock

---

[8] See "CO_2 Applications," available from Coherent Radiation Laboratories, 932 East Meadow Drive, Palo Alto, California, 1969.

samples indicate that the specific energy requirement is competitive with jackhammer and electron beam techniques, and superior to flame jet piercing. Provided these performance characteristics can be upscaled to higher power levels and larger rock samples, the CO_2 laser thermal fracture of rocks could be used for large scale rock crushing and tunnel boring.

V. Lasers and Industrial Processing

Pulsed and continuous lasers have found a wide variety of applications in the processing of material commonly used in industry. It appears that by now almost every type of material has been thrust into the focused beam of a high power laser, and the gross characteristics of various laser effects are well established. Recently several comprehensive reviews have appeared (Cohen and Epperson, 1968; Gagliano et al., 1969) which contain extensive bibliographies of the laser: materials-processing literature, and descriptions of specific applications in some detail. The reader is referred to these surveys for an introduction to laser techniques presently being applied in industry. Rather than attempt to duplicate these effeorts, the present treatment will consider a few of the more general concepts of material processing with concentrated heat sources. Laser and electron beam sources are considered to be equivalent, in that both serve to deposit large amounts of concentrated thermal energy onto the workpiece. For many applications the effects of incident beam energy can be assessed using the classical heat flow equations applied to rather simple physical models. Several of these models will be described, and where they are inadequate more suitable physical models will be discussed.

A. Surface Reflectivity

Many materials would appear to be unsuitable for laser processing because of their high reflectivity at certain laser wavelengths. Table III summarizes the nominal reflectivity of several metals at laser wavelengths of interest (American Institute of Physics Handbook, 1967). In particular, most metals are so highly reflecting at the 10.6 μ carbon dioxide wavelength that only a few percent of the incident beam energy is transmitted into the material. On this basis CO_2 lasers have been traditionally eliminated for most metalworking applications, and the Nd^{3+} and Cr^{3+} wavelengths have been favored. Indeed, pulsed ruby and glass lasers have encountered great success in welding small metallic pieces, and it is certain that the lower surface

TABLE III

REFLECTANCE OF SEVERAL METALS FOR NORMAL INCIDENCE
OF LIGHT AT COMMON LASER WAVELENGTHS

Wavelength (μ)	Au	Cu	Mo	Ag	Al	Cr	Fe	Ni
0.4880 (Ar II)	0.415	0.437	0.455	0.952	—	—	—	0.597
0.6943 (Cr^{3+})	0.930	0.831	0.498	0.961	—	0.555	0.575	0.676
1.06 (Nd^{3+})	0.981	0.901	0.582	0.964	0.733	0.570	0.650	0.741
10.6 (CO_2)	0.975	0.984	0.945	0.989	0.970	0.930	—	0.941

reflectivity at these wavelengths has been the determining factor. Table III illustrates the desirability of having high power ArII lasers available for certain metals.

Surface finish and the dynamics of material removal, however, greatly affect the absorption of energy within a material. Gagliano et al. (1969) demonstrated that the reflectivity of polished copper at 694.3 nm could be reduced from ~95% to less than 20% by oxidizing the surface, and that surface roughness on the order of the laser wavelength greatly increased the depth of energy penetration. Once some absorption of energy has occurred, handbook reflectivity data become almost meaningless. At high power densities a plasma plume of ejected vapors is formed, and the absorption of laser energy in the vapor can significantly reduce the effective reflectivity. The removal of surface material by the initial pulse of laser energy forms a small crater which "traps" the incident light within the hole; this entrapment of radiation also increases the effective absorption rate at the surface. Thus published reflectivity data can be employed to estimate absorption in smooth, uncontaminated surfaces at low power levels, but should not be extrapolated to high power densities where craters and plasma plumes are formed.

B. ABSORPTION

Incident energy which is not reflected at the surface is absorbed as the light propagates into the medium. This absorption is described by Lambert's Law, which states that

$$I(x) = I(O) \exp(-\alpha x) \qquad (1)$$

where $I(x)$ = light intensity in watts after propagation of x meters; $I(O)$ = light intensity at $x = 0$, in watts; α = absorption coefficient in meters^{-1}; and, x = propagation distance in meters.

Thus most of the energy propagating into the material is absorbed in a few e-folding "skin depths" δ, where

$$\delta = \alpha^{-1} \tag{2}$$

It can be shown (Ditchburn, 1963) that for normal incidence materials which strongly reflect light are highly absorbant as well. For most metals the skin depths δ are less than 0.1 μm for visible and infrared wavelengths, and for most organic compounds far infrared 10.6 μ CO_2 radiation is absorbed in less than 1 μm. Therefore laser absorption may be considered to be a surface effect in most materials of interest, with energy propagating into the bulk primarily through heat conduction. Energetic electrons can penetrate much farther into solid materials; 150 kV electrons dissipate most of their kinetic energy within a distance of ~ 100 μ in a target like rock (Schumacher and Taylor, 1969). In this case energy propagation can occur at a rate substantially greater than that given by heat conduction, providing the molten material can be removed rapidly enough. At very high beam energy densities both laser and electron sources can remove material through vaporization and sputtering, continuously exposing a new surface to beam irradiation. Thus for pulsed irradiation and machining applications, simple heat conduction models are often not adequate. However, heat conduction from the irradiated surface is usually the dominant energy transfer mechanism for pulsed and continuous welding operations. Several simple heat conduction models will be considered in the following sections.

C. Heat Conduction from a Surface

Heat flow in an isotropic solid is described (Carslaw and Jaeger, 1959a) by the following relation:

$$\vec{f} = -K\nabla T \tag{3}$$

where $\vec{f} =$ directed heat flux in joules $\sec^{-1}$ cm^{-2}; $K =$ coefficient of thermal conductivity in watts cm^{-1} $^\circ K^{-1}$; and $T =$ absolute temperature in $^\circ K$.

Thus heat flow is proportional to the thermal conductivity K and the temperature gradient, and is in the direction of maximally decreasing temperatures. The energy conservation law may be expressed as

$$\nabla \cdot \vec{f} + \rho c(\partial T/\partial t) = 0 \tag{4}$$

where $\rho =$ mass density in gm cm^{-3}; $c =$ specific heat in joules gm^{-1} $^\circ K^{-1}$; and $t =$ time in seconds. This merely states that the net flow rate of heat into an elemental volume is equal to the rate of increase of heat within the volume.

Combining Eqs. (3) and (4), it follows that

$$\nabla \cdot (-K\nabla T) + \rho c(\partial T/\partial t) = 0$$

or

$$\partial T/\partial t = \kappa \nabla^2 T, \tag{5}$$

where the thermal diffusivity κ is defined as

$$\kappa \equiv K/\rho c \tag{6}$$

The units of κ are cm^2/sec, and this material constant determines the rate at which heat diffuses into an isotropic solid. Equation (5) is the familiar diffusion equation for temperature T, and it can easily be shown that the same equation applies for the heat flux $\bar{f}$; i.e.,

$$\partial \bar{f}/\partial t = \kappa \nabla^2 \bar{f} \tag{7}$$

If heat is produced within the solid at a rate S joules $sec^{-1} cm^{-3}$, Eq. (5) becomes

$$\rho c(\partial T/\partial t) = K\nabla^2 T + S \tag{8}$$

or

$$\partial T/\partial t = \kappa \nabla^2 T + S/\rho c$$

In the steady state time derivatives vanish, and

$$\nabla^2 T = -S/K \tag{9}$$

and for no heat sources the familiar Laplace's equation applies:

$$\nabla^2 T = 0 \tag{10}$$

It is instructive to solve the diffusion equation for one-dimensional flow in a semi infinite medium. Assuming that the initial temperature throughout the medium is zero, and that the surface $x = 0$ is maintained at T_0 for $t > 0$, Carslaw and Jaeger (1959b) give the solution

$$T(x, t) = T_0 \text{ erfc } (x/2\sqrt{\kappa t}), \tag{11}$$

$$\text{erf } z \equiv 2/\sqrt{\pi} \int_0^z e^{-\xi^2} d\xi \tag{12}$$

$$\text{erfc } z \equiv 1 - \text{erf } z$$

$$= 2/\sqrt{\pi} \int_0^\infty e^{-\xi^2} d\xi \tag{13}$$

$$\text{ierfc } z \equiv \int_z^\infty \text{erfc } u \, du$$

$$= e^{-z^2}/\sqrt{\pi} - z \text{ erfc } z \tag{14}$$

These error functions appear frequently in heat flow and probability and are tabulated in several references (Carslaw and Jaeger, 1959c). For temperature $T(x, t)$ to increase half way to the wall temperature T_0, $T(x, t)/T_0 = 0.5$, and from Carslaw and Jaeger's table of complementary error functions (Carslaw and Jaeger, 1959c),

$$x/2\sqrt{\kappa \pi} = 0.523 \tag{15}$$

Penetration of the $T(x, t)/T_0 = 0.5$ isotherm to a depth of 1 cm would require a time

$$t \text{ (sec)} = 1.114/\kappa(\text{cm}^2/\text{sec}) \tag{16}$$

Table IV lists these penetration times for a few materials, using published

TABLE IV

CALCULATED PENETRATION TIMES FOR THE $T/T_0 = 0.5$ ISOTHERM
INTO VARIOUS THICKNESSES OF COMMON METALS

Material	Thermal diffusivity (cm²/sec)	Penetration time (sec)		
		$x = 0.1$ cm	$x = 1.0$ cm	$x = 10$ cm
Aluminum	0.91	0.0122	1.22	122
Chromium	0.20	0.0557	5.57	557
Copper	1.14	0.0098	0.98	97.8
Gold	1.18	0.0095	0.95	95
Silver	1.71	0.0065	0.65	65
Titanium	0.082	0.136	13.6	136
(Soil, concrete)	0.005	2.37	237	23,700

thermal diffusivities (Gagliano *et al.*, 1969). It is seen that even materials of high thermal diffusivity like silver possess characteristic isothermal penetration times of $\lesssim 1$ sec for a 1 cm thickness and that chromium and titanium require ~ 10 sec for comparable penetration.

Heat flux incident upon the surface of a semi-infinite medium causes a temperature rise given by Carslaw and Jaeger (1959b), as

$$T(x, t) = (2F_0/K)\{(\kappa t/\pi)^{1/2} \exp(-x^2/4\kappa t) - (x/2) \text{ erfc } (x/2\sqrt{\kappa t})\} \tag{17}$$

At the surface $x = 0$, the temperature rise is

$$T(x, t)|_{x=0} = [2F_0/K](\kappa t/\pi)^{1/2} \tag{18}$$

where F_0 is the constant heat flux in joules sec^{-1} cm^{-2}. Thus the time required to reach the melting point on the surface of a material may be

. the material properties and incident power ...g points and thermal conductivities of several ...ated times required for surface melting to occur at ...an incident flux of 10^4 W/cm^2, melting temperatures are ...ne surface in ~0.1 sec for Cr, Au, and Ag, but ~0.01 sec for Ti. ...melting time is inversely proportional to the square of the incident power density, so that at 10^6 W/cm^2 melting times are reduced to between 10^{-5} and 10^{-6} sec. Even if only 1% of the incident power is absorbed on the surface, it is apparent that beam densities of $\gtrsim 10^6$ W/cm^2 are capable of producing surface melting of these metals in times $\gtrsim 0.1$ sec.

TABLE V

CALCULATED TIME REQUIRED FOR SURFACE MELTING TO OCCUR IN SEVERAL METALS
IRRADIATED WITH A CONSTANT HEAT FLUX

Material	Thermal conductivity[a] (W cm^{-1} °K^{-1})	Diffusivity (cm^2 sec^{-1})	Melting temp.[b] (°K)	Melting time (sec)	
				$F_0 = 10^4$ W cm^{-2}	$F_0 = 10^6$ W cm^{-2}
Aluminum	2.38	0.91	933	4.24×10^{-2}	4.24×10^{-6}
Chromium	0.87	0.20	2176	1.4×10^{-1}	1.4×10^{-5}
Copper	4.0	1.14	1356	2.03×10^{-1}	2.03×10^{-5}
Gold	3.11	1.18	1336	1.15×10^{-1}	1.15×10^{-5}
Silver	4.18	1.71	1234	1.22×10^{-1}	1.22×10^{-5}
Titanium	0.20	0.082	1941	1.45×10^{-2}	1.45×10^{-5}

[a] *American Institute of Physics Handbook*, p. 4–90.
[b] *Ibid.*, p. 4–172.

A more realistic approximation to laser beam irradiation is the heating of a circular area of radius a on the surface of a semi-infinite medium. Carslaw and Jaeger (1959d) give the solution for a point on the z axis; that is, the axis perpendicular to the plane of the heated circle, and passing through its center. This is

$$T(z, t) = (2F_0 \sqrt{\kappa t}/K)\{\text{ierfc}\,(z/2\sqrt{\kappa t}) - \text{ierfc}\,([z^2 + a^2]^{1/2}/2\sqrt{\kappa t})\} \quad (19)$$

for an incident heat flux F_0 W/cm^2 and a distance z into the medium from the spot center. At the center of the spot ($z = 0$), the temperature rise for a flux F_0 is

$$T(z, t)|_{z=0} = (2F_0 \sqrt{\kappa t}/K)\{1/\sqrt{\pi} - \text{ierfc}\,(a/2\sqrt{\kappa t})\} \quad (20)$$

since ierfc $0 = 1/\sqrt{\pi}$. The second term of this expression vanishes for infinite argument, so that Eq. (20) for circular disk heating approaches the expression in Eq. (18) for complete surface heating as $(a/2\sqrt{\kappa t}) \to 0$. In fact, this second term is reduced to 10% of the first term in 3.42×10^{-3} sec for $a = 0.1$ cm in copper having $\kappa = 1.14$ cm²/sec. Thus for heat fluxes below $\sim 10^4$ W/cm² at $a = 0.1$ cm, Eq. (18) for complete surface heating is adequate; above $F_0 \sim 10^6$ W/cm² or for a < 0.1 cm, the complete Eq. (20) should be employed. Simple calculations on the basis of complete surface heating can be useful for continuous heating in large spot diameters.

D. Hole Penetration in the Steady State

Klemens (1968) has considered the problem of a deep hole bored into a material by a narrow beam of electron or laser energy in the steady state. If the hole is deep and narrow, conduction of heat away from the hole determines its depth. The heat conduction for a hole of length D through a cylinder of inside diameter l and inside temperature T_M, and outside diameter L and temperature T_0 is given by

$$W_I = 2\pi D K[(T_M - T_0)/\ln (L/l)] \tag{21}$$

Here W_I is the incident beam power and K the material thermal conductivity. Klemens argues that for the steady state little error is involved in approximating D by $L/2$, and assuming that

$$\ln (L/l) \simeq \ln (2D/l) \approx 4 \tag{22}$$

The dependence upon l is very slight in any case, since it enters Eq. (21) logarithmically. Thus the hole depth, for deep and narrow penetrations, is given by

$$D \simeq 4W_I/2\pi K(T_M - T_0) \tag{23}$$

and is approximately independent of the hole diameter. For a 1 kW laser beam penetrating into a metal such as copper ($T_M = 1356°$K, $K = 4.0$ W cm^{-1} °K^{-1}), the calculated hole depth is 0.151 cm. Table VI indicates the calculated steady-state hole depths for several materials for 300°K ambient temperature. It is seen that a 1 kW unit can produce narrow holes of ~ 1 mm in high conductivity metals such as Ag and Cu, and holes of ~ 16 cm depth in a material like rock. Thus continuous beam powers of at least 10^4 W would be required to produce welds of several centimeter depth in metals, whereas narrow holes of several centimeter depth can be made in rock with $\gtrsim 10^3$ W.

It should be noted that this computation is only approximate, and assumes that no energy is lost from the incident beam except that carried away in the material by conduction. Although energy loss by radiation is

TABLE VI

CALCULATED DEPTHS OF HOLES IN SEVERAL MATERIALS FOR A
CONSTANT INCIDENT BEAM FLUX, ASSUMING LONG NARROW HOLES

Material	Conductivity (W cm^{-1} °K^{-1})	Melting temp. (°K)	Depth D (cm)	
			$W_I = 10^3$ W	$W_I = 10^4$ W
Aluminum	2.38	933	0.423	4.23
Chromium	0.87	2176	0.391	3.91
Copper	4.0	1356	0.151	1.51
Gold	3.11	1336	0.198	1.98
Silver	4.18	1234	0.124	1.24
Titanium	0.20	1941	1.64	16.4
Rocks (avg.)	0.02	~ 2000	15.9	159.0

negligible, considerable energy can be carried away from the hole by emerging vapors. This loss increases as the square of the hole diameter, and is negligible only for long, thin holes. If the beam power is less than the loss by vapor flow, no deep hole is drilled at all; the beam gradually penetrates into the material surface, leaving a relatively wide depression. This process continues until D is comparable to l and the depth of penetration is governed by the rate at which material evaporation occurs.

If the workpiece moves with velocity v (cm/sec) during beam irradiation, the penetration depth is decreased. This occurs because a portion of the beam energy is now required to heat the wake of molten material behind the hole. Since less beam energy is available for hole penetration, less conduction losses (i.e., lower D) are required for energy balance. Klemens (1968) has computed that the velocity v_c at which hole penetration is halved is

$$v_c = 2\pi K/3l \qquad (24)$$

Thus for a typical metal, $\kappa \simeq 1$ cm^2/sec and $l \sim 0.2$ cm, and this velocity is $v_c \simeq 10$ cm/sec. For a poor conductor like concrete ($\kappa \simeq 0.005$ cm^2/sec), the velocity is $v_c \simeq 0.05$/sec.

E. RATE OF HOLE PENETRATION

At very high beam intensities ($\gtrsim 10^7$ W/cm^2) the heating is so rapid that conduction into the interior of the solid can be neglected. The incident radiation is absorbed in a thin layer of material at the surface, and rapid vaporization of the material occurs. This skin depth is ~ 100 μm for electron beam devices, and $\gtrsim 1$ μm lasers. Consequently the surface of the material recedes with a velocity dx/dt as material is vaporized. If the vapor is removed rapidly enough so that it does not interfere with the incident beam, the rate of vaporization is quite simply related to the incident flux F by

$$F = dx/dt \cdot C \tag{25}$$

Here C is the amount of energy required to vaporize a unit volume of material, and for most metals is on the order of 3×10^3 J cm^{-3}. Thus for unimpeded vaporization an incident flux of 3×10^7 W/cm^2 would result in a surface recession rate of $\sim 10^4$ cm/sec. However, this transient condition of unimpeded vaporization does not persist for a very long time. Vapor is produced in a time t_0 on the order of

$$t_0 \sim l(dx/dt) = lC/F \tag{26}$$

where l is the approximate skin depth of energy penetration. For l as large as 10^{-4} cm, $F = 3 \times 10^7$ W cm^{-1}, and $C = 3 \times 10^3$ J cm^{-3}, $t_0 = 10^{-8}$ sec. Thus vapor is created very rapidly for high incident fluxes and the effects of energy absorption by the vapor must be considered.

After a volume of material has been evaporated a period of time elapses before this vapor can be ejected from the irradiated volume. During this time it has about the same density as the solid, and therefore continues to absorb energy incident upon it. The vapor expands more rapidly than it would otherwise, and extracts beam energy which would otherwise be used for vaporization. Consequently, less material is removed. Klemens (1968) has shown that for low values of F the removal rate varies directly with F according to Eq. (25), but for high fluxes $(dx/dt) \alpha F^{1/3}$. The creation of a vaporization plume at high power densities substantially reduces the erosion rate.

VI. Conclusions

Lasers are well established as industrial processing tools in certain applications (Gagliano et al., 1969) such as resistor trimming, microcircuit welding, diamond die drilling, and semiconductor dicing. The availability of reliable commercial laser equipment has been a large contributing factor in the practical utilization of laser techniques, for in all cases the laser must compete economically with existing methods. It is certain that in coming years these devices will be available in more efficient, powerful, and reliable versions. Pulsed lasers have already achieved peak powers and irradiance exceeding any other known source of energy, and further increases in these capabilities seem likely. However, it is in average power capability that significant improvement is to be anticipated. Most of the problems associated with high average power units are component failures induced by excessive heating or discharge sputting, or the technical difficulties of building physically large units. As laser rods, pump lamps, mirrors, and engineering design improve, very high power devices will result. YAG and ArII lasers of increased power should find wide application in medium and heavy processing. The CO_2 laser, however, will probably prove to be the workhorse of the industry in future years as its cw power capability is pushed beyond 10 kW. Such devices might largely supplant conventional methods of cutting, slitting, heating, cracking, drilling, and welding in heavy industry. The electron beam welder appears to be particularly useful for vacuum welding of metals, and the CO_2 laser might never be able to compete in this area. It is likely that the emerging CO_2 laser and electron beam technologies will produce units capable of machining and welding almost all materials. Directed energy sources are still in a period of rapid growth and innovation, and we might expect the coming years to be as eventful as the past years.

ACKNOWLEDGMENTS

The author wishes to express his gratitude to colleagues at the Westinghouse Research Laboratory, in particular K. B. Steinbruegge, W. N. Platte, R. D. Haun, Jr., and J. C. Brown and to T. A. Osial of the Westinghouse Industrial Equipment Division. The advice of P. G. Klemens, Westinghouse consultant, on hole penetration models is also gratefully acknowledged.

REFERENCES

American Institute of Physics Handbook. (1967). (D. E. Gray, ed.), p. 6–107, 6–120. McGraw-Hill, New York..

Adams, M. J. (1968). *Weld. Inst. Res. Bull.* **9**, 1.

Banse, K., Boersch, H., Herziger, G., Schaefer, G., and Seelig, W. (1969). *Z. Angew. Phys.* **26**, 195.

Beaulieu, A. J. (1970). *Appl. Phys. Lett.* **16**, 504.

Bennett, W. R., Jr. (1965). Chemical Lasers, *Appl. Opt. Suppl.* **2**, p. 3.

Bennett, W. R., Jr., Knutson, J. W., Mercer, G. N., and Decht, J. L. (1964a). *Appl. Phys. Lett.* **4**, 180.

Bennett, W. R., Jr., Kindlmann, P. J., Mercer, G. N., and Sunderland, J. (1964b). *Appl. Phys. Lett.* **5**, 158.

Bod, D., Brasier, R. E., and Parkes, J. (1969). *Laser Focus* **5**, 36.

Bowness, C., Missio, D., and Rogala, T. (1962). *Proc. IEEE* **50**, 1704.

Bridges, W. B. (1964). *Appl. Phys. Lett.* **4**, 128.

Bridges, W. B., and Chester, A. N. (1965). *IEEE J. Quantum Electron.* **1**, 66.

Bronfin, B. R., Boedecker, L. R., and Cheyer, J. P. (1969). *Bull. Amer. Phys. Soc.* **14**, 857.

Browell, T. P., and Hetherington, G. (1964). *J. Brit. Soc. Sci. Glassblowers* **3**, 1.

Carslaw, H. S., and Jaeger, J. C. (1959a). "Conduction of Heat in Solids," Ch. 1. Oxford Univ. Press (Clarendon), London and New York.

Carslaw, H. S., and Jaeger, J. C. (1959b). "Conduction of Heat in Solids," Ch. 2. Oxford Univ. Press (Clarendon), London and New York.

Carslaw, H. S., and Jaeger, J. C. (1959c). "Conduction of Heat in Solids," Appendix II. Oxford Univ. Press (Clarendon), London and New York.

Carslaw, H. S., and Jaeger, J. C. (1959d). "Conduction of Heat in Solids," Ch. 10. Oxford Univ. Press (Clarendon), London and New York.

Chesler, R. B., Geusic, J. E., and Karr, M. A. (1969). *IEEE J. Quantum Electron.* **5**, 345. (Abstr.)

Chester A. N. (1968a). *Phys. Rev.* **169**, 172.

Chester, A. N. (1968b). *Phys. Rev.* **169**, 184.

Church, C. H., and Liberman, I. (1967) *Appl. Opt*, **6**, 1966.

Ciftan, M., Luck, C. F., Shafer, C. G., and Statz, H. (1961). *Proc. IEEE* **49**, 960.

Cohen, M. I., and Epperson, J. P. (1968). *In* " Electron Beam and Laser Beam Technology " (L. Marton and A. B. El-Kareh, eds.), *Advan. Electron.* Vol. 4, Suppl., pp. 139–186. Academic Press, New York.

Collins, R. J., and Kisliuk, P. (1962). *J. Appl. Phys.* **33**, 2009.

Cool, T. A., and Shirley, J. A. (1969). *Appl. Phys. Lett.* **14**, 70.

Deutsch, T. F., Horrigan, F. A., and Rudko, R. I. (1969). *Appl. Phys. Lett.* **15**, 88.

Ditchburn, R. W. (1963). " Light," p. 553. Wiley (Interscience), New York.

Dowley, M. W. (1968). *Appl. Phys. Lett.* **13**, 395.

Evtuhov, V., and Neeland, J. K. (1965). *Appl. Phys. Lett.* **6**, 75.

Fein, M. E., Verdeyen, J. T., and Cherrington, B. E. (1969). *Appl. Phys. Lett.* **14**, 337.

Gagliano, F. P., Lumley, R. M., and Watkins, L. S. (1969). *Proc. IEEE* **57**, 114.

Gerry, E. T. (1970). *Laser Focus* **6**, 27.

Gobeli, G. (1969). *Electronic News* **14**, 72.

Gordon, E. I., Labuda, E. F., and Bridges, W. B. (1964). *Appl. Phys. Lett.* **4**, 178.

Hagan, W. F. (1969). *J. Appl. Phys.* **40**, 511.

Haun, R. D., Jr. (1968). *IEEE Spectrum* **5**, 82.

Haun, R. D., Jr., Osial, T. A., Weaver, L. A., Steinbruegge, K. B., and Vaerewyck, E. G. (1968). *IEEE Trans. Ind. Gen. Appl.* **4**, 379.

Herziger, G., and Seelig, W. (1969). *IEEE J. Quantum Electron.* **5**, 364, (Abstr.)

Hill, A. E. (1968). *Appl. Phys. Lett.* **12**, 324.

Hill, A. E. (1971). *Appl. Phys. Lett.* **18**, 194.

Hocker, L. O., Kovacs, M. A., Rhodes, C. K., Flynn, G. W., and Javan, A. (1966). *Phys. Rev Lett.* **17**, 233.

Horrigan, F. A., Rudko, R. I., and Wilson, D. (1968). *Quantum Electronics Conf. Miami, Florida.* Paper 10J-4.

Klemens, P. G. (1968). *Int. Conf. Electron Ion Beam Sci. Technol. 3rd Boston, Mass.* 291

Koechner, (1969a). *Optical Society of America Meeting, Chicago, Ill.* Paper TuE12. p. 11.

Koechner, W. (1969b). *Laser Focus* **5**, 29.

Liberman. I. (1969). *IEEE J. Quantum Electron.* **5**, 345 (Abstr.)

Liberman, I., Larson, D. A., and Church, C. H. (1969). *IEEE J. Quantum Electron.* **5**, 238.

McClung, F. J., and Hellwarth, R. W. (1962). *J. Appl. Phys.* **33**, 828.

Moavenzadeh, F., Williamson, R. B., and McGarry, F. J. (1968). M.I.T. Dept. of Civil Eng., Rept. for the U.S. Dept. of Transport, Washington, D.C., Contr. C–85–65.

Nelson, D. F., and Boyle, W. S. (1962). *Appl. Opt.* **1**, 181.

Nighan, W. L., and Bennett, J. H. (1969). *Appl. Phys. Lett.* **14**, 240.

Patel, C. K. N. (1964a). *Phys. Rev. Lett.* **13**, 617.

Patel, C. K. N. (1964b). *Phys. Rev. A* **136**, 1187.

Platte, W. N., and Smith, J. F. (1963). *Weld. J.* (*New York*) **42**, 481.

Schumacher, B. W. (1968). *Int. Conf. Electron Ion Beam Sci. Technol.* 3rd Boston, Mass.,
    p. 447.
Schumacher, B. W., and Taylor, C. R. (1969). *Rec.* **10th** *Annu. Symp. Electron Ion Laser
    Beam Technol.*, *Gaithersburg*, **1969**, p. 271.
Shapiro, S. L., and Duguay, M. A. (1969). *Phys. Lett. A* **28**, 698.
Smith, J. F. (1969). *Laser Focus* **5**, 32.
Smith, R. G., and Galvin, M. F. (1967). *IEEE J. Quantum Electron* **3**, 406.
Snitzer, E. (1961). *Phys. Rev. Lett.* **7**, 444.
Soffer, B. H. (1964). *J. Appl. Phys.* **35**, 2551.
Sullivan, A. B. J., and Houldcroft, P. T. (1967). *Brit. Weld. J.* **14**, 443.
Tiffany, W. B., Targ, R., and Foster, J. D. (1969). *Appl. Phys. Lett.* **15**, 91.
Williamson, R. B., Moavenzadeh, F., and McGarry, F. J. (1968). M.I.T. Dept. of Civil
    Eng., Rept. for the U.S. Dept. of Transport, Contr. C-85-65.
Young, C. G., (1967). *Laser Focus* **3**. 21.
Young, C. G. (1969). *Proc. IEEE* **57**, 1267.

LASER COMMUNICATIONS

Monte Ross

McDonnell Douglas Astronautics Company
St. Louis, Missouri

I. Introduction

Laser communications may be divided into four general application classes: (a) terrestrial short-range paths through the atmospheres, (b) closed-pipe systems for sending high data rate between and within major metropolitan centers, (c) near-space communications for relaying high data rates, and (d) deep-space communications from the outer planets.

The division into the four classes is due to differences in path length, data regimes, line-of-sight requirements for laser links, and weather effects.

Obviously, in space line-of-sight can be billions of miles, whereas on the earth, line-of-sight is restricted to less than 100 miles. Line-of-sight requirements and weather effects can be overcome over long distances on earth by use of relay stations, forward scatter techniques, and closed pipe systems. However, many applications over short earth links can be met without resorting to these additional complications.

Each class has its own particular problems and solutions. In this paper, we review the fundamentals of laser communications, analyze each application, describe certain attractive design solutions, and indicate trends in laser communications.

II. Basic Advantages of Laser Communications

The advantage of laser communications over other technologies such as microwaves lies in (1) the attainable directivity with small "antennas" and (2) the wide bandwidths available and easily utilized.

The importance of the directionality factor can be noted by stating that the beamwidth of a electromagnetic signal is given by the diffraction limit as $\theta = 1.27 \lambda/D$, where λ is the wavelength and D is the transmitting aperture. Since λ is 10^3 to 10^4 smaller at optics than microwaves, D may be 10 cm to achieve beamwidths less than 10 μrad. The power required for transmission due to the directionality factor is much less than microwaves as given by the ratio of

$$\begin{matrix} \text{Less} \\ \text{power} \\ \text{required} \\ \text{(due to} \\ \text{beamwidth)} \end{matrix} = \left[\frac{(\lambda_L/D_L)}{(\lambda_M/D_M)} \right]^2 \tag{1}$$

where subscripts L and M refer to laser and microwave wavelengths.

In microwaves the antenna gain is established by consideration of $(\lambda/D)^2$. In antenna gain terms, a 10 cm aperture at optics can achieve antenna gain of 109 dB. At microwaves ($\lambda = 3$ cm), D would have to be 4×10^5 inches to equal this gain.

In Fig. 1 we plot diffraction-limited beamwidth for different transmitter apertures as a function of wavelength. The higher antenna gain of lasers does not result in direct system improvement by the ratio given in (1) due to different noise considerations at optical frequencies as compared to radio frequency (rf). This difference in noise aspects also results in signal design difference from that of rf. These areas are explored later in the text.

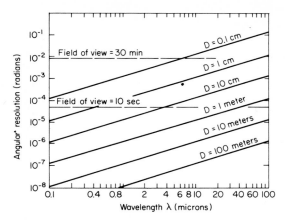

FIG. 1. Diffraction limited beamwidth as a function of wavelength. D = diameter of limiting aperture.

The second advantage of wide bandwidth is presently being realized in two ways: (1) use of short subnanosecond pulses and (2) analog cw modulation. The bandwidth generated by short pulses would take up the spectrum at microwaves but create no interference problems at optics since so much bandwidth is available. It is hard to visualize even multichannel high data rate laser systems making a slight "dent" in the total spectrum.

At present, the widest optical bandwidth communication system being considered utilizes 30 psec pulses which uses a bandwidth of approximately 30 GHz. At the laser wavelength of approximately 3×10^{14} Hz, 30 GHz is but 10^{-4} of the optical carrier frequency. One thousand such channels along the same path would only increase the bandwidth utilized to 10% of the carrier frequency. Yet, the 30 GHz presently being used in experiments exceeds the total rf and microwave spectrum. Further, the directionality factor of the laser would easily allow overlapping of spectrums for different links without interference problems.

III. Basic Types of Laser Links

There are two basic types of laser communication systems. The basic block diagrams are shown in Figs 2(a) and (2b). The heterodyne communication system is directly analogous to typical rf communications. The components work on different physical principles, but the system concept and techniques are direct transfers from established rf and microwave concepts. The laser signal is modulated, either by orthogonal phase-shift modulation with

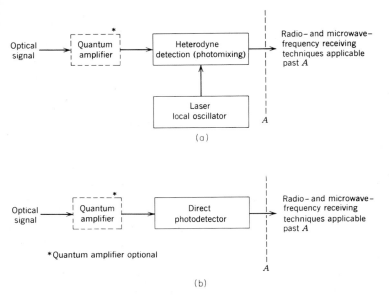

FIG. 2. Basic block diagrams of (a) photomixing (optical heterodyne) receiver and (b) direct detection receiver. Quantum amplifier generally neither practical or available.

circular output polarization, or by FM or pulse-code modulation. The received signal is mixed with a local oscillator, and the beat frequency passes through the intermediate frequency (IF) to a second detector, where the signal is recovered.

In direct detection, the system is more analogous to a crystal video detector at rf. The laser transmitter is intensity modulated, and the received energy is collected and focused on a photodetector (most likely a photomultiplier). The receiver responds only to the carrier's intensity changes (not to the phase). The signal is amplified within the photomultiplier so that at the output the signal is much larger than any thermal noise. The sensitivity limitations are signal-quantum noise and background noise.

To understand the limitations of direct detection and heterodyning we will review the basic operations of laser receivers. In either technique we could utilize an optical amplifier, known as a quantum amplifier, in front of the photomixer or photodetector. Figures 2(a) and (b) illustrate these two possibilities. Note that before the advent of the laser, only direct photodetection could be employed.

There are a number of receiving techniques (much as in rf receivers) that can be used once past the front end; these are usually peculiar to the particular system requirements. For example, if we are sending a microwave subcarrier, we require a microwave mixer, and an IF amplifier after detection. However, this technique is applicable to either front-end configuration of photomixing or direct photodetection. It is to be emphasized that, since the similarity to rf receivers becomes essentially identical after the optical front end, the discussion of receiving techniques will be primarily confined to the front end. However, the relative value of amplifiers, detectors, and heterodyne receivers has been changed by inclusion of quantum effects, so that conclusions valid at rf are not necessarily valid at optics.

It is of value to discuss direct photodetection first, since until recently this was the only available technique. The technique consists simply of detecting the incident energy within the spectral response of the detector, with the resultant detected signal being able to follow the amplitude variations induced by the incoming signal modulation. In direct photodetection, all optical frequency and phase information is lost. The detector cannot respond to frequency or phase modulation of the optical carrier. It will reproduce amplitude variations of the incident power, as long as the rate of the variations is less than the frequency response of the detector.

The direct photodetector can make no distinctions between signal photons or nonsignal (background) photons that are within the relatively broad spectral response characteristics. It has no special arrival angle requirement, except that the photon be intercepted by the photosensitive area. Thus, to achieve spectral discrimination we must insert an optical filter; similarly, if we are to achieve spatial discrimination, we must reduce the field of view by optical means.

Because of the laser's narrow spectral line, it has become possible to obtain mixing action at optical frequencies between two laser sources, one of which can be considered the signal and the other a local oscillator. Thus, it is possible to build an optical heterodyne or homodyne receiver. (Operation is called homodyne when the local oscillator is the same frequency as the optical carrier.) Figure 3 illustrates the photomixing technique. Complex experiments prior to laser development indicated that photomixing action can occur; however, the lack of a sufficiently narrow spectral source with

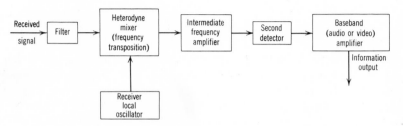

FIG. 3. Photomixing receiver system.

adequate power made measurements extremely difficult. Photomixing offers certain advantages as a receiving technique compared to direct photodetection. There are also a number of additional complexities to utilization of a photomixing system. Photomixing is best understood by considering the wave nature of light. This is consistent with the dual nature of radiation, represented by waves and particles. Photomixing, as in the rf heterodyning processes, is a form of coherent detection, whereas direct photodetection can be regarded as noncoherent detection. In noncoherent detection there is no negative output, the detector functioning as a rectifying element. The noncoherent detector response can be expressed as an even infinite series, as follows:

$$e_0 = ae_1{}^2 + be_1{}^4 + ce_1{}^6 + \cdots \tag{2}$$

Generally, we can ignore the higher order terms and get a good approximation of the action by assuming that $e_0 = ae_1{}^2$, i.e., that the rectifier is a square-law detector. Most photodetectors are ideal square-law devices in that higher order terms are not present.

The spatial requirements for photomixing have been shown to be much more severe than for microwave mixing (Ross, 1966). The basic reason is that the light wavelength is small compared to the photomixing area. Consider Fig. 4. The local oscillator and signal should be in phase across the

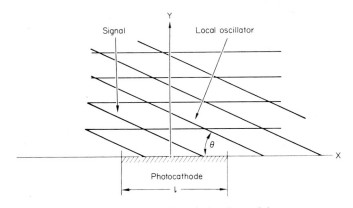

FIG. 4. Spatial relationship in photomixing.

whole photosurface. If they are not, beat currents at one part of the surface will be out of phase with beat currents at another part of the surface, resulting in signal loss. Since λ is of the order of 10^{-4} cm and the photosurface might be about 1 cm, it turns out that the angle between oscillator and signal must be less than 10^{-4} so as not to reduce the term involving the difference frequency.

The stringent spatial requirements on photomixing given above lead to serious practical problems in a receiver system, which differ considerably from the problems connected with the use of photomixing as an experimental laboratory tool. The atmosphere, for example, creates corruption of the phase front, making it most difficult to perform heterodyning, especially at visible wavelengths.

It is clear that many factors must be considered in deciding which receiving technique is more useful for a particular application. It would be fruitful, however, to present some fundamental comparisons between the two with the realization that any judgment must depend on how the comparison applies to a particular use. Table I is a summary of the comparisons.

TABLE I

COMPARISON BETWEEN PHOTOMIXING AND DIRECT PHOTODETECTION

Photomixing	Photodetection
Needs laser local oscillator	No local oscillator required
Spatial phasing requirements (superposition)	No spatial phase problem
Expected Doppler shifts require wide optical bandwidth and cause I–F problems	Expected Doppler shifts only require wider optical bandwidth
Phase distortion limits effective receiver area	Restriction several orders of magnitude less severe (effective receiver areas can be built much larger)
3 dB less noise (hfB) theoretically possible than in photodetection	Minimum noise is 2hfB
Large Conversion gain possible with no decrease in input SNR	Post detection secondary emission multiplication with no decrease in input SNR, current gains of 10^5 to 10^6
Background directional and frequency discrimination without use of optical filter. Additional discrimination with optical filter	No frequency discrimination in photodetection without use of optical filter.
Medium can affect system through loss of coherence	Medium not as critical. Loss of coherence not catastrophic

First, the fundamental difference is that photomixing requires a laser local oscillator. In some radarlike systems where transmitter and receiver are at the same physical location, it may be possible to utilize the same device as both transmitter source and local oscillator. In communication systems, however, it is clear that a laser must be used in a photomixer receiver, although one is not necessary in direct photodetection. Use of a laser local oscillator requires the same precision discussed earlier to avoid additional noise and interference, that is, a stable narrow linewidth source.

Another requirement of photomixing not necessary for direct photo-detection is that the local oscillator energy arrive at the photomixing surface in spatial phase with the signal energy. This requirement in turn puts constraints on how large a photon collecting area one can use, i.e., lens or parabolic mirror size. Optical techniques will restrict the receiver lens or reflecting parabola to the size at which phase distortion begins to become appreciable. When the path lengths from points on the collection area to the photocathode become significantly different by the order of the wavelength of the optical frequency, spatial phase coincidence with the local oscillator will be lost and rapid deterioration in photomixing performance will occur. Hence, for systems in which large collecting areas are possible, photodetection offers the ability to gather more useful signal photons.

The possible large Doppler shift at the optical frequencies can present serious problems in a photomixing system subject to large velocity changes. As the radial component of velocity changes, the Doppler shift frequency changes, causing a different frequency. In some cases, either the IF must be extremely broad or it must be tunable over a broad range, or the laser local oscillator must be tunable over the necessary range. There is, generally, a great amount of complexity and difficulty in tuning the local oscillator.

The heterodyne signal-to-noise ratio (SNR) given, for cw signals, is a factor of two better than direct detection, in the most sensitive condition of being signal photon limited (Oliver, 1961). However, as we will discuss, it is not good modulation design to use cw signals with direct detection. By using short pulses, substantial improvement in performance is possible. This has been under analytical and experimental study for some time, and in the following pages we treat some of the possible formats and error rate results. It is appropriate and more accurate to discuss digital communications in error rate terms rather than SNR. In the following section we consider signal and noise aspects of laser communications.

IV. Basic Signal and Noise Considerations

At optical frequencies, quantum noise becomes significant compared to the situation in the microwave region (Oliver, 1965). In Fig. 5, a plot of thermal and quantum noise is given as a function of frequency. The thermal noise optical radiation decreases sharply with frequency whereas the quantum noise increases linearly. The quantum noise results from the particle nature

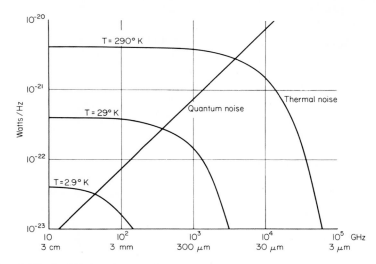

FIG. 5. Thermal and quantum noise as a function of wavelength. At $f = 3 \times 10^{14}\text{H}_z$, $\lambda = 1 \ \mu\text{m}$, $hf = 2 \times 10^{-19}$ watts/H_z.

of radiation. Since each photon of electromagnetic energy has energy hf, where h is Planck's constant and f, the frequency, the higher the frequency, the more energy in each photon. There is a basic statistical fluctuation due to the uncertainty principle in the numbers of photons. At microwave frequencies, because the thermal energy kT is high and the photon energy is low, thousands of photons need to be received before the signal is above the thermal noise. Since the rms fluctuations in the numbers of photons received is proportional to the square root of the number of photons received, one finds that photon or quantum noise at rf is insignificant (i.e., if it takes a signal made up of 10,000 photons to be above the thermal noise, then a fluctuation of $(10,000)^{1/2} \approx 100$ is of no consequence).

In the optical region this no longer is true—quantum effects predominate. Thus, 100 photons may be detected as a signal; however, there will be a statistical rms fluctuation of $(100)^{1/2}$ which must be considered noise since it is a random uncertainty. Various authors have shown that at optical frequencies the quantum noise hf is analogous to the thermal noise kT in that it is limiting the sensitivity. Resultant signal-to-noise ratio includes hf in place of kT as follows.

The heterodyne SNR is given, for cw signals, by

$$S/N = P_s/hfB = \bar{n}/B \tag{3}$$

where $\bar{n}$ is the numbers of photoelectrons per second and B, the information bandwidth (noting $P_s = \bar{n}hf$). In direct detection, in the most sensitive condition of being signal photon limited, we obtain for cw operation

$$S/N = P_s/2hfB = \bar{n}/2B \qquad (4)$$

The signal current, i_s, is given by $i_s = q\bar{n}$ where q is the electron charge, 1.6×10^{-19} coulombs. The signal power is $i_s^2 R$. The quantum noise power can be expressed in terms of the signal current fluctuations as $2qi_sBR$. This is the shot noise power resulting from the quantum noise. For direct detection systems, the SNR can be expressed as (see Ross, 1966)

$$S/N = i_s^2/2qi_s B \qquad (5)$$

When we consider all major receiver noise sources, in addition to the signal quantum noise, we have the ratio of signal power to signal, background and internal shot noise power given by

$$S/N = i_s^2/[(2qi_d B + 2qi_s B + 2qi_b B)(R) + KTB] \qquad (6)$$

where i_d and i_b represent average dark and background currents.

A major consideration is the detector thermal output noise power. Any reduction in R will reduce the ouput signal power, but will not affect the thermal noise power in the output resistance, which is independent of the value of R.

The advantage of detectors with inherent postdetection gain can be seen from analysis of this equation. If i_s is the output current which has been multiplied by postdetection gain, it improves the SNR over no postdetection gain and improves it dramatically in the cases where the thermal noise is greater than the total shot noise.

The shot noise is not discriminated against by postdetection gain, since it also is amplified. The thermal noise at the output is not amplified by the detector, however, and in this fact lies the advantage of postdetection gain such as occurs in photomultipliers and, to some extent, in avalanche photodiodes.

In many low-level applications, the thermal noise will be much greater than the output signal power unless detectors with postdetection gain are employed or a quantum amplifier is employed before the photodetector.

V. Modulation Techniques

In order to communicate one must modulate the carrier. Therefore, one should establish a modulation format that is desirable, then find a method of modulation which can implement that format. In practice, a compromise between the two occurs because the requirements of most efficient format implementations are difficult to meet at the present state of laser system technology.

To determine the merits and limitations of each modulation format it is necessary to consider the effects of optical signal and noise statistics. The analysis of rf modulation techniques properly assumed thermal noise as the primary system noise source. However, at optical frequencies, quantum noise predominates. Thus, the conclusions regarding system modulation effectiveness for rf frequencies are not necessarily valid at laser frequencies. In fact, consideration of the quantum effect in conjunction with optical detection techniques leads one to derive modulation techniques for laser communications that would be of questionable advantage at rf. High-data-rate laser communication concepts employing short pulses at high peak powers and at low duty cycles are particularly appealing (see Ross, 1967; Karp and Gagliardi, 1967, 1968; Champagne, 1966).

Laser radiation statistics are the subject of continuing analysis and investigation, since the laser is neither a black-body nor a completely coherent source. However, it is generally assumed that Poisson statistics can be employed in photodetection at a receiver far enough away from a laser source operating well above lasing threshold.

It also is generally assumed that the signal energy and the nonsignal energy are emanating from two disjoint sources, and that the number of photons received from either source is governed by a Poisson distribution. Under certain combinations of coherent signal and incoherent background some deviation from the Poisson distribution may result as shown by Lachs. (1965, 1967, 1968). For parametric values essential to efficient low-error-rate, short pulse communications, these deviations should not be significant. Error rate measurements have confirmed that Poisson statistics are satisfactory (Ross et al., 1970).

Fundamentally, the efficiency of a direct detection visible laser communications system depends upon (1) achieving system sensitivity with a high probability of signal detection, and (2) reducing the background noise level in the receiver to minimize the probability of false detection without significantly affecting the signal required to achieve a high probability of signal detection.

The noise in an optical communication system falls into two general categories: internal system-generated noise and external background radiation. The main internal optical noise sources are (a) the statistical fluctuation of the signal, (b) a finite extinction ratio in the optical modulator, and (c) receiver noise.

We consider three general types of noise discrimination: spectral, spatial, and temporal. The background noise level can be appreciably reduced by using a narrow filter at the receiver input. This is not a unique feature of short pulse modulation; it is common to all optical communication systems. Likewise, spatial filtering—minimizing the field of view of the optical receiver —is not unique to the short pulse system. However, temporal discrimination, which can be achieved by optical receiver pulse-gating techniques, is very powerful and is uniquely applicable to short pulse, low duty cycle modulation formats.

The effect of temporal noise discrimination techniques on communication efficiency is dependent upon the modulation format used in the system. In general, it can be stated that the shorter the sampling interval, the greater the noise discrimination. This is true because fewer background photons are received in the shorter interval. This reduces the probability that statistical fluctuation of the background level would exceed a present threshold in the receiver and introduce false detection errors.

Poisson statistics for low-level detection show that a decrease in background level causes an extreme decrease in the probability of false detection. Therefore, it is generally advantageous to have the sampling interval as short as possible, limited only by the constraints of pulse width, pulse gate time, and pulse resolution time.

As the result of the statistical fluctuations of the laser signal itself, there remains a minimum signal level necessary to ensure a high probability of pulse detection. The introduction of background noise at the receiver requires an increase in the signal level to achieve results equivalent to the "no background" case.

Background can be discriminated against by use of short pulse laser modulation techniques. This enables achievement of the most sensitive condition, that of signal-photon-limited system performance. Another potential advantage to short pulse modulation is that M-ary techniques can be employed where each signal pulse contains more than a single bit of information.

In general, for visible and near-infrared laser systems it is desirable to utilize short pulse laser modulation techniques. Several system concepts have evolved that are in this category. They are pulse-interval modulation (PIM), pulse-gated binary modulation (PGBM), pulse-polarization binary modulation (PPBM), and pulse-position modulation (PPM), as shown by Lee and Holt (1970) and Kinsel (1970). Some formats such as pulse amplitude modulation (PAM) are very poor choices.

Pulse-gated binary modulation is similar to normal cw binary PCM in that one bit per pulse is transmitted by a " 1 " or " 0 " output. The difference is that, in PGBM the laser operates at a low duty cycle in which the pulse width is only a small fraction of the interpulse spacing. A significant feature of PGBM is the fixed pulse spacing, which is compatible with the inherently regular-spaced pulse output of a mode-locked laser. Pulses are gated " on " or

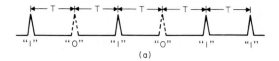

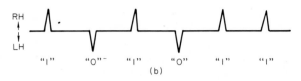

FIG. 6. (a) Pulse gated binary modulation (PGBM) waveform; (b) pulse polarization binary modulation (PPBM) waveform.

"off" with a high speed electrooptic modulator to provide coding. In addition, a fixed pulse spacing permits the use of a pulse-gated optical receiver for noise discrimination. These two features, coupled with the low duty cycle operation, make PGBM a powerful and efficient modulation technique for high data rates. The waveform is shown in Fig. 6(a).

Pulse-polarization binary modulation is identical to PGBM except for the method of modulation of the "1" and "0" pulse output. Instead of gating the mode-locked laser pulses on and off as in PGBM, the polarization of the laser pulse radiation is rotated in PPBM for "1" and "0" differentiation. The advantage of PPBM is that a signal is expected in every time interval at the receiver. The disadvantage is that the receiver must have a dual channel, one for each polarization. The waveform is shown in Fig. 6(b).

Pulse-interval modulation is an M-ary process in which one pulse conveys information representing many bits in an ordinary binary system (Ross, 1967). The normal interpulse time interval is divided into M discrete time slots. One and only one pulse is sent in the time interval of M slots (see Fig. 7). The specific time slot in which a pulse occurs is representative of a code symbol. The number of bits transmitted per pulse is therefore $\log_2 M$.

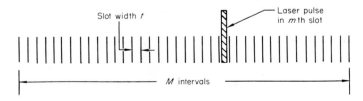

FIG. 7. Pulse interval modulation (PIM) waveform.

By using short pulses, many time slots (M large) are possible in a given time interval, thereby achieving many bits per pulse. Noise discrimination results from discrete sampling of each narrow time slot in the optical receiver. Very low duty cycle ($1/M$) is achieved because only one pulse occurs in the M time slots.

PIM, like PGBM, utilizes analog-to-digital conversion prior to encoding the laser pulsed output. However, in PIM a further conversion of the binary digital information into PIM format is required. The advantages of many bits per pulse and temporal noise discrimination make PIM an extremely efficient pulse modulation format. However, state-of-the-art high speed encoding and decoding electronics technology limits the achievable bit rate.

Pulse-position modulation is useful for direct analog information inputs. The technique is similar in form to the PIM technique, except that pulses are not assigned digital time slots and rates must be at least twice the information bandwidth to meet sampling theory requirements. Pulses are sent with interval spacing which are the discrete value of the sampled analog information to be conveyed. The analog information is handled without format processing; hence high speed analog-to-digital conversion is avoided.

For high information efficiency, it is most desirable to have a large M, short pulse system such as PIM, where M can be extremely large because of its digital discrete nature. It illustrates vividly the advantages of short pulse, low duty cycle, high peak power laser modulation. It is desirable to present this system concept in more detail. As we have discussed, the advantage of a short time period for a measurement is that few background photoelectrons are present, thus providing dramatic improvements in pulse detection probability.

In the receiver, the decision is made as to whether signal is present or not. The probability of receiving m photoelectrons in a time interval t is

$$P_t(m) = a^m e^{-a}/m! \tag{7}$$

where a is the average number of photoelectrons received in the time interval t.

There exists in the decision-making receiver a threshold level n_t above which it is decided a signal has been received. Obviously, by appropriate raising or lowering of the threshold one can change the probabilities o exceeding the threshold. An analysis shows (Curran and Ross, 1965) that an optimum threshold exists for each combination of signal, nonsignal, and duty cycle as given by

$$n_{\mathrm{opt}} = \bar{n}_s + \log\left[P(0)/P(1)\right]/\log\left[1 + (\bar{n}_s/\bar{n}_b)\right] \tag{8}$$

where n_{opt} = the optimum threshold value (optimum is defined as reducing the likelihood of an error to a minimum); $P(0)$ = the probability of transmitting a zero "0" (i.e., no signal set); $P(1)$ = the probability of transmitting a one "1" (i.e., signal sent); $\bar{n}_b$ = the average number of nonsignal photo-electrons per second, where nonsignal includes both internally and externally generated photoelectrons that are not from the signal source—thus, $a = \bar{n}_b t$ where there is no signal; $\bar{n}_s$ = the average number of signal photoelectrons in a single pulse. Thus, if one signal pulse is present within a measurement period t, $a = \bar{n}_b t + \bar{n}_s$.

An equal weighting of errors, i.e., an error of false detection costs as much as an error of no detection, is assumed in Eq. (8). However, we may arrange our system such that in time T we have M equal periods of duration t. If there is only one pulse to be transmitted in M periods, each of time t, the probability of transmitting a zero will be $(1 - 1/M)$; for $M \gg 1$, this will essentially be unity.

When we are making a decision every t, Eq. (8) can be written

$$n_{\text{opt}} = \bar{n}_s + \log M / \log [1 + (\bar{n}_s M / \bar{n}_b T)] \tag{9}$$

Thus, the threshold value will be a function of the number of short intervals in which a signal pulse might be present. Short pulse transmission will enable easier signal detection, but since there are more of these periods in which to make a decision, is it not likely that more frequent false detection might result?

The Poisson statistics are such that quite contrary results occur. There are fewer false detections because of the enormous gain in signal detection capability. This can be accomplished by raising the threshold [as given in Eq. (9)], thereby reducing the false detection probability each interval t to a low value.

Figure 8 shows the small signal increase necessary to attain the same error probability per pulse for much larger M values. This improves the error rate per bit in comparison with the long pulse (high duty cycle) case since many bits per pulse can be conveyed. Table II illustrates the bits per pulse sent for different M values since as we showed in Fig. 7 each slot can represent a unique number. If we restrict our system to only one pulse occurring in the M intervals in time T (a so-called M-ary system), then each pulse represents $\log_2 M$ bits. If we send on the average F pulses per second, we have that the bit rate R is given by

$$R = F \log_2 M \quad \text{bps} \tag{10}$$

The number of intervals M is not independent of the pulse rate once a pulse width is established. Given a pulse time interval t we have

$$R = (1/Mt) \log_2 M \quad \text{bps} \tag{11}$$

We can establish for PIM the amount of information per unit of signal energy received (bits/J) for fixed error rate per bit as a function of duty cycle.

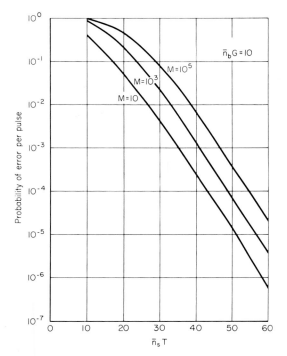

FIG. 8. Error probability per pulse for different M values.

TABLE II

PIM Relationships of Pulse Interval, Duty Cycle and Bits/Pulse[a]

M Intervals	Duty cycle[b] 1/M	Bits/pulse
10^4	10^{-4}	13.3
10^5	10^{-5}	16.6
10^6	10^{-6}	20.0
10^7	10^{-7}	23.3
10^8	10^{-8}	26.6

[a] Bits/pulse $= \log_2 M$.
[b] It is assumed the pulse width τ equals the pulse intervals t.

We note that the signal energy per pulse is $E = hf\bar{n}_s$, where h is Planck's constant $(6.62 \times 10^{-34}$ J-sec) and f is the optical frequency. The average signal power is given by $P_{av} = E_s F$. Thus, we have using Eq. (11) and the above (using $\lambda = 1$ μm),

$$R/P_{av} = 5 \times 10^{18}[(\log_2 M)/\bar{n}_s] \quad \text{bits/J} \tag{12}$$

We have determined Eq. (12) as a function of duty cycle $(1/M)$, keeping the error rate per bit fixed. We have fixed the bit rate and nonsignal power so that the only independent variable is duty cycle. The requirement of fixed error rate per bit will force $\bar{n}_s$ to change as a function of duty cycle. Calculations have been made for a variety of conditions and one set of data is plotted in Fig. 9.

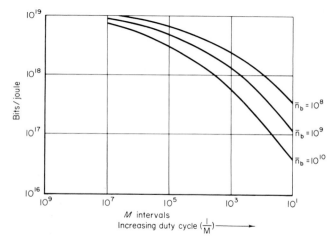

FIG. 9. Information efficiency as a function of duty cycle for PIM. Bit rate $= 1.3 \times 10^6$ bps; error rate/bit $= 10^{-4}$; background received power $= 2 \times 10^{-9}$ $\bar{n}_b$ watts.

Because PCM is a common form of pulse-time modulation used in communications, it is of value to compare PIM with PCM. We will consider the PCM system to be a simple on–off type of 50% duty cycle. Energy sent represents a "1," energy not sent represents a "0," and the noncoherent detector as in PIM must discriminate between "1"s and "0"s. Each pulse interval in PCM represents one bit. In this comparison, for simplicity, we assume all pulse intervals contain information. Thus, for a bit rate of R, the PCM system pulse interval is $1/R$.

The large improvements of the PIM systems over PCM type systems are illustrated in Table III. If we design a PIM system of error rate per bit of 10^{-4}, we find that for the same average power and average background

TABLE III

COMPARISON OF PIM[a] AND PCM[b] SYSTEMS INFORMATION RATE

	System bit rate					
	I 260 bps		II 20,000 bps		III $1.3 \cdot 10^6$ bps	
	PIM	PCM	PIM	PCM	PIM	PCM
(A) Error rate/bit same average power and same average background	10^{-4}	0.5	10^{-4}	0.5	10^{-4}	0.49
(B) Relative increase in PCM power to equal PIM error rate/bit	1	10^4	1	10^3	1	85

[a] PIM system: pulse width = 1 nsec. I. 10 pps, duty cycle 10^{-8}; II. 1000 pps, duty cycle 10^{-6}; III. 10^5 pps, duty cycle 10^{-4}. [b] PCM—50% duty cycle.

levels the PCM signal level is so deep in the noise that the error rate is near its maximum 0.5. If we wish to obtain the same error rate per bit for the PCM system as for PIM, then we must increase the PCM average power by the levels indicated in Row B.

PIM is limited in data rate capability, however, since it uses large amounts of time to send information although the pulse itself is short. For very high data rates, PGBM and PPBM, using interleaved mode-locked pulse trains, offer great promise. A Nd: YAG mode-locked train of 30 psec can support a time-multiplexed 30 Gbps data stream. Many technical aspects remain to achieve these data rates, however, significant progress in this direction has been achieved. A 224 Mbps system was demonstrated by Kinsel and Denton (1967).

Experiments in short pulse optical communications have been performed at high data rates (10^7 bps) with M-ary modulation formats and, using a subnanosecond internally gated receiver, at very high data rates (2×10^8 bps) with binary modulation formats to experimentally verify the potential of short pulse low duty cycle direct detection formats (Ross et al., 1970).

Pulse-gated binary modulation (PGBM) error rate experiments have been performed at 200 Mbps. In Fig. 10 we show the system block diagram. In Fig. 11 we show the error rate results and compare them to theoretical results. Multiplexed TV pictures have also been sent in digital mode-locked

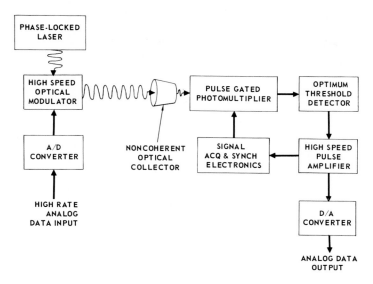

FIG. 10. Block diagram of a PGBM high data rate communication system.

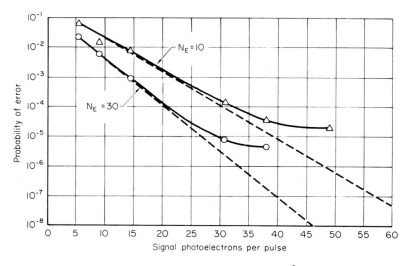

FIG. 11. Error rate data, analytical and experimental, of a 200 Mbps PGBM system. $\bar{n}_b G = 0.5$ photoelectrons per gate width; $N_E =$ extinction ratio. ---, theoretical. o—o, experimental.

pulse trains. Results demonstrate the capability of short pulse laser communication systems to discriminate against background light and to efficiently convey information. Subnanosecond gating of the receiver was achieved in the 200 Mbps experiments. Pulse-interval modulation (PIM) experiments were performed involving error rates measurements and TV pictures. In these M-ary experiments, as many as 12 bits per pulse were transmitted using 4095 digitally selected 1 nsec time slots. The system block diagram is shown in Fig. 12.

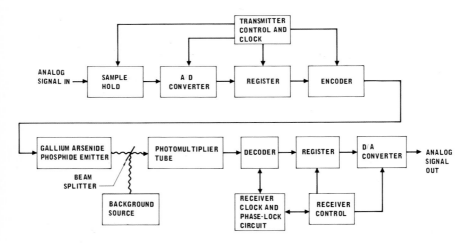

FIG. 12. Pulse interval modulation system experiment.

Photographs of single frames on the slow scan TV were taken with the video signal processed through the PIM system over the optical link under different signal and background conditions. Typical signal levels were 25 photoelectrons per pulse; the continuously present background was varied up to 10 photoelectrons in each pulse width time. Several photographs with the various system parameters as noted are shown in Fig. 13. The white dots represent "false detections." The average signal level is determined by considering the pulse rate and the numbers of signal photoelectrons per pulse. In these preliminary tests we used a 5 nsec pulse, due to modulator and detector restrictions. As an example, average background to average signal ratio for 5 background photoelectrons per pulse time (i.e., average background of 10^9 photoelectrons per second) at a repetition frequency of 100 kHz and 25 signal photoelectrons per pulse, is given by $10^9/5 \times 10^6 = 200$ if we count each sync pulse as signal energy. (In an operational system, there is no need for sending a sync pulse for each data pulse.)

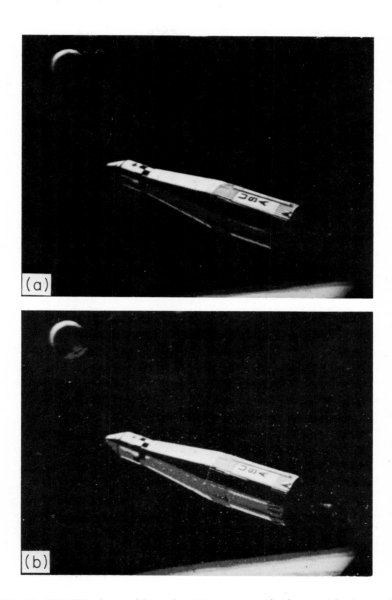

FIG. 13. PIM TV pictures illustrating *M*-ary communications and background discrimination; 25 signal photoelectrons detected per pulse, 10^7 bit rate, 8 bits/pulse. (a) Zero background; (b) 2×10^9 photoelectrons/second background.

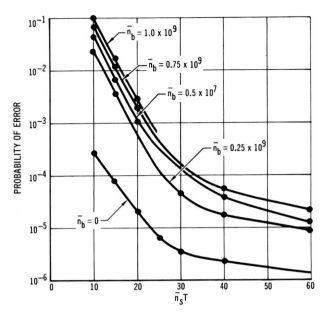

Fig. 14. PIM experimental error rate data for different background levels. M = 4095; bit rate = 2.5×10^6 bps.

Figure 14 shows plots of probability of error versus signal level ($\bar{n}_s T =$ signal photoelectrons per pulse) for average background levels ($\bar{n}_b$) from 0 to 10^9 photoelectrons per second. These curves show consistent results (similar curve shapes), and the expected increase in probability of error as the background level is increased. The data rate corresponding to these curves was 2.5×10^6 bps (2.08×10^5 samples per second at 12 bits per sample). Experiments were also conducted at 10^7 bps (1.25×10^6 samples per second at 8 bits per sample) with very similar results. In every case, the experimental data was within 25% of the theoretical predictions for signal levels below 20 photoelectrons per pulse. As the signal level increases, the difference between theoretical predications and experimental data increases because the experimental data approaches a limit imposed by the hardware.

Pulse position modulation experiments were also performed in another test of M-ary systems. Quantitative rms error measurements and TV pictures were taken.

Figure 15 shows representative plots of the measured rms time error as a function of the background level for signal levels of 14, 21, 28, and 42 signal photoelectrons per pulse time. The video bandwidth for this test was

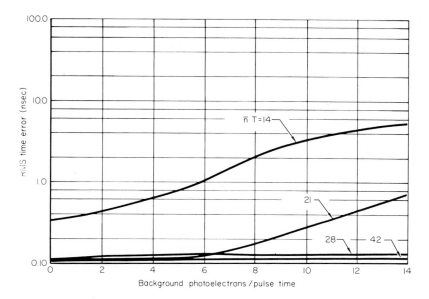

FIG. 15. Pulse position modulation (PPM) experimental rms error data. Sampling frequency = 2.5 MHz; video bandwidth = 1 MHz; 2 V peak to peak; 0-FS time span = 65 nsec.

0.16 MHz and the sampling frequency 0.4 MHz. It can be seen from the plots that background noise up to 14 photoelectrons per pulse has very little effect on the system for signal levels above 28 photoelectrons per pulse, since rms time error is almost constant at the system quiescent level. For low signal levels such as 14 photoelectrons per pulse the rms time error increases rapidly for backgrounds above 1 photoelectron per pulse. It should be noted that the ratio of average background to average signal is quite high as in PIM. The greater the number of possible positions or intervals relative to the transmitted pulse width, the greater the possible background discrimination.

Field experiments in short-pulse direct detection low-duty-cycle optical communications such as Montgomery (1969), indicated that the atmosphere could support short pulses over short horizontal paths. No error rate experiments with short pulses have yet been performed through the atmosphere. Laboratory error rate measurements demonstrate the beneficial effect of gating and the capability of the complete receiver to function with high performance at a low number of signal photoelectrons per pulse and high data rates (200 Mbps).

VI. Desirable Laser Characteristics

To attain highly information efficient modulation formats in the visible and near-IR using direct detection, the laser transmitter must be capable of a unique set of characteristics (Ross, 1968b). The laser transmitter should be capable of

(1) Being pulsed with accurate time control
(2) Generating short pulses
(3) Generating high peak powers
(4) Generating high repetition rates
(5) Being pulsed such that the interpulse spacing may vary considerably from pulse to pulse
(6) High power efficiency
(7) Diffraction-limited operation for narrow-beamwidth generation
(8) Operation without energy waste between short pulses.

Continuous-ware output-type laser cannot meet these requirements because the combined requirements define a laser transmitter that is internally modulated to achieve efficient, very low duty cycle operation. A cw laser, for example, that is externally modulated to attain characteristics through (5) would be extremely wasteful of pumping power. Thus we establish that we need an internally modulated, pulsed transmitter. We need pulsed capability that can be obtained through Q switching and time variable reflection (TVR) techniques. These are discussed in the following pages. We need to accomplish this at high repetition rates for high data rates and with individual pulse control from pulse to pulse. Mechanical Q-switching techniques are unsatisfactory for interpulse spacing control because they would not meet requirement (5).

Each type of laser may meet some requirements but it is lacking in others. This results in a different "best" laser choice depending on the application. Semiconductor lasers, for example, might meet all except (3) and (7), but these characteristics are critical to an efficient communication system. If narrow beamwidths cannot be generated effectively, the average transmitter's power requirements become very large because of the space loss. This is very important for long distance space paths but not critical to a short-range Earth link.

The laser that comes closest to meeting all requirements appears to be a mode-locked YAG, but it is lacking in pulse-spacing control and in high power efficiency. For deep space, the energy in each pulse is too little. In near space, however, the natural high rep rate and short pulses offer valuable features in data rates > 200 Mbps.

For deep space, an attractive approach may be to operate with semiconductor pumping of a Nd–YAG laser, in which case the Nd–YAG can be pumped up just prior to "giant pulsing." This would enable the laser to be off nearly all the time; this could be called a "rapid pump and dump" technique, by which short pulses at high rep rates are attained. Figure 16 illustrates this technique.

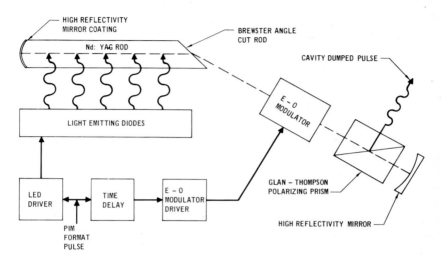

FIG. 16. "Cavity dumping" system for efficient short pulse *M*-ary communications.

Practical advantages occur from using solid-state lasers with the pulse-interval modulation concept in deep-space laser communications. Present solid-state lasers are capable of enormous peak powers. Gigawatts of peak pulse power have been obtained in solid-state lasers using giant pulse (Q switching) techniques at 1.06 μm. The second harmonic falls into the most sensitive region of photodetection capability. Also, the efficiency of second-harmonic generation is known to increase with peak power. In fact, 100% has been reported at the 1W level (Geusic *et al.*, 1968).

Typically the output "pulse" generated in a laser excited by a flashlamp consists of a series of narrow spikes which occur within the "pulse" time envelope. Therefore, the output energy of the laser is shared by the spikes, and the peak power output is diminished over what could be reached if the entire laser output was contained within a single spike.

Also, for given conditions of pulsed operation, the spiked output is not repeatable from pulse to pulse even though the average power output might be the same. Under the proper conditions, however, the laser operation can be modified to produce a single, giant output pulse, and the usually random pulses can be synchronized to an external control device.

Q switching is the name applied to the method of obtaining giant laser pulses (McClung and Hellwarth, 1962). The procedure is to introduce losses into the optical cavity during the pumping operation that produces population inversion. Emission occurring spontaneously during this time produces a few photons, but these are insufficient to stimulate laser action within the laser material so long as the cavity losses are high enough.

In the meantime, energy is still being stored in the laser material through the population inversion process. Hence, if the losses are suddenly removed and the optical cavity is restored to its original quality, the entire population inversion is stimulated at one time, and the output is a large, single pulse of coherent photons. Careful timing in this procedure allows the pumping operation to go to completion before any photons are coupled out of the cavity.

There are several methods of introducing losses into the cavity. The first experimental attainment of Q switching used a Kerr cell shutter placed within the cavity between the laser rod and one of the end mirrors. A typical procedure is to choose the output polarization in such a manner that when the Kerr cell is energized no radiation can pass to the end reflector. First, the flashlamp is fired, allowing the inversion process to begin. A few hundred microseconds later, the Kerr cell is suddenly deenergized, opening the optical path to the end mirror and allowing stimulating feedback into the laser material. It is necessary to merely delay switching off the Kerr cell until the maximum inversion is attained.

Organic dyes were used in Q switching as early as 1964 (Sorokin *et al.*, 1964). This method makes use of the saturable absorption property of certain substances. These materials absorb radiation to a certain point, then become transparent when the transitions responsible for the absorption are used up. Delay in the output is a function of the concentration of the dye which can be varied to get maximum output.

Ultrasonic control of Q switching also has been achieved (DeMaria *et al.*, 1963). The experimental arrangement consisted of a Fabry–Perot optical cavity with one mirror tilted away from parallelism with the other. A quartz ultrasonic cell is placed between the tilted mirror and the laser rod. Shortly after initiation of optical pumping, the cell is shock excited, generating an acoustic wavefront which moves through the quartz crystal. For an instant a condition prevails in which the light being refracted by the acoustic waves emerges from the cell at the angle normal to the nonparallel mirror. This completes the optical path and allows stimulating radiation to reflect back to the laser rod. Refracted light striking the nonparallel mirror other than normal is simply reflected out of the cavity.

Methods of Q switching discussed so far have related to pulsed operation of lasers. The rate at which these giant pulses can be generated is therefore limited by the time constant for recharging the flashlamp supply circuit.

Smith and Galvin (1967) demonstrated a repetitively Q switched, continuously pumped Nd^{3+}: YAG laser with peak power of 1 kW at repetition rates up to 500 per second. The Q-switching device in this case was a rotating mirror used as one of the cavity reflectors. During rotation, the cavity is aligned when the mirror axes were coincident and identical. This condition occurs exactly once during each rotation, and for other positions of the moving mirror the cavity is highly lossy.

It was found that the position of the mirror is critical to within 0.2 mm for stable Q switching. The lifetime of the energy level in Nd^{3+}: YAG from which lasing occurs is 230 μsec, so that repetition rates greater than 4.3 kHz result in the laser being just as well continuously pumped. With acoustic-optic Q switches, rep rates up to 50 kHz have been achieved.

Hook et al. (1966) demonstrated obtaining giant laser pulses that differ from Q switching, and this technique is called time variable reflectance (TVR). The elements of the cavity are the laser rod, two end reflectors, a calcite prism, and a Pockels cell. The prism, cell, and end mirror taken as a unit constitute the variable reflectance in the sense that the effect of the prism is a function of the voltage on the cell.

First, the cell is biased to prevent lasing action, allowing the pump energy to be stored. Then the cell is shorted out, opening the normal laser path to the mirror and allowing the stimulated radiation energy to build up within the cavity. Finally, the cell is biased so that the polarization is suddenly rotated 90 degrees. Since the refractive index of the calcite prism for the new polarization is different, the light is refracted out of the cavity. In this way, the laser light does not pass through a coated output mirror, and the cavity can be operated without damage at an energy density much higher than that allowed by other giant pulse techniques.

Control of the random spiking in pulsed laser output also have been done ultrasonically. In this case, the experiment is the same as the one discussed before, except standing acoustic waves are set up in the ultrasonic cell. The result is that the condition for an open optical path between the tilted mirrors occurs periodically in time, not just once as with the shock excited case. As the pumping excitation begins to build up, an open condition occurs, and laser action commences, only to be abruptly shut off as the open condition passes.

If the pumping excitation is correct, the level of excitation previous to the last laser output is reached before the open conditions occurs again, and lasing action is repeated. This process of periodically interrupted lasing continues throughout the duration of the pumping cycle, and for the case of uniform pumping the output is a series of pulses of equal amplitude spaced at the frequency of the standing acoustic wave.

The optical laser cavity is a resonant cavity that can support more than one mode of oscillation. It can produce undesirable effects. The coupling between some of these modes is so weak they are nearly independent. The result is that their phase match is not exact, so the laser output is less coherent than ideal. Also, these modes normally fluctuate randomly in phase and amplitude so that the resultant spectral output fluctuates in amplitude. The modes also compete for the avilable energy, so pumping efficiency is not optimum.

DiDomenico (1964) predicted that laser modes could be locked together in phase by modulating the internal cavity losses at a rate $c/2L$, where L is the cavity length. The number $c/2L$ is characteristic of the frequency separation of the axial modes.

It has been shown that some of the characteristics of mode-locked lasers are (a) frequency separation equal to $c/2L$, (b) pulse halfwidths proportional to the inverse of oscillation linewidth, and (c) peak power equal to the average nonmode-locked laser power times the number of coupled modes.

Very short duration optical pulses have been produced by taking advantage of the second characteristic. Solid-state lasers have inherently larger oscillation linewidths than gas lasers. Nd^{3+} : YAG lasers actively mode-locked have generated pulse widths as low as 30 psec in continuous operation by DiDomenico *et al.* (1966) and Osterink and Foster (1968).

Narrow pulses can be obtained by using a passive mode-locking element. These elements are saturable absorbers similar to those previously discussed except that their absorption is nonlinear with input intensity. After passing several times through the dye cell, the pulse reaches a minimum width with all modes in phase. The mode-locked pulses are simultaneously Q switched so only a few pulses are obtained.

Techniques have been developed for selecting a single pulse out of the mode-locked burst. A variable reflectance technique is used to shunt one pulse out of the cavity. Experiments have been performed with Nd^{+3} glass rods which produced 20 psec wide pulses of 40 GW peak power. Timing synchronization is difficult to achieve because of the short times involved. A typical experimental setup for producing simultaneous mode-locked, Q-switched pulses is shown in Fig. 17. The Glan–Thomson prism allows one polarization to remain in the cavity optical path, but shunts the 90-degree polarization out of the cavity. The electrooptic cell acts as the polarizer.

High-data-rate pulse communications require that digital signals be generated at high frequency. Thus, production of narrow pulses from lasers is important when discussing their application as transmitters. Continuous-wave modelocked lasers are especially attractive because of their high data rate and capability of being time-multiplexed to form even higher data trains.

Thus far, we have discussed lasers for pulsed communications. However, cw lasers can be useful in many cases. The same characteristics of high

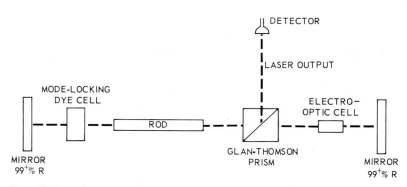

FIG. 17. Experimental setup for simultaneous mode-locking and cavity dumping.

directivity is desirable in all cases. Other characteristics become important depending on the modulation technique. In the visible and near-IR, we assume direct detection only and at 10.6 μm, we assume heterodyne detection only since the system disadvantages of alternate methods are so great. Continuous-wave lasers in the visible and near-IR can be externally pulsed and do not need spectral purity. If analog modulation is employed, it is wise to place the information on an FM subcarrier first. Changes in laser amplitude, nonlinear operation of the modulator, and atmospheric amplitude effects are then reduced in importance. However, for more than one subcarrier, the laser should be single mode and single frequency to avoid intermodulation effects between subcarrier channels due to multiple laser frequency outputs. This restriction is difficult to attain in practice due to etalon effects inside the laser cavity and the wide gain line of the laser which supports multiple frequency outputs. In the case of Nd : YAG, for example, 5 GHz linewidths can support many frequency outputs, including outputs dependent on the distance between reflections in the cavity.

For heterodyne detection systems very high frequency stability and coherence is also required. CO_2 lasers must have this capability to operate single mode, single frequency to be useful for communications in order that effective photomixing be achieved (McElroy *et al.*, 1970). Significant progress in this direction has been attained. In space long life, high reliability is a requirement. A 5 mW He–Ne laser has been space-qualified (Bridges and Kolb, 1969), and CO_2 lasers (Carbone, 1968) and Nd : YAG lasers (Allen *et al.*, 1969) are being developed toward space use for communications. The CO_2 and He–Ne lasers are gas types, whereas the Nd : YAG can be completely solid state if diode pumped rather than lamp pumped. Sun pumped Nd : YAG is also being developed. Diode pumping of Nd : YAG is presently being accomplished by light emitting diodes of GaAsP (Ostermaier, 1970) and GaAlAs (Farmer, 1970); however, laser diode pumping, the possibilities of which have been demonstrated in experiments, may be the best choice (Ross, 1968a) especially for deep space where high pulsed Nd: YAG powers at lower rep rates are highly desirable.

In short-range terrestrial or closed pipe systems, solid-state diodes, either laser or noncoherent types, can be highly attractive. They are capable of short pulses, low cost, and pulse powers commensurate with short ranges. Present restrictions on rep rate with laser diodes may be coming to an end owing to recent advances using double heterojunction techniques. This should enable wide bandwidth capability for short links with inexpensive systems.

VII. Modulators

Laser modulators are quite often the most difficult components in the system. In this section we discuss the characteristics of modulators and how they work. The ratio of the velocity of light in a vacuum to its velocity in a material medium is called the refractive index of the medium; it is unity or greater. A medium in which the velocity of light does not depend on the direction of propagation nor the state of polarization is referred to as isotropic; examples of such materials include glass, gases, liquids, and cubic crystals.

Crystalline media are generally anisotropic. Thus, the velocity of light through them depends on the direction of propagation and the state of polarization. In the absence of optical activity, light propagates in an anisotropic medium as two mutually orthogonal, linearly polarized waves which travel at different velocities; hence, they have different refractive indices. The difference between these refractive indices for two orthogonal polarizations is known as the birefringence in the direction of propagation.

Birefringence occurs naturally in many crystals of calcite; it can also be induced by external agents. For example, the refractive indices of a material can be altered by temperature changes, applied stresses, applied magnetic fields, and applied electric fields.

The application of an electric field to crystals can induce a birefringence that produces retardation as a function of the field. Crystals in which the retardation is proportional to the first power of the electric field are said to exhibit a Pockels effect. Materials in which the retardation is proportional to the square of the electric field are said to exhibit the Kerr effect. In both cases the constant of proportionality is referred to as the electrooptic coefficient. Kaminow and Turner (1966) and Blumenthal (1962) describe the basis of electrooptic modulation. Materials exhibiting a Pockels effect include crystals of ammonium dihydrogen phosphate (KDP), and deuterated potassium dihydrogen phosphate (KD*P). Modulator materials include lithium niobate, barium sodium niobate, strontium barium niobate, and potassium tantalate niobate (KTN). These show relatively large electrooptic coefficients; this means that smaller applied fields are necessary to get equivalent values of retardation. Geusic *et al.* (1967) discuss many of these materials. Rice *et al.* (1969) discuss barium sodium niobate in detail.

Modulation operations require that crystals be able to withstand high power densities and be of excellent optical quality. These demands are difficult to meet in most materials, and crystal growing and fabrication techniques have not overcome all problems satisfactorily. In modulators based on the electrooptic and magnetooptic effects, the polarization state of a wave propagating in the medium is altered by the external electric or magnetic field. External polarizing optics act upon this induced polarization change to control the intensity of light passed by the modulator. Polarization modulation can be accomplished by either the electrooptic or magnetooptic effects, and phase modulation can be accomplished by the electrooptic effect. Modulation also can be accomplished using acoustic-optic effects.

There are several basic modulator designs based on the electrooptic effect. A typical arrangement for using a Pockels effect crystal for amplitude modulation of light is shown in Fig. 18(a). Another configuration is shown in Fig. 18(b). The incident beam is polarized by the polarizing beam splitter

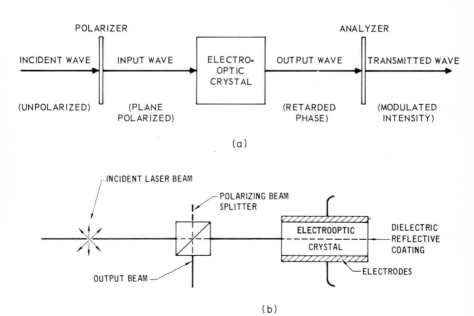

FIG. 18. (a) Basic electrooptic modulator; (b) double-pass modulator configuration.

prism and is focused into the crystal by the reducing optics where it strikes the crystal polarized at 45° to the z axis. Light propagating normal to the z direction will travel at one of two different refractive indices depending upon the direction of polarization: n_0 for light polarized normal to z and n_e for light polarized parallel to z. A light wave polarized at 45° to z is resolved by the crystal into two equal components polarized along and normal to the z axis, and since these two waves travel with different velocities, the slow wave is retarded more upon traversing the crystal. The beam is reflected from a dielectric coating on the end of the crystal and passes back through the crystal experiencing additional retardation.

The polarization of the transmitted beam will depend upon the net retardation between the fast and slow waves. No polarization change occurs when the retardation is an even multiple of π radians, but a 90° rotation of the polarization direction occurs when the double pass retardation is an odd multiple of π radians. If n_0 and n_e change by different amounts when a field is applied to the crystal, a net retardation change is induced and intensity modulation results when the reflected beam passes into the polarizing beam splitter prism. If no polarization change occurred in the crystal, the light will be totally transmitted back along the incident direction. If the polarization has been rotated by 90°, the reflected beam will be deflected out of the prism into the transmitter beam directing optics. The net induced retardation change $\Delta\Gamma$ is linearly proportional to the applied voltage and the length of propagation of the beam in the crystal: it can be expressed for a double pass by

$$\Delta\Gamma = (2\pi l/d)(V/V_\pi) \tag{13}$$

where l and d are the length and thickness of the crystal, and V is the applied voltage. The half-wave switching voltage V_π is a material parameter which represents the voltage that must be applied to a crystal having unity aspect ratio $(l=d)$ to induce a retardation of π and switch the crystal. The voltage necessary to optically switch if the aspect ratio is not unity $(l=d)$ is called the switching voltage V_s and is given by

$$V_s = V_\pi d/2l \tag{14}$$

The intensity of the transmitted beam I_T is given in terms of the retardation Γ by

$$I_T = I_0 \sin^2(\Gamma/2) \tag{15}$$

where I_0 is the incident intensity. Since Γ is the sum of $\Delta\Gamma$ and the passive retardation Γ_0, Eq. (15) applies equally well to $\Delta\Gamma$ when Γ_0 is adjusted to an even multiple of 2π radians. Since the temperature must be maintained within narrow limits to maintain a high extinction ratio, I_{on}/I_{off}, fine temperature control and an applied dc bias voltage are used to adjust the passive retardation. The passive retardation must be held to within 0.20 rad to maintain an extinction ratio of 20 dB.

The electrical characteristics of an electrooptic modulator crystal are generally frequency dependent and are quite complicated at frequencies near electromechanical resonances. In the simplest approximation, the electrical properties of an electrooptic modulator crystal resemble those of a lossy capacitor. This approximate model is quite good for useful materials, and suffices for the design of a modulator driver.

The crystal capacitance is an important factor in the design of high speed modulators since it limits the ultimate rise time. In the modulator, the electric field is applied only along the z direction, which means that the effective dielectric constant is the K_3 principal dielectric constant. For a crystal having a square cross section and a length l, the crystal capacitance C is given by

$$C = K_3 \varepsilon_0 l \tag{16}$$

where ε_0 is the permittivity of free space. The reactive energy stored E_R when the modulator is switched on from zero applied voltage is

$$E_R = (d^2/8l)K_3 \varepsilon_0 V_\pi^2 \tag{17}$$

in which a double pass configuration is assumed, and d^2 is the cross-sectional area of the modulator crystal. The reactive power can be defined as the product of this amount of energy and the average number of times the modulator is turned on per second:

$$P_R = Mf_L E_R \tag{18}$$

where M is the average duty factor and f_L is the repetition frequency of the mode-locked laser. For a "1" "0" "1" "0" repetitive code, and $M = 1/2$,

$$P_R(1010) = (f_L d^2/16l)(K_3 \varepsilon_0 V_\pi^2) \tag{19}$$

The material parameter $\varepsilon_0 K_3 V_\pi^2$ is called the energy product for a particular crystal, and is an important figure of merit for the material since it is proportional to CV_s^2. Dielectric losses occur only when the crystal voltage is changing, so losses depend upon the modulating waveform; however, the average power dissipated in a crystal driven from zero applied field by a sinusoidal peak to peak voltage of frequency f_L equal to $(V_\pi d/2l)$, the switching voltage, is given by

$$P_D = \omega_L d^2/32l \tan \delta(K_3 \varepsilon_0 V_\pi^2) \tag{20}$$

where ω is the angular frequency, $\tan \delta$ is the loss tangent, and P_D is the average power dissipated. This assumed waveform would be equivalent to a repetitive " 1 " " 0 " " 1 " " 0 " code applied to the modulator. The major portion of the power required by a high speed modulator, however, is the power dissipated in the driver itself. The drive power required (neglecting crystal dissipation) can then be approximated by the expression

$$P_L = \tfrac{3}{2} f_L C V_s^2 \tag{21}$$

assuming the 50% duty cycle due to equal likelihood of " 1 "'s and " 0 "'s. The drive power is the sum of P_L and P_D.

Imperfections and inhomogeneities in the crystal produce an output wave that does not have uniform retardation through the cross section of the wave. This causes a lowering of the extinction ratio. One of the most significant operational parameters of modulators is extinction ratio; that is, the ratio of light " on " when a pulse is sent to light transmitted when the modulator is "off." However, analytical and experimental results have both shown that extinction ratios as low as 13 dB do not seriously affect system performance. In the presence of any background noise of consequence, no significant improvement will occur for extinction ratios much greater than this value. A typical plot of error rate performance as a function of extinction ratio is shown in Fig. 19, where $\bar{n}_b G$ is the background photoelectrons in the gate time of the receiver and $\bar{n}_s T$ is the signal photoelectrons per pulse. High extinction ratios are feasible with the older modulator materials which require high switching voltages—such as KDP, ADP—but are quite difficult to attain in the newer crystal modulators, although this situation is changing with crystal growth improvement.

Another significant property of the modulator is the insertion loss, which is the absorption and reflection loss of the optical signal itself. It should be less than 1 dB. For high optical power inputs, any significant absorption will cause thermal lensing effects in the crystal. Good optical quality crystals can meet the 1 dB requirement readily.

Many of the commercially available Pockels effect electrooptic modulators are made from KDP or KD*P. These are dielectric-type crystals which exhibit a capacitance of the order of 30–50 pF to the driving source. They require voltage swings of several hundred volts to achieve 100% modulation of an incident light beam.

The relatively high capacitance and correspondingly high voltage swing make KDP or KD*P impractical for use at the very high speed operation required for wideband communication links. Presently available high speed switching devices cannot handle the power required to swing several hundred volts under steady-state conditions at high repetition rates. Solid-state circuits are limited in their voltage and bandwidth combination such that less than 50 V is required before speeds greater than 100 Mbps can be attained.

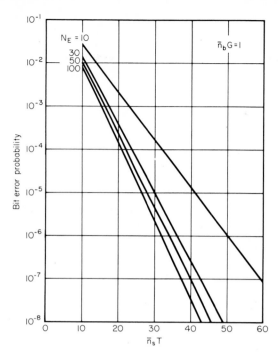

FIG. 19. Modulator extinction ratio effects on error rate. PGBM with finite N_E.

The newer crystals, which exhibit a Pockels effect with much lower half-wave voltages, appear to have great promise for practical wideband optical communications links. In Table IV we show various electrooptic materials,

TABLE IV

PROPERTIES OF HIGH SPEED ELECTROOPTIC MATERIALS

Material	V_π(100 MHz)	K_3(100 MHz)	Q(100 MHz)
LiNbO$_3$	3100V @ 0.633 μm	30	100
LiTaO$_3$	2900V @ 0.633 μm	45	Unavailable
KDP	12,000V @ 0.633 μm	32	>100
KD*P	3300V @ 0.633 μm	55	13
Ba$_2$NaNb$_5$O$_{15}$	2500V @ 0.633 μm	45	>50
Sr$_{.75}$Ba$_{.25}$Nb$_2$O$_6$ (SBN–75)	350V @ 0.633 μm (room temperature)	1100	2
Sr$_{.50}$Ba$_{.50}$Nb$_2$O$_6$ (SBN–50)	1700 @ 1.064 μm 780V @ 0.633 μm 570V @ 0.532 μm (room temperature)	265	25

including the newer materials. The half-wave switching voltages and the Q at high frequency are given.

A lithium tantalate electrooptic modulator, which is very practical from the standpoint of required drive power, has been utilized in broadband communication experiments at Bell Telephone Laboratories by Denton *et al.* (1966). The capacitance of the crystal and its mount was only 5.5 pF, and it only required a 30 V pulse to achieve full modulation. However, extreme temperature stability ($\pm 0.025°$ C) was required and crystal size was very small ($0.2 \times 0.2 \times 10$ mm) and fragile. As seen from Table IV and early experiments, strontium barium niobate (SBN) appears to be very promising.

It is very important that the modulator have low capacitance and low switching voltage. The problem of charging and discharging a typical electrooptic modulator capacitance load is formidable, especially at high rates. Modern solid-state devices are capable of solving the modulator drive problem given if the required switching voltage is not over 50 V.

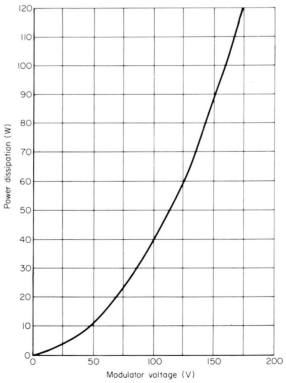

FIG. 20. Power requirements of modulators as function of switching voltage. 200 MHz pulse train; $P_{max} \approx C V_P{}^2/t_p$; $C = 20$ pf.

A plot of modulator driver power dissipation is a function of the square of required modulator voltage is shown in Fig. 20. In 200 MHz modulation rates, the modulator capacitance has been assumed to be 20 pF. Negligible dissipation occurs during full- or off-switch conditions. Dramatic improvements can be obtained by use of electrooptic cells requiring lower voltage. Other power losses to be considered are modulator crystal losses and rf radiation losses. It can be assumed that the modulator crystal losses will be small because the loss tangents of crystals most likely to be used are small. These factors normally account for less than 1 W.

Modulator materials discussed thus far have been use in the near-IR and visible. In the infrared at the CO_2 laser wavelength, gallium arsenide and cadium telluride are promising materials. The modulator power required can be in terms of megahertz per watt. For IR modulation, it requires more power than in the visible for equivalent modulation bandwidths. The most available of the two best materials, gallium arsenide, requires 0.5 MHz/W inside the laser cavity. Under the same condition, cadmium telluride is 2.0 MHz/W. If they were used outside the cavity, much more power would be required.

Efficient communications system design would necessitate careful study, since efficient transmitter development can be negated by large power requirements in the modulator. Improvements in transmitter efficiency will be lessened in importance unless improvements in modulator power requirements are also obtained.

VIII. Detector Receivers

Useful photodetectors in the visible and near-IR consist of photomultipliers, solid-state photodiodes, and photoconductors. For high speed and high sensitivity the most useful devices are photomultipliers and avalanche photodiodes. These devices, because of their internal gain, overcome thermal noise in the receivers.

Photomultipliers depend on the photoemissive characteristics of particular materials. The photoemissive materials are placed on a cathode, forming a photocathode. The photocathode will eject electrons when light falls upon it.

To understand devices which function by photoemissive action, we must first examine certain properties of photoemissivity. If a photon of frequency f interacts with an electron bound in the photocathode, the entire quantum energy hf will be converted into the kinetic energy of the electron. The kinetic energy enables the electron to leave the surface, i.e., to be ejected, with an energy

$$E = hf - q\phi \qquad (22)$$

where $q\phi$ is w, the energy required for the electron to overcome the binding forces of the metal, q is the charge of an electron, and the factor ϕ is known as the work function of the photocathode material.

It is seen that to leave the metal with energy zero or greater,

$$hf \geq q\phi \tag{23}$$

The wavelength at which $hf = q\phi$ is often called the threshold wavelength, since at lower frequencies, each photon possesses insufficient energy to liberate an electron from the cathode. In terms of wavelength and work function, this can be written as

$$\lambda_0 = hc/q\phi = 1.24/\phi \tag{24}$$

where λ is in microns. In general, for photoelectric surfaces the threshold wavelength lies between 0.6 and 1.2 μ.

It is important to note that the photoelectric action depends not on the total incident energy, but on the energy of individual photons. Hence photoemissive devices are photon detectors and not energy detectors. Yet, over the range where they are functioning as photon detectors, they can be considered power-sensitive devices in the sense that they throw away all phase information. The most important characteristic of a good photoemissive material is seen from all of the foregoing to be the possession of a high quantum efficiency ζ. The quantum efficiency is defined as the average number of electrons emitted per incident photon. An individual photon does or does not eject an electron. Taking the statistical average, however, each material has a particular quantum yield at a particular wavelength. The quantum yields or efficiencies vary from 30% down toward zero. With photoemissive devices, it would appear that the highest theoretical quantum efficiency is 1 or 100%; i.e., one electron out for each incoming photon.

Because of the variation in quantum efficiency for each material and wavelength, curves exist for each material, which plot quantum efficiency versus wavelength. These are shown in Fig. 21 along with photocathode sensitivity in microamperes per watt as a function of wavelength. These curves show the standard surfaces available in commercial tubes. Recent developments, including multiple reflective spaced and semiconductor photocathodes, are making available much higher quantum efficiencies in the near-IR. Quantum efficiencies as high as 2% at 1.06 μm have been reported. This makes the use of near-IR laser sources much more attractive than the curves of Fig. 18 would indicate.

The use of secondary emission in a vacuum tube makes possible construction of photomultipliers. Figure 22 illustrates schematically how the ordinary photomultiplier functions. The emitted photoelectron for the photocathode

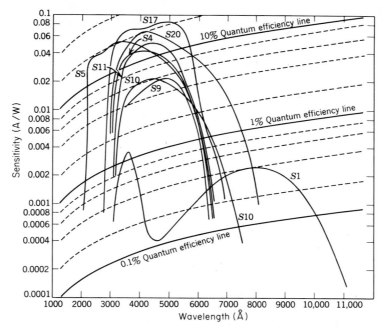

FIG. 21. Photocathode quantum efficiencies.

is accelerated by a voltage E_1 and focused upon an electrode, the dynode D_1, where each incident electron causes the emission of several secondary electrons. The secondary electrons are similarly accelerated by E_2 and focused upon dynode D_2, etc., until in the last step the electrons are collected by the positive anode A.

The photomultiplier current gain is thus a function of how many steps there are in the tube, and the secondary emission ratio δ is defined as the

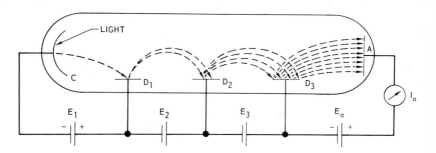

FIG. 22. Photomultiplier schematic.

number of secondary electrons emitted upon the impact of a primary electron. The value of δ will vary with the voltage between successive dynodes, with the geometry involved, and with the surface composition of the secondary emission material. The values of δ range up to 10, although most commercial tubes have much less than this. The current gain is specifically expressed as

$$G_c = \delta^M \qquad (25)$$

where M is the number of steps. Commercial photomultipliers are built with 9 to 14 stages and have gains of 10^5 to 10^7. As an example, a tube with 10 stages and a δ of 4 will have a gain greater than 10^6. Some tubes with much higher gains are available. One of the important photomultiplier construction considerations is in the focusing of the electrons on the dynodes. Although almost all the commercial tubes use electrostatic focusing systems, focusing of the electrons from one stage to the next can be accomplished with either magnetic or electrostatic techniques. Because the secondary emission ratio depends on voltage, the gain is very dependent on volts per stage.

Ordinary photomultipliers have a flat frequency response out to about 100 MHz. Transit time effects cause a rapid drop-off at about 100 MHz, although with special precautions, several hundred megahertz frequency response has been achieved. Actually, two effects can be observed to contribute to the frequency limitations: (1) a time delay between input and output signal, and (2) a spread in transit time. The time delays are due to the finite transit time of the electrons through the tube; the time dispersion is due to differences in the initial velocities of the emitted photoelectrons, and differences in path lengths of the electrons.

Very high speed photomultipliers are achieved by use of crossed magnetic fields enabling controlled electron trajectories. Two particular devices are

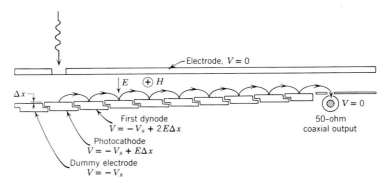

FIG. 23. Static crossed field photomultiplier schematic.

the static crossed-field photomultiplier (Miller and Witwer, 1965) and the dynamic cross-field photomultiplier (Gaddy and Holshouser, 1963; Leverenz and Gaddy, 1970). The static cross-field photomultiplier is shown in Fig. 23. The static cross-field device has separate dynodes, each one spaced slightly closer to the zero voltage electrode as shown. The alignment of each dynode can be critical. High dc voltage is used for the static field and several hundred gauss is the magnetic field. Commercial static crossed-field units are available which go beyond 4 GHz with gains over 10^5. The active photocathode area is quite small (~ 4 mm^2) due to the tight geometrical requirements.

The dynamic crossed-field photomultiplier (DCFP) possesses the essential characteristics for a high-data-rate optical communications receiver detecting a mode-locked laser PCM stream.

(1) Sensitive photodetection in the visible region
(2) High electron multiplier gain to overcome postdetection amplifier noise
(3) Subnanosecond response
(4) Subnanosecond gating to reject background and internal noise
(5) Large photocathode area to minimize the optics requirements.

Both the static and dynamic cross-field devices offer the first three advantages. The dynamic crossed-field structure offers the combined advantages of all these essential characteristics. Experimental results (Ross *et al.*, 1970) confirm background discrimination.

Detection of light is achieved in the DCFP by sampling the photoelectrons generated at the photocathode at the frequency of the rf driving field, bunching these electrons, and then multiplying the electrons in each bunch in successive steps by means of secondary emission. The electron bunches are focused in position, time, and phase so that large current gains are achieved without overlap.

The DCFP operation is illustrated in Fig. 24.

The DCFP consists of two parallel metal strips between which an rf driving electric field is applied along with a dc biasing electric field. A static magnetic field is applied normal to the electric field, and normal to the length of the strips, so that an electron in motion between the strips is accelerated along the direction of the strips. The lower strip has a photocathode near one end, a collecting hole near the other, and is coated with a good secondary emitting surface. Photoelectrons generated at the photocathode are accelerated towards the top strip during the positive half cycle of the rf drive, and the magnetic field will cause them to curve in a cycloidal path towards the collector end of the assembly. On the opposite half cycle the electrons are returned to the lower strip with sufficient energy so that each electron will generate several secondary electrons. These secondary electrons repeat this process until reaching the collecting hole near the end of the lower

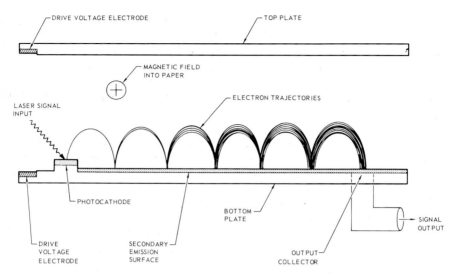

FIG. 24. Dynamic crossed field photomultiplier schematic.

strip. After passing through the collecting hole, the multiplied secondary electrons strike the collector or anode which is held several hundred volts above the potential of the lower plate. Figure 25 is a photograph of a 200 MHz experimental DCFP shown without shield or magnetic field.

Only photoelectrons which are generated during the proper portion of the.rf drive cycle will enter into the phase-focusing secondary multiplication sequence, hence the gating effect of the DCFP.

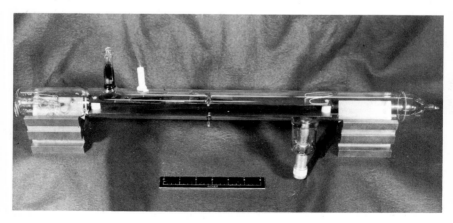

FIG. 25. Experimental 200-MHz dynamic crossed field photomultiplier.

The rf electric field between the plates of the DCFP supplies the energy which causes the electron multiplication. A primary task is supplying rf power to the DCFP to develop this driving field. The most efficient and convenient way to facilitate this is to resonate the capacitance of the DCFP plates with an external inductance at the driving frequency. Power is then coupled in at an appropriate point to achieve a good impedance match. Resonating the drive circuit in this way, with components having high Q, insures economy of driving power.

Avalanche photodiodes offer potential advantage in the near-IR where photocathode quantum efficiency of photomultipliers is very poor. The choice between avalanche photodiode and photomultipliers at 1.06 μm is difficult. Improved photocathode sensitivity due to semiconductor photocathode progress may swing the choice to photomultipliers, although diodes have the advantage of small size.

Solid-state photodiodes are often useful in short-range systems even if they do not have the sensitivity of avalanche photodiodes. Solid-state photodiodes have quite high quantum efficiency but are limited in sensitivity because of the lack of internal gain. In cases where background noise is higher than internal noise, this deficiency is not critical. However, for high sensitivity, it is required that background be sufficiently reduced by optical filters, narrow field-of-view, and temporal techniques such as pulse gating, that the remaining background noise is small compared to the thermal noise of a detector amplifier following a photodiode.

The operation of solid-state photodiodes can be described as follows. The voltage–current characteristics are shown in Fig. 26. With no light the device has a simple rectifier characteristic. As light increases the reverse current increases sharply, and hence it is this third quadrant that photodiodes are operated. Photodiodes speed is dependent, not only upon capacitance which is also related to photosensitive area, but upon laser wavelength. Germanium photodiodes are better than silicon at the 1.06 μm wavelength for detection of short pulses due to the lower absorption coefficient of silicon.

Avalanche photodiodes are made of similar materials as ordinary photodiodes such as germanium and silicon. Biard and Schaunfield (1967) indicate gain bandwidth as high as 10^{10}; internal gains of 100 at 1 GHz appear feasible. Operation occurs in an avalanche mode to achieve this behavior. Very precise biasing and threshold detection is required to achieve reliable performance at high sensitivity and high speed. Gain of an avalanche photodiode does not approach that of photomultipliers but is sufficient given low noise amplifiers following the detector to overcome thermal noise—given several hundred to a couple of thousand photons received per pulse. This is equivalent performance to very poor quantum efficiency photomultipliers. High speed avalanche photodetectors have small photosensitive areas which makes

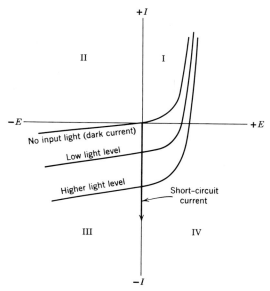

FIG. 26. Solid-state photodiode operation.

optics alignment more difficult generally than with photomultipliers. Wider area avalanche photodiodes are obtainable but at a reduction in speed of response. The power supply requirements of photodiodes are substantially less than photomultipliers because of the lower supply voltages.

IX. Beam Deflectors

For fixed stations, electronic beam steering or deflection is not important. However, in many applications, especially space, fast beam steering is necessary. In addition to conventional beam pointing by means of gimballed mirrors, fine beam steering can be accomplished by piezoelectric devices known as bender bimorphs. A mirror is mounted on a bimetallic strip which is driven at volts ranging up to 500 V. One kHz scan rates over 400 resolution elements in each dimension has been achieved in commercial units. In space application sync satellites of $\pm.1°$ attitude stability are being built; electronic beam steering enables fine beam control within $\pm.1°$ to the fraction of the laser beamwidth itself. For example, $\pm.1°/400$ is approximately ± 4 μrad which should enable use of a 10-μrad beam.

Other devices such as electrooptic crystals have been used for beam steering. However, it is difficult to achieve a high number of resolution elements at sufficiently high scan rates without excessive power requirements at present. With some of the newer electrooptic materials, this approach may be satisfactory and lead to better system performance than the bender bimorphs.

X. Optical Collectors

With direct detection, large aperture optics become possible. On earth, very large collectors can be used for receiving space signals. In space, 1–3 ft optical collectors can be readily used because they can be lightweight and do not require the accuracy, resultant quality, and structural support of optical telescopes. In Fig. 27 is shown (Ross and Jackson, 1970) the weight of differ-

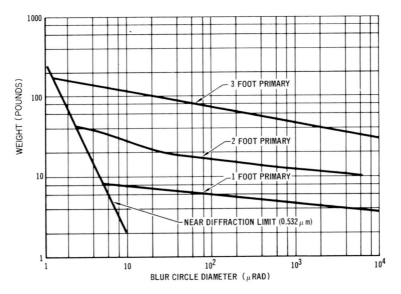

FIG. 27. Weight of optical collectors as function of surface accuracy.

ent size collectors if diffraction limited optics are not required. The blur circle is a measure of the optics quality. For direct detection systems, large blur circles are possible if proper attention has been given to (1) photosensitive area to be sure all signal light falls within the sensitive area, and (2) background considerations so that the resultant wider field of view does not allow background noise to increase the signal level required.

With direct detection, large-aperture optics on Earth becomes quite resonable. Figure 28 shows a 10-meter diameter optical collector. It has 248 segmented mirrors which can be individually aligned and is accurate to better than 20 arc minutes (Burke and Kirchhoff, 1968). For these collectors, the cost is much less than a half-million dollars compared to the multimillions of even a 2-meter optical telescope.

If one uses the system only at night, the major limitation is that the accuracy must be good enough to enable the full signal to fall on the photocathode surface. In daytime, the background problem is much more serious;

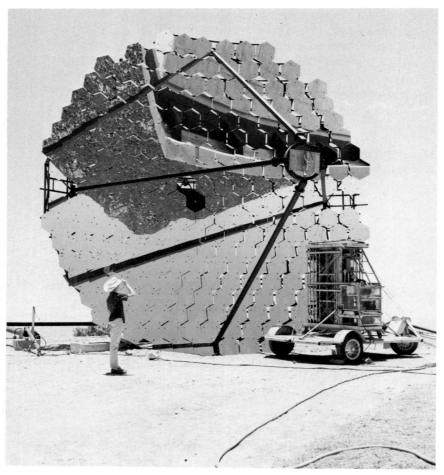

FIG. 28. Ten-meter diameter optical collector at Mt. Hopkins, Arizona suitable for direct detection of pulsed signals from space.

even with narrowband filters and use of short pulses, one must limit the field of view to reduce background energy. One needs a surface accuracy that will keep the background count per nanosecond sufficiently below the expected signal-pulse count. One cannot reduce the field of view by use of a field stop; this would prevent arrival at the photocathode of signal photons which have been imperfectly directed because of collector-surface deviation. Therefore, the surface deviation will essentially define the field of view which, in turn, will establish the background level that will be detected.

Cost and complexity of collectors are highly dependent on surface accuracies. Surface accuracies which result in one-arc-minute field of view for large collectors appear to represent a good trade between cost, complexity, and necessary background rejection. Improved system performance results from use of a large collector as the signal increases directly proportional to the area, and the noise resulting from background is increasing by the square root of the area. Such improvements are directly translatable into lower spacecraft-transmitted power or less stringent transmitter beamwidth and pointing requirements.

XI. Laser System Considerations

The laser communication system design is highly dependent on the application. This is especially so since compromise between component reality and system design is required for every application.

In short-range terrestial applications, the best choice would appear to be pulse modulated (PPM or PCM) direct detection systems to overcome as much as possible atmospheric scintillation effects. Use of He–Ne lasers for wide bandwidths are feasible but for video bandwidths, use of external modulators and higher power requirements make He–Ne systems more complex and expensive than semiconductor diode systems. Semiconductor laser diodes can readily internally be modulated with 50 nsec pulses which will enable video bandwidth to be sent given cw laser diodes. Noncoherent light emitting diodes can be used for very wideband video but suffer from directivity capability which restrict range. Turn-on time of light emitting diodes of 1 nsec has been achieved. Beamwidth is many degrees, however. Optics can reduce this to a few degrees but a significant loss in light output occurs.

For ranges of less than a few miles, laser diodes or noncoherent diodes are attractive transmitters, either singly or in arrays. Their simplicity, light-weight, small power requirements, easily modulatable properties, make them attractive where very narrow beams and high peak powers are not essential, and data rate requirements are not excessive.

In general, short-range systems are limited by direct line-of-sight, but recent experiments demonstrate that scattering of light by particles enable bouncing of the laser beam off clouds allowing communications over several miles. It is too early to tell the limitations of this technique. Obviously, higher powered lasers are required if forward scatter techniques are to be employed in lieu of direct line-of-sight.

Closed pipe systems have been investigated for a number of years. Although many techniques have been examined, no fully satisfactory one is apparent. Recently, glass fiber "pipes" to convey signals have been investigated and appear promising for short-range use within cities.

Long distance closed pipe systems will require very large bandwidth usage to make it economical to implement. These systems will need coherent lasers for narrow beamwidths and will likely use mode-locked lasers so that many pulse trains can be interleaved into a multichannel system (see Denton and Kinsel, 1968). With use of 30 psec 200 MHz, YAG mode-locked lasers, 100 channels can be multiplexed to provide greater than 10^{10} bps data transmission.

Laser space communications research and development in the recent past has traveled two main routes: (1) 10.6 μ heterodyne systems, (2) short pulse visible or near-IR direct detection systems. There have been very good reasons for the specific choices. Carbon dioxide lasers at 10.6 μm are, of course, reasonably efficient, capable of diffraction limited performance, and sufficient power is achievable. Heterodyne detection is required to enable signal quantum-limited sensitivity, since heterodyne action provides both conversion gain to overcome detector noise limitations and background noise discrimination. Direct detection systems can provide background noise discrimination by spectral, spatial, and temporal discrimination. The value of temporal discrimination, which can be achieved through use of short pulses, was not fully recognized until the last several years. In addition, short pulses offer certain coding advantages which enable efficient communication concepts. In order to make deep-space laser communications practical and a viable alternative to rf, the weight, power, and size of the onboard transmitter must be reasonably small. Coding techniques, efficient modulation formats, novel system concepts are required to achieve these goals.

The CO_2 laser must be exceptionally stable in frequency since a heterodyne system depends on a known local oscillator frequency and a known carrier frequency. Single mode diffraction-limited performance is required to achieve the narrow beamwidth necessary for long-range communications. Useful aperture sizes for heterodyne detection is limited on the earth because of the atmosphere. This restricts the number of photons collected. This limitation, due to phase corruption of the wave by the atmosphere, is a significant disadvantage for deep space since the received beam will be weak and one needs all the intercepting area one can reasonably attain. Direct detection systems do not suffer from phase corruption of the atmosphere since the phase of the optical signal is of no consequence. Because of this, one is not limited by a coherent aperture as in heterodyne systems. The collector is essentially what has been referred to in the literature as a "photon bucket." There are limitations on this kind of collector, but receiving apertures much larger than coherent apertures can be achieved before these limitations take place. The coherent aperture for CO_2 wavelength is approximately 1–1.5 meters (Fried, 1967) for visible wavelengths it is a few inches (Hodara, 1968). The improvement in coherent aperture size at 10.6 μm is approximately 20, the ratio of the wavelengths (Monroe, 1968). At present, it appears that noncoherent detection apertures can be greater than 15 meters.

XII. Near-Space Systems

In near earth orbital missions of mid and late 1970's a primary objective of each mission will be the return to earth of large amounts of data, primarily pictorial data. Conventional radio frequency techniques may become less attractive for relaying the huge amounts of information that will be gathered by reconnaissance and earth resources satellites. During the 1970's and 1980's the numbers of satellites to be deployed will increase the data relay load to many real time television channels. At data rates greater than 10^8 bps, even the newer rf techniques, such as millimeter waves and solid-state power sources, find it increasingly difficult to compete for spacecraft weight and power.

For near-space (earth orbiting) and synchronous satellite communications, both CO_2 heterodyne and direct detection visible and near-IR laser systems appear feasible. Decisions as to which is more desirable depend on the particular mission, data rate, technology development, and experimental verifications.

A CO_2 (10.6 μm) laser communication system was to be tested on the synchronous satellite ATS-F in 1973 (McAvoy et al., 1968). The experiment was to consist of receiving a 5 MHz video signal via rf techniques from another satellite and transmitting it down to the earth over the CO_2 laser link. The CO_2 laser communication system for ATS-F planned to use a 400 mW single mode cw output, and uses 5-in. diameter optics at each end of the link. Engineering difficulties unfortunately, have postponed this experiment.

Although the CO_2 laser has high efficiency and high coherence, photomixing with a cooled photodetector is required for sensitive detection. This necessitates radiative coolers aimed at cold space. This would suffice in synchronous orbit but creates a severe system problem for a low orbit satellite receiver. Doppler shift in heterodyne systems is also a significant problem. The peak Doppler shift for 10.6 μm is calculated to be approximately 675 MHz. Communication experiments at 10.6 μm have demonstrated in ground tests its performance potential (Goodwin and Nusswaier, 1968).

For information bandwidths as great as 50–100 MHz, a technical problem of modulator performance arises. Although some interesting approaches have been indicated, no satisfactory solution to CO_2 laser modulation at 100 MHz has been demonstrated. As noted in Section VII (Modulators), if internal cavity modulation is applied, at best 2.0 MHz/W of modulation bandwidth can be achieved (using cadmium telluride). However, modulation internally is limited by the linewidth of the CO_2 laser to bandwidths not much above 50 MHz. Beyond this value, external cavity modulation, which inherently requires more power, must be employed.

In direct detection systems in the visible and near-IR, as we have mentioned, mode-locked lasers appears very attractive since they generate short pulses, lower duty cycle, at a high pulse rate. A pulsed laser communication system which appears most suitable for data regimes above 10^8 bps is denoted as Pulse Gated Binary Modulation (PGBM). For this system, the laser transmitter consists of a mode-locked, frequency doubled Nd : YAG laser pumped with solid-state light sources, or possibly, the Sun itself. A mode-locking crystal causes the Nd : YAG laser 1.06 μm energy to be bunched in a sequence of 30 psec duration pulses which are radiated at typical rates of 200 million to 1 billion pulses per second. The exact rate is dependent on the laser cavity length. Another optical element called the frequency doubler converts most of the 1.06 μm energy to one half the wavelength, or 0.53 μm, a bright green color. While this frequency doubling operation is required to better match the spectral sensitivity of photomultiplier detectors typically used at the receiver end of the communication link, it is possible that with improved 1.06 μm photodetectors it will not be necessary. Finally, another electrooptic crystal is used to impress the message upon the laser pulse stream. Digital modulation is accomplished by transmitting the pulse to signify a binary one and by blocking a pulse to signify a binary zero.

At the receiver, the signal photons must be gathered and detected in competition with the background light coming from clouds, skies, or earth. Lightweight nondiffraction-limited optics may be used since direct detection is utilized eliminating the need for astronomical quality optics required for coherent detection.

Experimental validation of analytical results was obtained in laboratory optical link tests as described earlier. Applications in near space of these pulse laser communication techniques have been extensively studied. Specifically, high data rate earth orbital missions including low orbit to sync satellite links, sync satellite to sync satellite links, sync satellite to earth, and low orbit satellite to earth links have been examined. Detailed analyses of link constraints and requirements have been accomplished. Specific system configurations to best utilize the pulse visible communications within the link constraints have been devised (Ross and Jackson, 1970).

Potential transmitter and receiver parameters for a low orbit to sync satellite link are given in Table V for a data transmitter beamwidth of 10

TABLE V

LOW ORBIT SATELLITE TO SYNCHRONOUS SATELLITE[a]

	Size (in.)	Weight (lb)	Power
Low orbit satellite Transmitter incl. Beacon receiver	$6 \times 12 \times 23$	50	Less than 100 W
Synchronous satellite Receiver incl. Beacon transmitter	$12 \times 12 \times 24$	50	Less than 50 W

[a] 200 Mbps PGBM.

μrad. The data transmitter operates at the doubled frequency in the green, and the beacon aboard the sync satellite operates at the fundamental Nd: YAG frequency. Trades are possible between receiving optics, transmitter power, and transmitter beamwidth. The optimum choice of system parameters depends on exact mission requirements and spacecraft design and capability. A broad range of high data rate earth orbital system 200 Mpbs to 1 Gpbs, are feasible within the confines of 20 mW to 1 W transmitter power, 10 μrad to 100 μrad beamwidth, and 4 in. to 3 ft lightweight noncoherent receiving optical collectors. With available modulator technology, 200 Mbps data streams can be achieved, with straightfoward multiplexing approaches to achieve 1 Gbps or more. Further modulator advances are required and electronic device speeds have to be improved before direct data rates higher than a few hundred Mbps can be achieved. However, improvements in speed for space operation are occurring rapidly.

Wideband analog modulation techniques are also being developed for direct detection systems. Of interest is the system in which information is applied by frequency modulation of the subcarrier which amplitude modulates the carrier (Hance *et al.*, 1970). A block diagram is shown in Fig. 29. All analog systems avoid A/D and D/A conversion, and the technique appears to be of value where bandwidth beyond analog to digital conversion techniques can be accomplished. However, the inefficiency of subcarrier methods in the optical link make greater laser power required compared to an equivalent digital link data rate using baseband methods.

The conversion between analog bandwidth (MHz) and digital data rate in megabits per second is dependent on a number of factors, but typically a

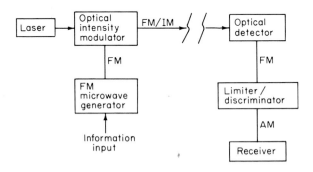

FIG. 29. Block diagram wideband FM-IM direct detection.

ratio of 1 to 12 is considered. A 100 MHz analog bandwidth equals a 1.2 Gbps digital data rate. Since visible and near-IR lasers are relatively inefficient, substantial increases in laser power mean considerable increase in prime power which is of prime importance in space systems, but much less important for terrestrial or ship based systems.

An efficient method of generating wideband data would be to operate a pulse position modulated signal from a mode-locked train. The difficulty of electronically delaying one pulse from another restricts this approach for the present, but the high information efficiency of *M*-ary systems such as PPM has been demonstrated. PPM requires sampling the analog bandwidth at least twice each cycle, thus a 2 GHz mode-locked pulse train of 30 psec could theoretically be pulse position modulated to convey 1 GHz analog bandwidth without A/D and D/A conversion.

At present, serious interest in Nd: YAG laser communications at 1 Gbps is being expressed by the United States Air Force for an experiment in space in 1975. NASA is planning a laser communication experiment on ATS-G in 1975. Lincoln Laboratories in their LES experimental satellite program may perform a low data rate ($\sim$ 1 MHz) space test in 1973.

XIII. Deep-Space Systems

In near space both CO_2 lasers and direct detection visible and near-IR lasers appear feasible. However, if one examines the deep-space problem one finds that two factors weigh heavily against use of CO_2 lasers in deep space; one is the limited coherent aperture on earth; the second is the longer wavelength which requires much larger, heavier optics to attain a beam the same width as with visible lasers. The limited collector size and weight force the CO_2 laser power for deep space use to such large values as to make it unattractive compared to other techniques.

In deep space, pointing and tracking becomes even more important than in near space due to the long transit times and the always large point ahead angles (compared to the transmitted beamwidth). Point ahead may be 70 μrad for example, compared to a 10 μrad beam.

The pointing and tracking problem for lasers has been shown to be

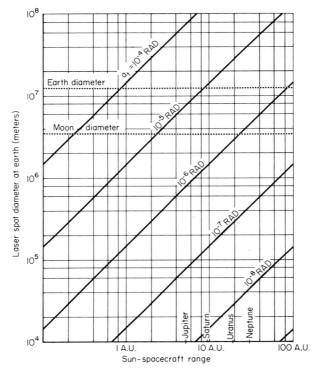

FIG. 30. Laser beam spot size at earth resulting from space transmitter beamwidths.

solvable in laboratory working models and in telescope results aboard the orbiting astronomical laboratory. Pointing and tracking to 0.1 arc-sec can be achieved if one is willing to pay the price in weight and size. Obviously less stringent pointing and tracking requirements are desirable. For deep space, it is advantageous to have the laser spot diameter cover the entire earth. This beamspread considerably simplifies the system, in that it is not required for the transmitter to know to which station on earth to point, or that weather changes require switching from one station to another. All earth stations are capable of receiving the signal. Figure 30 shows the transmitter beam spread on earth at different planet distances as a function of beamwidth.

Without the use of short pulse modulation techniques, this pointing simplification (and wider beam) results in excessively high laser transmitter powers aboard the spacecraft. However, the information efficiency achieved by techniques such as PIM yields feasible average power requirements for the grand tour missions.

Table VI shows the specifications for a deep-space PIM link from Neptune which is 30 astronautical units distant.

The use of short pulse modulation formats in the visible and near-IR combined with noncoherent detection and solid-state laser implementation offers a method of attaining high data rates from deep space that cannot be otherwise achieved with reasonable spacecraft size, weight, and power requirements. Success in system development would enable much more information per dollar expended and lead to much more information about our solar system within the next 20 years. The attractiveness and possibly even the success of future outer planet missions will depend on the communication capability we are able to achieve. Short pulse laser communications offers a way of achieving high information rates at high values of bits per pound, enabling smaller boosters and less expensive space probes to send back more information from deep space—and, in addition, sending it back in time to perform spacecraft guidance and sensor tacks to significantly aid mission success.

While it is premature to discuss outer space communications from beyond our solar system it is worth noting that the use of short pulse direct detection M-ary systems such as PIM are highly applicable to efficient communications at interstellar distances.

The difficulties of any communications at these distances are enormous but it becomes possible with direct detection, short pulse laser communication to gain the advantages of high directivity from the source, intense peak power very much greater than any star's background noise contribution, and large optical collectors on Earth to collect sufficient photons to detect the signal.

TABLE VI

DEEP-SPACE NEPTUNE–EARTH LASER LINK

	PIM System
Data rate (bps)	10,000
Transmitter antenna diameter	4 inch optics
Receiver antenna diameter or collector	16 meters
Laser pulsewidth	1 nsec
Laser peak power	1.2 MW
Rep rate	500 pps
Duty cycle	$<10^{-6}$
Average signal power	600 mW
Receiver field of view	1 arc-minute
Receiver spectral width	1Å
Receiver noise temperature	—
Laser system efficiency[a]	10^{-3} (losses due to non-ideal system)

[a] This includes laser transmitter efficiency, optics losses in transmitter and receiver, and quantum efficiency of photo detector.

Calculations indicate a laser transmitter 10 light-years distant of 10^4 J pulse and 1 μrad beam of 1 nsec pulse width can be detected on Earth with a 30-meter diameter optical collector receiver. The transmitter parameters are not too far removed from our own near-term technological capability and the receiver capability can be accomplished today, if required. In any examination of interstellar communication possibilities and likelihood, serious consideration should be given to laser communications using these techniques.

XIV. Final Note

This paper, of necessity, has been restricted to giving an overview and presenting some fundamental considerations for different applications for laser communications. For further information, in addition to the specific references given, Pratt, 1969, the IEEE special issue on Optical Communications, October 1970, and the report on the NASA-MIT 1968 Optical Communications Workshop, NASA report SP-217, are suggested for further reading and the many more additional pertinent references. The NASA report deals extensively with two areas not seriously treated here—atmospheric effects on coherent laser communications, and quantum mechanical treatments of optimum receivers for laser communications.

ACKNOWLEDGMENTS

This chapter was greatly aided by contributions by Dr. R. Rice on the discussion on modulators. I also wish to acknowledge the help and cooperation of McDonnell Douglas Astronautics Co., Eastern Division. A significant amount of the data presented has been accomplished in conjunction with my co-workers at McDonnell Douglas and partially under USAF Avionics Laboratory programs.

REFERENCES

Allen, R. B., Scalise, J. B., and DeKinder, R. E., Jr. (1969). *IEEE CLEA Conf., Digest, Washington, D.C.*, Paper 12–5.
Biard, J. R., and Schaunfield, W. N. (1967). *IEEE Trans. Electron Devices* **14** (5), 233
Blumenthal, R. (1962). *Proc. IRE* **50**, 452.
Bridges, W. B., and Kolb, W. P. (1969). *IEEE CLEA Conf., Washington D.C.*
Burke, J. J., and Kirchhoff, W. (1968). *Sky & Telescope* Nov., p. 284.
Carbone, R. J. (1968). *IEEE J. Quantum Electron.* **4** (3).
Champagne, E. B. (1966). *Appl. Opt.* **5**, 1843.
Curran, T., and Ross, M. (1965). *Proc. IEEE* **53**, 1770.
DeMaria, A. J., Gagosz, R., and Barnard, G. (1963). *J. Appl. Phys.* **34**, 453.
Denton, R. T., and Kinsel, T. S. (1968). *Proc. IEEE* **56**, 140.
Denton, R. T., Kinsel, T. S., and Chen, F. S. (1966). *Proc. IEEE* **54**, 1472.
DiDomenico, M., Jr.(1964). *J. Appl. Phys.* **35**, 2870.
DiDomenico, M., Jr., Geusic, J. E., Marcos, H. M., and Smith, R. G. (1966). *Appl. Phys. Lett.* **8**, 180.
Farmer, G., (1970). *Int. Electron Device Meet. Washington, D.C.*
Fried, D. L. (1967). *Proc. IEEE* **55**, 57.
Gaddy, O. L., and Holshouser, D. F. (1963). *Proc. IEEE* **51**, 153.
Geusic, J. E., Levinstein, H. J., Rubin, J. J., Singh, S. J., and Van Uitert, L. G. (1967). *Appl. Phys. Lett.* **11**, 269.
Geusic, J. E., Levinstein, H. J., Singh, S. J., Smith, R. G., and Van Uitert, L. G. (1968). *International Quantum Electronics Conf. Digest, Miami*, Paper 11K–3.
Goodwin, F., and Nussmair, T. (1968). *Int. Quantum Electron. Conf., Miami*, Paper 10J–5.
Hance, H. V., Ohlmann, R. C., Peretson, D. C., and Chow, K. K. (1970). *Proc. IEEE*, 1714.
Hodara, H. (1968). *Proc. IEEE* **56**, 2130.
Hook, W. R., Hilberg, R. P., and Dishington, R. H. (1966). *Proc. IEEE* **54**, 1954.
Kaminow, I. P., and Turner, E. H. (1966). *Proc. IEEE* **54** (10), 1374.
Karp, S., and Gagliardi, R. M. (1967). *IEEE Eastcon Conv.*, Washington, D.C.
Karp, S., and Gagliardi, R. M. (1968). *NASA Tech. Note* **NASA TN D-4623**.
Kinsel, T. S. (1970). *Proc. IEEE*, **58**, 1666.
Kinsel, T. S., and Denton, R. T. (1967). *Proc. IEEE*, **56**, 146.
Lachs, G. (1965). *Phys. Rev.* **138**, B1012.
Lachs, G. (1967). *J. Appl. Phys.* **38**, 3439.
Lachs, G. (1968). *J. Appl. Phys.* **39**, 4192.
Lee, G., and Holt, C. (1970). *National Telemetry Conf.*, Los Angeles.
Leverenz, D. J., and Gaddy, O. L. (1970). *Proc. IEEE* **58**, 1487.
McAvoy, N., Richard, H. L., McElroy, J. H., and Richards, W. E. (1968). *NASA Goddard Space Flight Center Preprint* X–524–68–206, *May.*

McClung, F. J., and Hellwarth, R. W. (1962). *J. Appl. Phys.* **33**, 828.

McElroy, J. H., McAvoy, N., and Richard, H. L. (1970). *Laser Journal* **2** (1).

Miller, R. C., and Witwer, N. C. (1965). *IEEE J. Quantum Electron.* **1**, 62.

Monroe, M. E. (1968). "Measurement of Spatial Coherence and Intensity Correlation Function of Atmospherically Distorted Laser Waves at .63 and 10.6 Mocrons." TR 2384–7. Ohio State Univ. Columbus, Ohio.

Montgomery, R. M. (1969). *IEEE CLEA Conf. Digest, Washington, D.C.*, Paper 13-5.

Oliver, B. M. (1961). *Proc. IEEE* **49**, 1960.

Oliver, B. M. (1965). *Proc. IEEE* **53**, 436.

Osterink, L. M., and Foster, J. D. (1968). *Int. Quantum Electron. Conf., Miami,* Paper 17Q–8.

Ostermaier, F. (1970). *International Electron Device Meet., Washington,* D.C.

Pratt, W. (1969). "Laser Communications," Wiley, New York.

Rice, R. R., Fay, H., Dess, H. M., and Alford, W. J. (1969). *J. Electrochem. Soc.* **116**, 62.

Ross, M. (1966). "Laser Receivers," Ch. 2. Wiley, New York.

Ross, M. (1967). *IEEE Trans. Aerosp. Electron. Syst.* **3**, Suppl., 324.

Ross, M. (1968a). *Proc. IEEE* **56**, 196.

Ross, M. (1968b). *Int. Conf. on Microwave and Optical Generation and Amplification, IEEE,* Hamburg.

Ross, M., and Jackson, J. (1970). *IEEE Electron. Aerosp. Cent. Rec. Washington, D.C.*, p. 86.

Ross, M., Brand, J., and Green, S. (1970). *Proc. IEEE* **58**, 1719

Smith, R. G., and Galvin, M. F. (1967). *IEEE J. Quantum Electron.* **3**, 406.

Sorokin, P. A., Luzzi, J. J., Lombard, J. R., and Pettit, G. D. (1964). *IBM J. Res. Develop.* **8**, 182.

AUTHOR INDEX

Numbers in italics refer to the pages on which the complete references are listed.

Brown, G. M., 44, *56*
Brumm, D., 11, *59*
Buck, A. L., 64, *129*
Buerger, M. J., 2, *56*
Buholz, N., 155, 192, *199*
Burch, J. M., 42, 51, *56*
Burckhardt, C. B., *57*
Burke, J. J., 284, *294*
Burr, R., 44, 45, 51, *56*
Burrell, G. J., 147, 164, 192, *199*

C

Candler, C., 69, *129*
Carbone, R. J., 267, *294*
Carruthers, J., 161, *199*
Carslaw, H. S., 229, 230, 231, 232, *236*, *237*
Carter, R. R., 128, *130*
Carter, W. H., 14, 15, 16, *56*
Catherin, J. M., 146, 156, *199*
Cavanaugh, L. A., 44, 45, 51, *56*
Chambers, R. P., 3, *56*
Champagne, E. B., 249, *294*
Chen, F. S., 35, *56*, 274, *294*
Cherrington, B. E., 153, *200*, 208, *237*
Chesler, R. B., 219, *237*
Chester, A. N., 204, 211, *236*, *237*
Cheyer, J. P., 209, *236*
Chodorow, M., 155, 192, *199*
Chow, K. K., 290, *294*
Chumichev, R. F., 154, *200*
Church, C. H., 218, 219, *237*
Ciftan, M., 216, *237*
Cohen, M. I., 202, 203, 223, 227, *237*
Collier, R., 42, *56*
Collins, R. J., 148, 150, 165, 183, 186, 187, 189, 190, *199*, 217, *237*
Collins, S. A., Jr., 192, *199*
Conte, S. D., 169, *199*
Cook, H. D., 82, *129*
Cool, T. A., 207, *237*
Cordelle, J., 53, *56*
Courtney-Pratt, J. S., 3, *56*
Croce, P., 55, *58*
Curcio, J. A., 112, *129*
Curran, T., 252, *294*

D

Davis, D. T., 128, *129*
Davis, D. T. M., Jr., 134, 138, 165, 148, 200
Decht, J. L., 210, 215, *236*
DeKinder, R. E., Jr., 267, *294*
de Lang, H., 148, 154, *199*
DeMaria, A. J., 264, *294*
De Mars, G. A., 165, 191, *199*, *200*
Denton, R. T., 256, 274, 286, *294*
Dess, H. M., 269, *295*
Dessus, B., 146, 156, *199*
Deutsch, T. F., 207, 208, *237*
DeVelis, J., 3, 7, *56*
DiDomenico, M., Jr., 266, *294*
Dijkstra, G., 148, 164, *200*
Dishington, R. H., 265, *294*
Ditchburn, R. W., 135, 144, *199*, 229, *237*
Doherty, E., 42, *56*
Dooley, R. P., 41, *56*
Dougal, A. A., 14, 15, *56*
Dowley, M. W., 204, *237*
Doyle, B., 192, 193, *199*
Doyle, W. M., 154, *199*
Drummeter, L. F., 112, *129*
Duguay, M. A., 212, 217, *238*
Dukes, J. N., 86, *129*
Durrett, R. H., 156, 165, 174, 176, 177, *199*
Dutton, E. J., 67, 105, *129*
Dyson, J., 2, *57*

E

Earnshaw, K. B., 108, *129*
El Sum, H. M. A., 2, 3, 4, 13, 40, *56*, *57*, *58*
Elterman, L., 112, *129*
Engelhard, E., 71, *129*
Engeling, P. D., 14, 15, *56*
Ennos, A. E., 42, 51, *56*, *57*
Epperson, J. P., 202, 203, 223, 227, *237*
Evtuhov, V., 215, *237*

F

Falconer, D. G., 11, *59*
Faller, J. E., 72, *129*

SUBJECT INDEX

A

Alignment, in laser applications in metrology and geodesy, 63–69
Argon ion laser, 209–212

B

Backscattering reduction, in laser gyro, 153–155
Beam deflectors, in laser communications, 282–283
Bubble-chamber photography, 27

C

Cameras, with Fraunhofer holography, 17–26
Carbon dioxide laser, 204–209
Communications, *see* Laser communications
Compensated interferometer, 73–76

D

Data processing, optical, 53–55
Data storage and retrieval
  holographic image formation in, 33–36
  holographic memories and, 34–35
  television tape player and, 36
Degrees of freedom, in interferometry, 81–82
Detector receivers, in laser communications, 275–282

D (continued)

Diffraction, in laser beam alignment, 65–66
Diffuse light, coherent detection of, 121–124
Dispersion method, atmospheric limitations and, 102–106
Doppler methods, optical, 119–120
Dynamic aerosol camera, 26

E

Electron beam particle size analysis, 28

F

Fizeau instrument, 106
Fizeau method, 102
Focusing, in laser applications in metrology and geodesy, 124–125
Fog droplet camera (laser fog disdrometer), 17–26
Fourier transform holograms, 11–12
Fraunhofer holograms
  application to small and large particles, 26–28
  far field, 7–8
Fraunhofer holography
  bubble-chamber photography with, 27
  dynamic aerosol camera in, 26
  electron beam particle size analysis and, 28
  microscopy using, 16–28
  particle size analysis in, 17–28
Fresnel holograms, near field, 6–7

G

Gain saturation, in laser gyro, 172–174
Gas jet-assisted laser cutting, 224–226
Gas laser systems, 203–212
Geodesy, laser applications in, 61–129
  see also Laser applications in
    metrology and geodesy
Geodetic instrument, prototype, 106–111
Geometrical attenuation, laser power and,
  111
Glass laser, 216–217
Gyro, *see* Laser gyro

H

Heat conduction, from surface, 229–233
Hole penetration
  rate of, 234–235
  in steady state, 223–224
Hologram(s)
  far-field Fraunhofer, 7–8
  Fourier transform, 11
  near-field Fresnel, 6–7
  optical data processing and, 53–55
  as optical element, 53–55
Hologram camera, 17–26
Holographic image formation
  holographic memories and, 34–35
  through irregular media, 36–39
  nonoptical holography and, 40–42
Holographic image formation applications,
  12–42
  contour generation, 51–53
  data storage and retrieval in, 33–36
  in microscopy, 13–16
  in microscopy using Fraunhofer holo-
    graphy, 16–28
  in photography, 31–33
  reference beam holography in, 28–31
Holographic interferometry, 42–51
  see also Interferometry
  double exposure, 44–47
  multiple exposure, 47–51
  single exposure, 43–44
Holographic lenses and gratings, 53
Holographic memories, 34–35
Holographic microscopy, interference,
  52–53

Holography

  see also Holographic image formation
    applications
  applications of, 8–56
  basic system concepts of, 4–12
  contour generation with, 51–53
  far field Fraunhofer holograms in, 7–8
  Fraunhofer, *see* Fraunhofer holograms;
    Fraunhofer holography
  history of, 2–3
  holographic image formation applica-
    tions in, 12–42
  in-line, 6–8
  interference microscopy in, 52–53
  near-field Fresnel holograms in, 6–7
  nonimage-forming applications in, 42–53
  nonoptical, 40-42
  off-axis, 8–12
  reference beam, 28–31

I

Industrial processing
  absorption and, 228–229
  lasers and, 227–235
  surface reflectivity and, 227–228
Interference microscopy, holograph and,
  52–53
Interference patterns, compensated
  interferometer and, 73–76
Interferometer
  active ring laser type, 137–139
  compensated, 73–76
  Sagnac, 134–137
  uncompensated, 76–80
Interferometry
  analysis of outputs in, 86–92
  degrees of freedom in, 81–82
  holographic, 42–51
  interference patterns in, 72–80
  lossy-beamsplitter method in, 86–88
  polarization method in, 88–92
  principles of, 69–72
  refractive index correction in, 94–95
  reversible counting in, 82–86
  three-dimensional applications in, 95–96
  wavelength stabilization and, 92–94
Irregular media, holographic image formation through, 36–39